Capturing COVID

MEDIA AND THE PANDEMIC IN THE DIGITAL ERA

KATHERINE A. FOSS

UNIVERSITY OF MASSACHUSETTS PRESS
Amherst and Boston

Printed in the United States of America

ISBN 978-1-62534-828-9 (paper); 829-6 (hardcover)

Designed by Sally Nichols
Set in Minion Pro
Printed and bound by Books International, Inc.

Cover design by adam b. bohannon
Cover photo by Proxima Studio
Multimedia video wall television broadcast.
Adobe Stock #182911572

Library of Congress Cataloging-in-Publication Data
A catalog record for this book is available through the Library of Congress.

Library of Congress Control Number: 2024951015

British Library Cataloguing-in-Publication Data
A catalog record for this book is available from the British Library.

REMEMBERING THE MILLIONS LOST

Contents

Acknowledgements

It takes a village to propose, write, and finish a book. Thank you to Matt Becker and the incredible team at University of Massachusetts Press.

To Cathy Sgambati, Andrew Oppmann, Jimmy Hart, and Gina Logue at Middle Tennessee State University, thank you for providing so many opportunities for me to share my thoughts and expertise. I am also grateful to every journalist, museum curator, public health authority, historian, medical professional, and individual who answered my questions and offered experiences that guided the writing of this text. I appreciate those that shared disease experiences for my blog, emails about articles I've written, and other communication about and during the pandemic.

At MTSU, I appreciate the continued support of Dean Beverly Keel, Associate Dean Zeny Panol, and Assistant Dean Jennifer Woodard. Thank you to Ken Blake for greatly aiding me in capturing coronavirus tweets in February 2020, long before this book project was conceived. I truly value you as a colleague.

I have enjoyed hearing opinions on this project and on pandemic life from the staff and faculty in the School of Journalism & Strategic Media. Thank you also to Leslie Shearon for sharing your perspectives and observations. A special shout out to all of my students I have had in class. Your stories influenced my perspectives on many facets of this book, directly and indirectly. I appreciate feedback on my presentations related to the work of this book: "COVID Narratives" at the Midwinter Conference at the University of Oklahoma and "Navigating the Cruise Ship Crisis" in the College of Media & Entertainment Research Series at MTSU. Thanks to Jan Lauren Boyles and the Association for Education in Journalism & Mass Communication (AEJMC) staff. I could not have made it through the pandemic planning of two virtual conferences without you.

As always, thanks to my writing partner, Tanya Peres Lemons, who keeps me accountable and shares in the ups and downs of the book process. I could not have finished a draft without Jennifer Handy, Kristi Wahlman, and my husband, Eric. Finally, kudos to my kids and my dogs, who joyfully distract me without any hesitation (one of you is playing a recorder as I write this, and the other wants me to watch a magic trick).

Preface

January 6, 2022

We have spent the last twenty-two months avoiding and escaping the virus. Now, after all of this time, it has arrived in our house. With a faint second line, the positive COVID test sitting on my bathroom counter represents so much more than what the results mean. Fortunately, my ten-year-old seems to be alright as she's bopping along to *Descendants 2*, despite a runny nose and a sore throat. Two years ago, similar symptoms would have simply warranted a day home from school and a brief pause of activities. Today's test stares at us, as I reassure my daughter that she will be okay, hasn't done anything wrong, and that her completed vaccination series offers protection. In a sea of unmasked faces, she had kept covered up. Thus, the information that the home laboratory kit simply provides notification that she needs to stay home. COVID had caught up with the Foss house for the first time. This is a moment filled with anxiety, built up from the past two years of fearing an invisible enemy that caused the world to turn upside down. And yet, as so many others have said, the Omicron situation was a far cry from the coronavirus of March 2020, especially in our vaccinated household . . .

◉ ◉ ◉ ◉ ◉

June 2023

I wrote the above paragraph in a cathartic attempt to reassure myself and to assuage my own guilt that my daughter had become sick. Over the next week, my husband also tested positive, though nearly asymptomatic. My then twelve-year-old and I remained negative, even with close contact with the contagious members in our family. Even with all that the world has learned about COVID, who specifically will become infected and who will not remain unclear. One year later, my oldest child and I tested positive and fortunately experienced mild cases, fairly similar to the effects I feel after each COVID booster.

For my last book on epidemics, *Constructing the Outbreak: Epidemics in Media and Collective Memory*, I worked hard to understand the epidemic experiences of the past, entering each moment in history trying to imagine how people back then felt, thought, and made decisions. This project has brought on the opposite issues. It has been *too* close to home. I cannot write about news diffusion without pondering my coronavirus introduction, first mentioned by an acquaintance at the climbing gym in January 2020. The chapter on the lockdown spurs my own frenzied thirst for information, memories of picking up my kids on March 13, 2020 (knowing that they wouldn't return anytime soon), and stress of juggling distance learning while improvising the online shift for my own classes. As I attempted to objectively analyze this period of time, I also reminisced about my desperate desire to be alone back then as I simultaneously tried to make life okay for my children with *Sound of Music* day (not well-received), the purchase a rubber boat for our little backyard pond, an in-town scavenger hunt, and other meager efforts to help our family navigate the uncertainty of March–May 2020.

What none of us knew was just how long the pandemic would impede life. Schools initially closed for only two weeks, which, of course, was then extended for the rest of the academic year. At multiple times, we thought that the pandemic had started to wane (summer 2020 and then up and down until the vaccine rollout. After that, Omicron and other variants stifled the resemblance of "normal"). Gradually, for different people in different places, life resumed, although some individuals, especially those higher at risk, are still distance learning, staying home, and masking in public. Officially, on May 5, 2023, the World Health Organization (WHO) ended the Public Health Emergency of International Concern (PHEIC).[1]

It is difficult to capture just how tense and publicly judgmental this period of time was. Online and in-person, we as a global society scrutinized each other's behavior and questioned our own. What seemed "acceptable" dramatically fluctuated. Every little action carried with it so much stress and anxiety. Small decisions, like buying milk, brought a flurry of questions that changed with time (i.e., should we order it online? Is it worth the risk to go to the store? Will the store have milk? Do we wear a mask? Which mask? Do we wear the mask outside before entering? Is it okay to touch a phone inside the store? Will others judge me for wearing a mask? For wearing the wrong mask? Did I hear a cough? How far am I from the cough? Will I get sick? Will I get my family sick?). And that was all for getting a carton of milk.

Bigger tasks were even more anxiety-inducing. Most parents had to decide when to send their kids back to in-person school at some point. For us in Rutherford County, Tennessee, this time came in Fall 2020 after the school board voted to offer parents a choice of in-person, fully masked, or online classes with the same teachers and classmates. Since my husband and I both had to work, we opted to send our kids (ages nine and eleven) in-person. After I shared a "first day of school" picture online, a childless acquaintance sent me a scathing email about our decision. Unless you experienced parenting children at home during the pandemic, you cannot truly understand just how difficult it was.

In August 2020, I was back teaching in a classroom full of college students. Well, sort of. The scheduling center had moved my introduction to media class into one of the student union ballrooms, with chairs spread six feet apart. The room was gigantic, we were all masked, and I had to use a microphone for students to hear me. Class met once a week, with the rest of the teaching shifted online. It was a strange experience. At the same time, we were so grateful to be cautiously together after the spring hiatus.

December 2020 brought joyful news of the vaccine approvals, but also marked our first holiday season alone without our extended family. To ease our loneliness, we began fostering puppies—another unusual experience I endorsed because of the circumstances.

Every single day from December 2020 to March 2021, I checked on the updated vaccine eligibility, watching as various groups were added, waiting for my turn to protect my family (particularly as I was also teaching large classes at that time). I advocated for educators to be included. I volunteered at the Red Cross Blood Bank and at the MTSU vaccination clinic. When I received my first dose, I cried happy tears. Likewise, as my children became eligible in May and October, I rejoiced, knowing what it meant for our family. The vaccination process was intensely emotional for me. As such, I did not and still do not understand anti-vaxxer rhetoric and decision-making, even as I study such discourse academically. This moment revealed the true divisiveness that permeates beyond geographic regions. Within my own extended family, I had to decide what battles to pick and which to let go.

In no way can I pretend to know and understand all experiences. The pandemic exacerbated existing stigma and injustice. How inhumane to refuse to serve an Asian-appearing customer for "fears" of the virus. While I absolutely empathize and stand behind the George Floyd protesters, I cannot begin to imagine the trauma of discrimination or feel the impact of the legislation against trans athletes slipped in during this time of turmoil. Yes, Spring 2020 put a lot of stress on our household, but at least we remained employed and our kids had stable Wi-Fi and the technology to tackle online assignments.

I write this book not just as another person who lived through the pandemic, but also as someone who critically commented and contributed media content. I spent much of the first year of the crisis using my blog and popular articles to counter misinformation online. The unexpected timing of my epidemics book (published in September 2020) made me a sought-after expert. I published numerous disease-themed articles, gave virtual and in-person public talks, and was quoted more than eighty times. This in itself was highly unusual. *Constructing the Outbreak* was my sixth book, but the first one that regular people wanted to talk about. This time in the limelight added a layer to my experience. I was publicly trying to help others make sense of the moment, while privately attempting to understand it myself.

During this time, I served as one of the primary planners and facilitators for our international professional association's annual conference. In May 2020, we (the board of directors) made the tough decision to shift the August conference online. Although I'm glad we pulled off the conference (twice—again in 2021), no one could have understood how stressful it was to lead that experience unless they were part of the planning. Professionally, I was happy to be interacting virtually with the public and my colleagues. Yet, I struggled personally with the lack of face-to-face interaction that took so long to return as I craved conversations with friends, colleagues, students, and even strangers. Even though we as a household were privileged in so many ways, I found it a bit traumatic to recall some of these experiences necessarily to write this book.

Globally, we will spend at least the next five to ten years attempting to recover from this pandemic. The families and friends of those lost to COVID may never completely come back from this tragedy. Although day-to-day life has returned to "normal" for most people, we are not in the same reality as we were in December 2019. The shift from pandemic mode back to regular life resembled almost a distorted universe, in which things are kind of like "the before" but with the intermingling of challenging emotional feelings and memories. Unlike the lapse in collective memory for the 1918 influenza pandemic, we cannot and should not write our experiences out of the history books. Around the world, our lives were turned upside down for a lengthy period of time. We must never forget. And yet, we've already started to lose some of these moments, thus the importance of writing them down.

Capturing COVID

CHAPTER ONE

The Unexpected Crisis in the Digital Era

"Pandemic is not a word to use lightly or carelessly. It is a word that, if misused, can cause unreasonable fear, or unjustified acceptance that the fight is over, leading to unnecessary suffering and death."[1]

On March 11, 2020, WHO Director Tedros Adhanom Ghebreyesus contextualized his declaration that the novel coronavirus, COVID-19, had indeed become pandemic. Within two weeks, much of the world had shutdown, as anyone who could work remotely was advised to "shelter in place." Unemployment skyrocketed as nonessential businesses temporarily closed. Traffic ceased. Streets became vacant. School hallways echoed with emptiness. New phrases flooded the everyday vernacular: "Flatten the curve," "social distance," "pod," "bubble," and "You're on mute."

Global media consumption soared as people turned to various sources and social media platforms for information, entertainment, and human interaction.[2] Although health crises have certainly occurred before, the COVID-19 pandemic was the first to occur in a digital era, enabling regular people to easily create and disseminate content capturing their experiences and perspectives, as well as share (mis) information—a crisis in itself that WHO labeled the "infodemic."[3] As a result, this emergency seemed much longer and more divided, with large groups of people resisting the recommendations and mandates of public health authorities. At the same time, in many ways, this moment resembled past epidemics, replicating patterns of disease coverage that favored the white, rich, and powerful, while stigmatizing othered groups.

Three years later, WHO declared that the PHEIC had ended, noting the shift of handling COVID from crisis to "an established and ongoing health issue."[4] Global deaths from COVID exceeded 6.9 million.[5] The United States had the highest death toll with over 1.1 million lives.[6] On the upside, 72.3 percent of the world had received at least one dose of the multiple effective vaccines developed during the pandemic.[7]

This book addresses the mediated discourses that shaped knowledge, perception, and behavior throughout the stages of the pandemic, examining the politicization of the crisis and its related divisiveness, stigma, inequality, and impact on daily life. Unlike past epidemics and pandemics, technology in 2020–2022 provided the quick, global diffusion of information, allowing the potential for preparation before the crisis and a transnational awareness of COVID's devastation. Early communication about the emerging threat translated to a much longer pandemic time frame than ever before, with "COVID fatigue" contributing to local government's decisions and public behavior that contradicted health recommendations, as evident by the resistance to masks, vaccines, and other public health measures.

Two objectives carry through this text. The first is to construct the mediated narratives of the COVID-19 pandemic from news and entertainment media, as well as citizen-produced posts, blogs, community boards, memes, songs, videos, and other shared content. Second, in itself, this book serves to document and capture moments, stories, experiences, and themes of this pandemic conveyed in media forms, thus preserving them in collective memory.

What Is COVID-19?

Scientists confirmed that the virus causing the "mystery pneumonia" out of Wuhan, China was, in fact, a new coronavirus: SARS-CoV-2, which WHO nicknamed "COVID-19."[8] Coronaviruses cause the common cold, as well as Severe Acute Respiratory Syndrome (SARS) and Middle East respiratory syndrome (MERS). COVID-19 has a lower case-fatality rate than SARS and MERS, but is much more contagious, spreading through respiratory droplets.[9] Incubation periods for COVID were initially unclear, as the Centers for Disease Control and Prevention (CDC) listed two–fourteen days.[10] Research showed a similar broad range, with a mean of 6.3 days.[11] A 2022 meta-analysis found that incubation periods decreased with the variants, from five days for Alpha to 3.42 days for Omicron.[12] Studies also suggested that incubation periods may vary by patient age and health.[13]

In March 2020, the CDC only listed fever, cough, and shortness of breath as possible COVID symptoms.[14] A month later, the CDC added muscle pain, headache, sore throat, chills, shaking, and loss of taste or smell to its website.[15] Later into the pandemic, digestive symptoms (diarrhea, vomiting, and nausea) also became associated with COVID.[16] Across the initial and variant strains, some people never experience symptoms.[17] On the other hand, COVID can become severe and even deadly. Like influenza, COVID can lead to pneumonia, cardiac and respiratory problems, organ failure, and secondary infections.[18] Additionally, COVID infections may result in blood clots, Multisystem Inflammatory Syndrome, paralysis, and other neurological effects in children or adults.[19] Age and certain health conditions significantly heighten the risk, especially cancer, diabetes, cystic fibrosis, and heart and respiratory conditions, compromised immune systems, and other chronic diseases.[20] Around 15 percent[i] of those infected develop long COVID—ongoing effects that may include fatigue, mental fog, respiratory and cardiac problems, neurological or digestive issues, or "symptoms that are not explained by tests or easy to manage."[21] Children are the least likely to be infected, hospitalized, or die from COVID. Risk of hospitalization and death significantly increases with age. People 50–64 years old are 60 times more likely to die from COVID than those age 18–29 and this gap widens with age.[22] Yet, people of all ages did and can die from COVID.[23]

When COVID first emerged, no vaccines or specific treatment

i This number has been difficult to accurately pinpoint and is still being studied.

existed for the disease. In December 2020, the US Food and Drug Administration issued Emergency Use Authorization for both the Pfizer and Moderna vaccines.[24] These vaccines provide significant protection against severe illness and death.[25] In the course of the pandemic, effective treatments were also developed for individuals with heightened risks. Anti-viral pills and intravenous infusions can shorten the duration of symptoms and decrease the likelihood of severe COVID.[26] From February to March 2020 and July to August 2022, case-fatality rates[ii] globally declined by 96.8 percent due to vaccination, improved treatment options, and stronger immunity against the virus.[27]

Pandemics Past and Present

The impact of disease can be so profound that it takes over competing events of the moment. Outbreaks, epidemics, and pandemics have been integral to the unfolding and telling of history—shaping migration, colonization, war, leadership, scientific discovery, education, public health, and everyday life.[28] Inoculation debates during the 1721 Boston smallpox epidemic led to the first democratic newspaper in colonial America. Philadelphia's 1793 yellow fever epidemic demonstrated the need for contingency plans in congressional meetings. Tuberculosis greatly influenced artistic works created in the Romantic era, profoundly bolstered sanitation, and sparked the study of climate and weather.[29] The timing of influenza transmission patterns in 1918–1919 shaped World War I.[30] Therapy for polio patients at Warm Spring contributed to modern rehabilitation techniques.[31]

Disease played an integral role in colonization, as Europeans carried smallpox, measles, and other contagions that decimated Indigenous populations.[32] Disease is political, as "fear of disease" has been used to justify discrimination and hate crimes against marginalized groups.[33] During the Black Death, Jewish people, Muslims, beggars, and other

ii The Case Fatality Rate has been difficult to accurately calculate since not everyone infected with COVID was formally diagnosed. See "Mortality Risk of COVID-19." *Our World in Data*, https://ourworldindata.org/mortality-risk-covid.

perceived outsiders were accused of spreading plague and murdered across Europe.[34] Immigrants have long been blamed for various diseases, stemming from what Alan M. Kraut referred to as "medicalized nativism."[35] Irish immigrants were blamed for cholera epidemics in 1832 and 1849.[36] Mary Mallon (more famously known as "Typhoid Mary") served as a public scapegoat largely in part because she was an Irish immigrant woman of lower socioeconomic class, despite hundreds of other known asymptomatic carriers at that time.[37] In the 1980s, the Reagan administration and mainstream media ignored and stigmatized Acquired Immune Deficiency Syndrome (AIDS) as a "gay disease."[38] HIV-positive Haitian refugees were turned away from the United States because of their status in 1992.[39] During the 2003 SARS epidemic, Asian Americans faced stigma in New York City even though no cases were recorded there.[40] Outbreaks amplify inequity, magnifying disparities, as marginalized communities are less likely to be able to flee town and have access to medical care. While epidemics draw attention, much of the news coverage (i.e., "Hong Kong Flu," HIV/AIDS, SARS, Ebola, and Zika) has been xenophobic and ethnocentric, othering and marginalizing disease as a scourge in far-off places or in certain groups of people.[41] Individuals of othered groups are far less likely to have their deaths memorialized and shared. At least in western discourse, the documented stories of disease are primarily from wealthy, white male leaders. Aside from a few exceptions (i.e., the writings of Richard Allen and Absalom Jones), the experiences of communities of color have been lost.[42]

Endemic describes the typical level of a particular disease in a particular population.[43] When a disease reemerges in a community, causes a surge in cases, or spreads to a new area, it constitutes an outbreak. Outbreaks have occurred, often simultaneously, throughout history, significantly shaping a community.[44] Epidemics typically refer to larger-scale outbreaks, while pandemics involve high disease transmission, infectiousness, and severity over multiple countries or geographic areas.[45] The formal designation for a potentially global-level disease crisis is a PHEIC, as determined by the WHO's International Health Regulations' set of factors (i.e., what disease is causing the crisis event, its potential impact, or its risk for spreading internationally).[46] WHO has declared seven PHEIC since 2007: H1N1 influenza (2009), Ebola in West Africa (2013–2015), poliomyelitis containment and eradication (2014–present), Zika (2016), Ebola in the Democratic Republic of Congo (2018–2020), COVID-19 (January 30, 2020–May 5, 2023), and monkey pox (July 2022–May 2023).[47] Until COVID, no PHEIC had directly impacted the United States in the twenty-first century.

CONTEXTUALIZING COVID

Many factors set the stage for how COVID would be covered, handled, and understood. Improved sanitation and vaccines eliminated raging infectious disease in most developed countries. In 2019, most people in the United States had never experienced contagious disease outbreaks, let alone epidemics. Seventeen years earlier, SARS plagued primarily mainland China and Hong Kong, with 8,098 cases and 774 deaths.[48] From 2014 to 2016, Ebola emerged in West African countries, exceeding 28,000 cases and causing 11,325 deaths.[49] North America, Europe, and Australia almost entirely escaped cases and deaths in twenty-first century epidemics. In the United States, no one had experienced a large-scale epidemic for more than fifty years. They may have read about concerns of H1N1 in 2009, but never truly lived through quarantines, mask-wearing, mass school closings, and the ever-present worry amplified in epidemic times. Adults had likely seen media coverage of Ebola, which was framed as a distant threat. Until the COVID-19 pandemic, disease was relegated to the "conquered" category in western media discourse. It had been decades since parents fretted about their children catching smallpox, diphtheria, polio, rubella, pertussis, mumps, and measles (other than outbreaks among unvaccinated groups). More likely, Americans could remember what were construed as "close-calls" or distant threats—warning about swine flu in the 1970s, media-driven panic of H1N1, and the possibility of Ebola outbreaks in the United States.[50] People frequently went to work sick and contagious.[51] This lack of firsthand epidemic experience meant that people did not fear disease as they had with polio.[52] Moreover, the minimalized coverage of past pandemics and epidemics in history books and popular culture had nearly erased these experiences from collective memory.[53]

Cultural conventions, values, and institutions shaped how various governments approached the pandemic, as well as how people responded. Individualism is deeply entrenched in US history and culture, in which responsibility for survival and success rests on individuals.[54] Linked to this flawed ethos is a health care model underscored by personal responsibility, connecting choices to health outcomes, ignoring genetics, environment, and other factors that contribute to the need for care.[55] The lack of free, accessible health care for all Americans means that many citizens make their health decisions based on cost. Although the 2010 Affordable Care Act dramatically reduced the number of uninsured, in 2019, 28.9 million people were still without health insurance, mostly due to cost—a group that was disproportionately Hispanic or Black.[56] People without insurance are less likely to have regular providers and more likely to postpone care and medication and to be hospitalized.[57] They experience poorer qualities of health and shorter life expectancies.[58]

The Pre-Pandemic Media Landscape

Much of what distinguished COVID from past crises stemmed from the contemporary media landscape, both directly and indirectly. Historical, political, cultural, and technological contexts set the stage for mis/disinformation to flourish during the COVID-19 pandemic. And while this book centers on the United States, this problem was certainly not geographically unique. Before the digital era, production and consumption of news were much more straightforward. News sources could be easily identified. All messages went through gatekeepers in order to reach a mass audience. The downside, of course, was that gatekeeping thwarted agency and voice in those without the connections or means to publish in newspapers.[iii] In the twenty-first century,

iii For example, during the influenza pandemic of 1917–1918, censorship during World War I impacted outlets available and what could be said.

the media landscape became much murkier. Individuals still trained in journalism schools, but the outlets and platforms had expanded exponentially. Any ordinary consumer with knowledge and access could create and disseminate content. Some unscrupulous individuals and groups were out to intentionally deceive, distorting factual content to support their own agendas, often presented as legitimate news sites. As a result, who was a journalist and what was news had become more difficult to discern, so much that most people were not confident in their abilities to identify credible information.[59]

Technology changed the production and reception of news, as consumption of traditional broadcasting and print news declined. A 2018 Pew Research survey asked adults for their main sources of information. Nearly half of participants said television, especially local TV news, followed by news websites (33%), radio (26%), social media (20%), and print newspapers (16%).[60] Yet, these source preferences varied significantly by age. Older age groups preferred television and print newspapers, while younger groups used social media and news websites.[61]

As more people switched their primary source of news to online formats, circulation for local newspapers declined by 40 percent and nearly 1,800 daily and weekly newspapers shutdown over a fifteen-year period, according to a 2018 report.[62] With nearly 200 counties lacking local newspapers, news deserts became much more common, especially in southern regions.[63] Rural counties with more individuals from lower socioeconomic brackets and rates of education had fewer newspapers.[64] Moreover, many of the papers that remained had been consolidated into larger news organizations, hindering both the depth and focus of local coverage.[65]

Digital technology radically changed how people consumed content. It became much easier to access a multitude of content from around the world. Smart phones, apps, and social media also made it simple to create and share content without having to work through gatekeepers to get published. Pre-pandemic, YouTube and Facebook were the most popular social media platforms, with 73 percent and 69 percent of adults using them in a 2018 Pew Research survey.[66] Adults' preferences for other social media platforms were as follows: Instagram, Pinterest, LinkedIn, Snapchat, Twitter, WhatsApp, and Reddit, ranging from 37 percent down to only 11 percent of participants.[67] Those between the ages of 18 and 24 preferred YouTube (90%), Instagram (75%) Facebook (76%), and Snapchat (73%).[68] Younger age groups also reported using social media sites more regularly than older groups.[69] TikTok was still fairly new and primarily used by teenagers and young adults.[70]

In moments of public health crisis, media keep people informed of rising cases, death tolls, and impacts on the town. Some patterns in media transcend time and technological shifts. News media set the tone for a rising crisis, provide fora for speculation and discussion of causality, prevention, and treatment, capture emotion and experience, and help to mourn the deceased. Across time and medium, the voices of those in power are most likely to be shared and preserved. In US history, "experts" have been mostly wealthy, white cis-men, and media messages have stigmatized and marginalized already-othered groups.[71] News stories on epidemics are gripping, receiving more attention than chronic disease. During the 2002–2003 SARS epidemic, news outlets disproportionately covered SARS more than heart disease and other health topics more prevalent in the population.[72] Ebola outbreaks in West Africa dominated Americans' top news interests.[73]

At the same time, expanding technology changed both the production and consumption of content in crises. It took months for people in 1918 to learn about the influenza pandemic. Email, cell phones, social media, 24-hour news cycles, and other tools provide instant delivery of information. Public health authorities can directly convey messages through social media channels. Posts from individuals have proven useful in identifying patterns of disease. Spikes in Google searches or posts about particular symptoms can indicate a spreading outbreak.[74] These channels can be used to crowdsource knowledge in a crisis.[75] Online messaging can also indicate public awareness and perception of an issue or rising crisis.[76] Communication is instantaneous and possible, even during quarantines and stay-at-home orders.

In past epidemics and pandemics, news and entertainment content flowed through a limited number of channels; therefore, most people (who had access) consumed from the same pool of information. For example, in October 1918, it is highly likely that most people in Lawrence, Kansas, read one of the many *Lawrence Daily Gazette* stories on rising influenza cases.[77] The fragmentation of twenty-first century media means that even in a small town, many people would have missed a similar article in their local papers. It's much more difficult to deliver a unified message that the majority of the public will receive.

Before the digital revolution, experts were more clearly defined and vetted. The only way to pass on information was either cutting out an article out of the newspaper and physically sharing the story or to verbally tell another person of the message. Widespread sharing from consumers did not occur outside of interpersonal connections. Social media platforms allow anyone with access and knowledge to write a post, share a story, or make a video. The downside is that Twitter (now called X), Snapchat, Facebook, Instagram, YouTube, TikTok, and other platforms have no gatekeepers, enabling the creation and sharing of content, no matter how incomplete, out-of-context, or completely fabricated it is. Moreover, social media's structure ("likes" and "shares") rewards extreme or clickbaiting types of messages.

The lack of gatekeeping and plethora of sites, videos, blogs, posts, and shares created a confusing online environment even before the 2020 pandemic. Most people struggled to identify credible information over other types of content. Only 27 percent of Americans indicated that they were "very confident" in identifying factual news from opinion or commentary.[78] Adding to this, people perceived social media platforms themselves to be news sources, not as vehicles for content produced by other entities.[79] Even before the expansion of platforms, people regularly shared articles and links on social media without reading the content.[80] The public's lack of understanding of news and credibility allowed the flourishing of *misinformation*—the unintentional spread of exaggerated or inaccurate information—and *disinformation*—deliberate sharing of dishonest, fabricated, and manipulative content.[81]

Political Context

The contentious 2016 election of Donald Trump exacerbated existing problems: of stigma and marginalization, the flawed emphasis on individualism, anti-science rhetoric, and flurries of misinformation spread by social media. Trump and his administration fueled a partisan divide, perpetuating anti-science ideologies and policies, while attacking mainstream media. An avid social media user before his 2021 Twitter and Facebook bans, Trump produced 11,887 tweets from January 2017 through October 15, 2019, to more than 66 million followers.[82] His messages sometimes conveyed presidential business, but more frequently attacked news organizations, Democrats, underrepresented groups, and others and spread conspiracy theories, while praising himself, Fox News, and conservative media. [83] Trump encouraged his followers to distrust mainstream media, using the phrase "fake news" at least 216 times from his inauguration through 2019.[84] "Fake news" has had multiple definitions. Historically, the phrase referred to parody/satire or as "fabrication"—"articles which have no factual basis but are published in the style of news articles to create legitimacy."[85] However, according to The Poynter Institute's *Politifact* from 2017, when Trump referred to "fake news," it meant "coverage that [was] unsympathetic to his administration and his performance, even when the news reports [were] accurate."[86] Such emphasis on "fake news" has been shown to decrease trust in media and make it more difficult to identify credible news.[87] As a result, Republicans, especially viewers of the Fox News cable channel,[88] were far less likely to trust media than Democrats.[89] Moreover, the Trump administration enhanced momentum for anti-science ideologies and in 2018 significantly reduced global health security funding.[90] Much of what unfolded in the pandemic had been previously established or taken away by Trump and his administration.

SCOPE AND OVERVIEW OF THE BOOK

As it would be impossible to study all media content in the pandemic, each chapter that follows focuses on the unfolding of specific scientific and cultural moments in the global health crisis. Press releases, reports, interviews, websites, blogs, social media posts, and other material made public are used to help define and construct these significant events as they unfolded in their particular time markers of the pandemic. This book also heavily draws from secondary sources—reports, *Google Trends*, surveys, and scholarly studies, especially for broad analysis of content (i.e., hundreds of thousands of tweets). A critical textual analysis was conducted on all materials, which involved the systematic analysis of language (i.e., word choice—"mysterious pneumonia" or "coronavirus"), visual aesthetics (i.e., emojis, graphics, photos, video), production/delivery (i.e., source, organization/outlet, platform), and mise-en-scène (all components taken together). This qualitative approach situates media content within "wider social and cultural practices."[91] Social construction of reality underscores this book, with the understanding that media messages help to shape a meaningful reality.[92] Thus, to examine forms of media produced during and about the pandemic provides a greater understanding to the cultural, economic, and political contexts of the moment. Specific mass communication and media theories are introduced as relevant to individual chapters.

Media content produced by news industries, public health authorities, organizations, individuals, and others significantly impacted how people thought about, perceived, and behaved leading up to and during the COVID-19 pandemic. Dis/misinformation and conspiracy theories rampantly inhibited many people's beliefs in the severity of COVID and their subsequent willingness to isolate, mask, get vaccinated, and adhere to other mitigation strategies. Although it is necessary to touch on how and for whom misinformation prevailed, myths and conspiracy are deliberately not at the center here. Since this book aims to preserve narratives and not distort them, specific lines of fabrication about COVID origins, transmission, and the vaccines will not be repeated in this text. In a similar vein, the use of racist statements as examples, including those quoted in social media, will be minimized as to not further stigmatize the many people hurt by such content.

This book moves somewhat chronologically through the COVID-19 pandemic, focusing on the United States, but also bringing in reference points from other countries and regions. Chapter 2 traces the diffusion of the new virus, from its first discoveries in Wuhan 2019 through the end of January 2020, when most of the world knew about the emerging threat. In chapter 3, mediated narratives of the quarantined *Diamond Princess* cruise ship are explored, contextualizing how news and social media messages debated at this moment set the stage for the pandemic. Chapter 4 examines the Spring 2020 "lockdown" period, highlighting COVID's immediate impact on work, school, and everyday life. Specifically, this chapter contrasts constructions of the "essential worker" with those sheltering at home, creating a unique mediated climate. Then chapter 5 captures how existing stigma and racism fueled and escalated during the pandemic, from anti-Asian blame through the protests against injustice and police brutality after the murder of George Floyd.

Chapter 6 details news and social media's coverage and reception of the COVID-19 vaccine rollout, from the vaccine trials to the widespread distribution of multiple approved vaccines. In chapter 7, fictionalizations of COVID responses are analyzed, exploring how various television programs incorporated (or did not incorporate) the global health crisis into their storylines. Chapter 8 concludes the book and the discussion of mediated COVID narratives, exploring the long-term economic, environmental, social, cultural, and global impacts of the pandemic.

CHAPTER TWO

Diffusion from Wuhan

FROM "MYSTERY PNEUMONIA" TO COVID PANDEMIC

Fall 2019 resembled "normal life," "the before," a pre-crisis time in which we blew out birthday candles, sat shoulder-to-shoulder in packed stadiums, and took public health for granted. Coronaviruses weren't talked about much or searched for online. That December, #coronavirus referred to virology studies and Middle East Respiratory System cases in Qatar and Saudi Arabia. #Corona denoted town-specific news and events, including an earthquake in California and a New York Santa Claus Bike Ride. This hashtag also highlighted artist SheebyDeeb's dystopic webtoon, the latest discoveries about the sun's surface by solar physicists, and new rendering software. Of course, #Corona was also used for the popular beer brand, marketing twelve pack sales, promoting an open bar at a holiday party, and for drinking selfies, such as a tweet featuring a half-full bottle with the message "Sunday night essentials after 14 hours in the slammer."

Unbeknownst to most people, the crisis that would change everything began brewing in early December.[1] No one knows exactly how this coronavirus entered the human population, although the most likely possibility is that it jumped species from other animals.[2] It spread without detection for weeks. Once the burgeoning crisis was identified in Wuhan, western media's initial framework of the disease as a far-off threat set the stage for a delayed response, anti-Asian stigma, conspiracies theories, and misinformation that would hinder and undermine trust and mitigation strategies throughout and beyond the pandemic.

This chapter traces the dissemination of information, from the pre-crisis stage to WHO's declaration of the PHEIC on January 30, 2020. Names for the disease reflected the moment, from the initial use of "mystery pneumonia" to SARS-CoV-2 (January 5, 2020), novel coronavirus, coronavirus, and, finally, COVID-19—the WHO's abbreviation announced on February 11, 2020. Uncertainty shrouded the first months of the developing crisis. What is pieced together here remained largely disconnected at the time, with scientists, journalists, and consumers alike bombarded with fragmented information and speculation. Much of what is known about the initial emergence of the virus was discovered in later studies, especially during the 2021 WHO clinical review of China's National Notifiable Disease Reporting System (NNDRS) data and extensive testing of lab samples.[3]

THE DIFFUSION OF NEWS

Even in a digital age, news isn't constructed, disseminated, received, and understood instantaneously. Everett M. Rogers first defined diffusion as "the process by which an innovation is communicated through certain channels over time among the members of a social system."[4] Studies into the diffusion of news explore how new information, particularly of an event or crisis, travels through mass and interpersonal communication channels.[5] In 1945, sociologist Delbert C. Miller first examined the diffusion of news, looking at the rate and means by which people found out about President Franklin Delano Roosevelt's death.[6] Of his college students who had heard the news, 91 percent had found out within 30 minutes of the radio announcement and told an average of seven people each.[7] Miller's research and other studies on diffusion of shocking events generalized that (at least before smartphones), timing of an announcement impacts how people will receive the news (type of medium or from other people). Moreover, the perceived salience or importance of an announcement impacts the likelihood that people will tell others about it.[8] Social media outlets expand the ways that individuals spread information, allowing them to directly share and comment on news stories that they deem important. Consumers can also interact with government agencies and others in the midst of crises to stay updated and ask questions.[9]

Outbreaks and epidemics differ from assassinations and other tragic, sudden events. During health crises, a time lag generally occurs from the first cases of what would become epidemic to media coverage of the emerging crisis. And, before technology rapidly sped up information distribution, news of an outbreak was generally limited to a particular geographic area. For example, in the 1793 yellow fever epidemic, nearly a month passed between the first cases and coverage in the Philadelphia papers.[10] During the 1918–19 influenza pandemic (the misnamed "Spanish Flu"), only local papers addressed the spring 1918 outbreaks, creating a misperception that the disease came from overseas over the summer. In other words, epidemic and pandemic coverage used to be almost entirely local until the crisis reached such a level that it could not be ignored.

In a digital era, online content and social media posts become both channels of information dissemination and a means of public surveillance. Google keyword searches capture patterns of public interest in particular topics and sometimes, provide epidemiological clues into outbreaks.[11] Tweets and social media posts can be used to indicate increases in disease activity, as demonstrated for H1N1, Ebola, tuberculosis, and outbreaks of tropical diseases.[12] Spikes in web content about possible symptoms, risks, and other aspects of current epidemics reflect media coverage at the time.[13] Because news outlets tend to be ethnocentric, coverage is more likely with regional or national cases of a disease (as opposed to present in another country). For example, American news content, Google searches, and social media posts about Ebola skyrocketed only after the first confirmed case in the United States.[14]

Moreover, the collective memory of an epidemic sets the stage for media constructions of future epidemics. Specifically, the 2002–2003 SARS epidemic shaped mitigation efforts, public perception, news diffusion, and media constructions for the COVID pandemic. SARS first emerged in southern China as an unknown, severe form of pneumonia in November in 2002 (but was not reported to WHO until February 2003).[15] In March, the new disease became epidemic, sparking WHO and other public health agency responses, travel restrictions, and other measures. By December 2003, 8,096 probable cases, with 774 deaths occurred over 29 countries.[16] The United States had eight confirmed plus nineteen likely cases. Western media largely othered the SARS epidemic, using a framework of difference to downplay risk and provide reassurance.[17] Such discourse perpetuated blame and stigmatization on Asian countries, which carried over to the discrimination of Asian Americans and UK refugees and migrants.[18] The not-too-distant memory of SARS and its devastation was well woven into early discourse of what would be later identified and abbreviated as COVID-19.

DECEMBER 2019: A MYSTERY PNEUMONIA IN WUHAN

On December 8, 2019, an individual in Wuhan, China began having symptoms in what would later be confirmed as the first case of a new virus.[i] According to the WHO's 2021 clinical review of the China's NNDRS,[ii] onset of symptoms for several other Wuhan individuals were noted December 11–16 and then surged in the second half of December.[19] At the time, doctors had yet to notice any abnormalities in their respiratory patients. Analysis of social media posts from this time period, however, suggests an uptake in mild infections. In

i The WHO report notes that three possible cases, one with an onset date of December 1, 2019, have been since ruled out. Furthermore, retroactive testing of thousands of samples before this time also tested negative for SARS-CoV-2.

ii The "WHO-convened Global Study of Origins of SARS-CoV-2: China Part" conducted a series of investigations in attempts to pinpoint when the virus first emerged in the Wuhan population, including studying lab samples from 2019 and early 2020, monitoring cold medicine purchase rates, changes in mortality, which did not spike in the 65 and older population until late January. WHO also conducted case-searching for mild coronavirus symptoms that possibly predated the Wuhan outbreak.

mid-December, many social media users in Wuhan turned online for information on respiratory symptoms, searching "Feidian" (translated as severe acute respiratory syndrome), "coronavirus," "shortness of breath," "dyspnea," "diarrhea," and "SARS" in the Chinese *WeChat* app.[20] This unusual online activity suggested that local people had taken notice of the emerging illness among them and were possibly sick themselves.

It wasn't until December 26 that health professionals noted anything unusual. At the Hubei Hospital of Integrated Chinese and Western Medicine, pulmonologist Dr. Zhang Jixian noted that the CT scans of an elderly couple presenting with what "looked like flu or common pneumonia"[21] did not resemble lungs infected with SARS or common viruses.[22] Even though the couple's son had no symptoms, his scan revealed similar issues, as did the images of a fourth patient ill with a cough and a fever.[23] In an April 2020 interview, Zhang recalled, "We've had patients with ground-glass opacities in their lungs caused by virus infection, but his were a lot more and larger than we had seen before."[24]

Zhang alerted the hospital's head, who notified the Jianghan District Center for Disease Control. She later explained, "We said we suspected something wrong, but we didn't know what it was."[25] At the same time, Zhang isolated the four patients, created a nine-bed isolation ward, purchased protective gear online, and encouraged care providers to also use more protection.[26] The female patient had connections to the Huanan Seafood Market, initiating the focus on the market as a potential site of origin.[27] As investigations began, four more patients arrived with similar pneumonia and were linked to the same market.[28]

On December 29 at 1:00 p.m. China Standard Time, the hospital's vice president sent a report on the situation to the provincial and municipal health and Health Commission, prompting an immediate formal epidemiologic investigation.[29] This work led the Wuhan Municipal Health and Health Commission to produce two documents, translated as "Urgent Notice on Reporting the Treatment of Unexplained Pneumonia" for medical institutions (posted online twelve minutes after its release) and "Emergency Notice on Doing a Good Job in the Treatment of Unexplained Pneumonia," which included plans for an investigation into the South China Seafood Market as possibly connected to the outbreak of pneumonia (posted online at 19:00, ten minutes after distribution).[30]

In the short window between the documents, Dr. Li Wenliang, an ophthalmologist at Wuhan Central Hospital, warned a private *WeChat* group of fellow doctors about SARS cases linked to the South China Fruit and Seafood Market, advising them to guard themselves against infection.[31] Li's messages and the two Health Commission documents began circulating online, becoming the first correspondence to the outside world of the emerging crisis.[iii] For his messages, Dr. Li was later apprehended by police, reprimanded for posting online, and forced to sign an admonishment statement about distributing false information potentially disruptive to the public order.[32]

Pictures of the announcements about the "unexplained pneumonia" circulated on the Chinese social media platform Sina Weibo.[33] Panda@DCheng36387164 was one of the first to bring the images to Twitter, tweeting (translated from Chinese), "SARS/Suspected SARS outbreak in Wuhan, China."[34] RadioFreeAsia@RFA posted, (translated):

> [Pneumonia of unknown cause appears in Wuhan]
>
> The Wuhan Municipal Health Commission issued an emergency announcement on the 30th, stating that according to the emergency notification from superiors, 'unexplained pneumonia' appeared one after another in the Huanan Seafood Market in Wuhan City. The Wuhan Municipal Government is mobilizing all personnel to respond well. Patients with unexplained pneumonia with similar characteristics have been treated for one week.[35]

---

iii Dr. Li returned to work as a doctor. He became feverish on January 10, 2020, contracting the coronavirus from an ill patient. On February 7, 2020, Dr. Li died of the virus he warned others about, becoming one of the first health care heroes memorialized in media coverage. Shortly after his death, American author Francesca Cavallo documented the story in the children's book *Doctor Li and the Crown-wearing Virus* (2020). Seven other people were also accused of spreading false information.

With the Wuhan announcements leaked to Weibo and then Twitter, news of the "Wuhan unexplained pneumonia," had spread beyond the borders of China. Dr. Marjorie Pollack, Deputy Editor of *ProMed*, the Program for Monitoring Emerging Diseases, received a tip from a reliable contributor about an emerging outbreak shared online.[36] Once the information was confirmed and more details gathered, ProMed published a post[37] to approximately 83,000 email subscribers at 11:59 p.m. CST on December 30 (1:59 p.m. on December 31 in China), conveying that the Medical Administration and Medical Administration of Wuhan Municipal Health Committee had issued "an urgent notice on the treatment of pneumonia of unknown cause."[38] The memo continued, "It is understood that the 1st patient with unexplained pneumonia that appeared in Wuhan this time came from Wuhan South China Seafood Market."[39] *ProMed's* email caught the attention of the China Country WHO Office, spurring an Incident Management Support Team to address the rising crisis.[40]

At the same time that Pollock and her team were preparing the *ProMed* post, at 1:38 p.m. China Standard Time on December 31, 2019,[iv] the Wuhan Municipal Health Commission published its "briefing on the current situation of pneumonia in our city" (in its entirety, translated from Chinese):

> Recently, some medical institutions have found that many pneumonia cases received are related to Huanan Seafood City. After receiving the report, the Municipal Health Commission immediately carried out case searches and retrospective investigations related to Huanan Seafood City in the city's medical and health institutions. Twenty-seven cases have been found, of which seven are in serious condition, the remaining cases are stable and controllable, and two cases have improved and are scheduled to be discharged in the near future.
>
> The clinical manifestations of the cases were mainly fever, a few patients had difficulty breathing, and chest X-ray showed

iv 11:38 p.m. CDT in the U.S.

infiltrative lesions in both lungs. At present, all cases have been isolated and treated, the follow-up investigation and medical observation of close contacts are in progress, and the hygienic investigation and environmental sanitation disposal of South China Seafood City are in progress.

Wuhan City organized clinical medicine, epidemiology and virology experts from Tongji Hospital, Provincial Center for Disease Control and Prevention, Wuhan Institute of Virology, Chinese Academy of Sciences, Wuhan Infectious Diseases Hospital, and Wuhan Center for Disease Control and Prevention to conduct consultations, epidemiological investigation, preliminary laboratory testing and other aspects of the analysis that the above cases are viral pneumonia. So far, the investigation has not found obvious human-to-human transmission, and no medical staff infection has been found. The detection of the pathogen and the investigation of the cause of infection are currently underway.

Viral pneumonia is more common in winter and spring, and can be sporadic or outbreak [*sic* as translated]. The main clinical manifestations are fever, body aches, a small number of dyspnea, and pulmonary infiltrates. Viral pneumonia is related to the virulence of the virus, the route of infection, and the age and immune status of the host. Influenza virus is the most common virus causing viral pneumonia, and others are parainfluenza virus, cytomegalovirus, adenovirus, rhinovirus, and coronavirus. The diagnosis depends on the etiological examination, including virus isolation, serological examination, and virus antigen and nucleic acid detection. The disease can be prevented and controllable. In terms of prevention, keep indoor air circulation, avoid closed, airless public places and crowded places, and wear masks when going out. The clinical treatment is mainly symptomatic, and bed rest is required. If you have the above symptoms, especially if the fever persists, you should go to a medical institution in time.[41]

At 4:31 p.m. in China, *RedNet.cn*, a Hunan news website, was the first to break the news story in China. The lengthy article, "Sudden unexplained pneumonia? Don't panic! All you need to know is here" repeated content from the Wuhan public announcement, reassured readers that officials were investigating Seafood City, and specified prevention, including guidelines for mask-wearing.[42] Four criteria needed to be met for identifying the "Pneumonia of unknown cause": fever, specify types of lung images, affected white blood cell count, and no improvement from antibiotics. The story concluded with the Hunan Province's 12320 Health Service Hotline number.

At 4:32 p.m. China Standard Time, *The People's Daily*, China's newspaper of the Communist Party Central Committee, published a brief article on the rising crisis from the Xinhua News Agency. "Viral Pneumonia Cases Reported in Central China" stated that twenty-seven cases of pneumonia had been diagnosed, ending with "The commission said all cases were found to be related to a seafood market, and there were no clear signs of human-to-human transmission."[43] *Twenty-first Century Business Herald 21* and *The Beijing News* were also two of the earliest newspapers to break the story, both suggesting the outbreak's connection to the South China Seafood Market.[44] Neither Dr. Zhang, nor the initial patients, were mentioned in any of the official announcements or news coverage.

China's state-affiliated media outlets (Chinese citizens are prohibited from using Twitter[v]) produced social media content about the emerging crisis. The English-language Chinese cable network @CGTNOfficial posted the "latest news" logo with "Local authorities have confirmed cases of pneumonia of unknown cause in Wuhan, central China's Hubei Province. A team of national experts has been sent to conduct virus testing. The patients, from a local seafood market, are in quarantine." Likewise, @globaltimesnews (an English-language newspaper) tweeted, "Several patients ailing with the 'unknown' pneumonia in Wuhan are

---

v Despite China's ban on Twitter for its citizens, millions of tech-savvy Chinese people work around restrictions to use this platform and others. Ng, Kate. "Despite Being Blocked, Twitter Estimates It Has About 10 Million Users in China." *Techwire*. July 11, 2016, https://techwireasia.com/2016/07/blocked-twitter-10-million-users-china/.

seafood retailers, and the cases cannot be determined as SARS, as of yet: reports," retweeted a link to its own story, with an image of a masked person next to a very sick person in a hospital bed. CCTV Asia Pacific tweeted a similar message in Mandarin and English, repeating, "27 cases of viral pneumonia reported in Central China's Wuhan City."

Regular Twitter users also began sharing the information. Hong Kong journalist Alok Gupta@alok227 tweeted, "#Pneumonia outbreak reported from Wuhan, Hubei province in China. The patients reportedly workers from a local seafood market have been quarantined, says local media." @YaxueCao (founder and editor of ChinaChange.org in DC) tweeted, "Health authorities in Wuhan warn cases of mystery pneumonia. Netizens said SARS patients have been identified and quarantined" (retweeting @DCheng36387164's Weibo image). @catsfaith (from Anchorage) simply stated, "from notes there a pneumonia outbreak in a seafood market in Wuhan China, further information later." A handful of other people, primarily from Hong Kong, passed on the Wuhan news:

> @typicalHKer: "There are quite a number of pneumonia cases in Wuhan, China, please stay safe and avoid going to mainland China."
>
> @ThoughtsHk: "Several cases of unidentified pneumonia in Wuhan, a city in central China. As a guy from a city which experienced SARS, I'm highly concerned about this news."
>
> @Dystopia (from Hong Kong): "Warning sign #China's plague outbreak in #Wuhan
>
> —Unknown #pneumonia, till last week at least 7 infected, rest people isolated.
>
> Remember the epidemic #SARS in 2003 which took 299 lives in #HongKong?
>
> Wear Mask, Stay Safe & Healthy"
>
> @benjaminqiu: "Rumors running wild in China now that there are new cases of suspected SARS (officially referred to

> as "pneumonia of unknown reasons") in, well, Wuhan." (This tweet included a 2017 story about the 2002 SARS epidemic).
>
> @xxkkxxLL: "Unknown pneumonia has appeared in Wuhan, China, everyone must be careful."

On December 31, *ProMed* issued a second post on Wuhan with the updated information, adding, "Whether or not it is SARS has not yet been clarified, and citizens need not panic."[45]

Meanwhile, still on December 31, the Government of the Hong Kong Special Administrative Region issued a press release, stating that "a number of pneumonia cases related to a local seafood market was recently reported in Wuhan."[46] The notice advised surgical masks for travelers to the area and suggested caution in handling poultry and other birds. On the same day, *South China Morning Post* published the article (translated) "Hong Kong takes emergency measures as mystery 'pneumonia' infects dozens in China's Wuhan city," stating:

> Hong Kong health authorities are taking no chances with a mysterious outbreak of viral pneumonia in the central Chinese city of Wuhan, warning of symptoms similar to SARS and bird flu as they step up border screening and put hospitals on alert.[47]

While the pattern wasn't known at the time, the WHO study identified possible 174 cases of the virus in December 2019, 100 of which were later confirmed by lab testing.[48] For the cases with known history, 44.6 percent had no connection to Chinese markets.[49] Slightly more than half of these cases had exposure to any market, with 32 percent linked to Huanan market.[50] Despite government and media framing of the initial outbreak, Huanan and the other markets were not definitively shown to be origin sites for the pandemic.[51]

"27 TO 44 INFECTIONS": JANUARY 1–5, 2020

On January 1,, 2020, authorities in Wuhan closed the Huanan Seafood Wholesale Market.[52] Around the world, media began to cover the outbreak, repeating the same limited information, that "27 infections" had been reported in Wuhan, connected to the Huanan market. The Canadian *Globe and Mail*, *France 24*, *Reuters*, *AFP*, *The Liberty Times* (Taiwan), *The Philippine Star*, *China Daily*, *The Daily Mail* (UK), and other news outlets shared the story. Nearly all coverage from this early time period mentioned the 2002–2003 SARS epidemic. On January 1, *The Independent* (London) used an AFP/Getty photo of two mask-wearing Chinese women and a baby from June 2, 2003, with the caption "Online rumours say it is the Sars virus but experts think this is unlike" for its story on the emerging disease: "Mystery illness in Chinese city affects nearly 30 people."[53] The brief article began "Health chiefs in China are investigating an outbreak of a respiratory illness that some people have likened to the 2003 Sars epidemic that killed nearly 800 people."[54] Similarly, a *SCMP* story from January 3 stated, "The outbreak, which emerged last month, has revived memories of the 2002–2003 SARS epidemic that started in southern China and killed more than 700 people in the mainland, Hong Kong and elsewhere."[55] Memories of this past devastation were then used to explain Hong Kong's implementation of temperature checks and other measures to reduce transmission. Social media furthered speculation about the reemergence of SARS, with many posts mentioning a possible return of the virus.

On January 4, the US Associated Press produced a widely distributed story on the crisis, "Cases of mystery respiratory illness in China rise to 44," referring to a "new type of viral pneumonia linked to a food market in Central China."[56] This article noted that the disease likely was not SARS. Adding to the content distributed on this date, *The Garden Island* paper in Hawaii noted that the "mysterious infectious disease" may have spread to Hong Kong.[57] At this point, news articles about the rising epidemic were brief—repeating the information from the Associated Press (including the seafood market), did not contain images, and, at least in US papers, were placed deep in the news section and toward the bottom of pages/news sites. Aside from the temperature checks in Hong Kong and notes about screening travelers from Wuhan, mitigation was not part of the discussion.

In the beginning of January 2020, social media messages about the emerging epidemic primarily stemmed from scientists, journalists, public health authorities, and those connected to Wuhan, recirculating the scarce information known about the crisis. Those outside of Asia paid little attention to the rising crisis. Tweets referred to "27 cases" in Wuhan, the seafood market, and concerns that the "mystery pneumonia" (not yet called coronavirus) may be connected to SARS. January 4 marked the first tweet from the World Health Organization: "#China has reported to WHO a cluster of #pneumonia cases—with no deaths—in Wuhan, Hubei Province. Investigations are underway to identify the cause of this illness." The following day, WHO tweeted additional background information, stating, "On 31 December 2019, WHO was informed of cases of #pneumonia of unknown cause in Wuhan City, #China. A total of 44 cases have been reported: 11 patients are severely ill, while the remaining 33 are in stable condition" (paired with the WHO *Disease Outbreak News* graphic).

The Wuhan situation had become enough of a crisis to initiate WHO's *Disease Outbreak News* (DONs)—briefings for the general public that offer "information on confirmed acute public health events or potential events of concern."[58] WHO published its first *Disease Outbreak News* on the "pneumonia of unknown etiology" on January 5, 2020, outlining the timeline and events from the China Country Office's initial alert on December 31, 2019, and the response measures taken thus far (closure of the seafood market, contact tracing, ongoing "pathogen identification" investigation, and improved sanitation). In the briefing, WHO did not "recommend any specific measures for travelers," other than monitoring individual symptoms of respiratory illness.[59] Along with the linked report, WHO posted a series of five

Disease Outbreak News tweets, updating the number of cases in Wuhan, briefly explaining coronaviruses, and stating that the cause was still unknown. Most of the WHO content for the general public, however, continued to be on regular health topics, including suicide awareness, pollution risks, and cervical cancer screening.

The Wuhan Municipal Health Commission released another update on "the unexplained viral pneumonia."[60] The report listed the current case total at fifty-nine patients in the city with no deaths, and overall, strong connections to the Huanan Seafood City (South China Seafood Wholesale Market). Moreover, "preliminary investigations have shown that no clear evidence of human-to-human transmission has been found."[61] Despite evidence suggesting the steady increase of cases, coverage was nearly absent from Chinese media. From January 1 through January 5, *The People's Daily* only ran a link to one story on its homepage: news of the virus emerging in Hong Kong, which contained no description or images.[62]

"A NOVEL CORONAVIRUS": JANUARY 6–12

News organizations outside of China continued to publish brief, buried articles about the "mysterious virus" in Wuhan, noting increasing numbers, repeating the possible link to the seafood market, and stating that the virus was not SARS.[63] On January 6, the *New York Times* ran its first article: "China Grapples with Mystery Pneumonia-like Illness," which also appeared in the *Washington Post* and other papers.[64] The accompanying photo featured a "health surveillance" worker screening mostly unmasked passengers at a Hong Kong airport.[65] Although media from around the world covered the outbreak, this coverage drew from a relatively small pool of information, repeating the Wuhan origin, possible seafood market connection, and other facts known at this point.

On January 7, the China CDC first isolated the novel coronavirus, verified by the National Health Commission as the source of the epidemic the next day.[66] The *Wall Street Journal* published the initial news that Chinese scientists had concluded genetic sequencing of the virus, finding it to be a novel coronavirus, according to an unnamed source in China.[67] *ProMed* was again quick to share the news, emailing subscribers that a novel coronavirus had been found (citing the *Wall Street Journal*).[68]

China Central Television posted a transcript interview with team leader Xu Jianguo from the Xinhua News Agency out of Beijing. Xu Jianguo stated:

> As of 21:00 on January 7, 2020, a new type of coronavirus was detected in the laboratory, and the whole genome sequence of the virus was obtained. A total of 15 positive results of the new type of coronavirus were detected by nucleic acid detection methods, from 1 positive patient. The virus was isolated from the sample and showed a typical coronavirus shape under the electron microscope.[69]

Jianguo was also quoted in the *South China Morning Post* story on January 9, which repeated the information. Its story highlights read, "New strain is found in 15 of the patients from Wuhan. Experts urge need for further investigation after some of the 59 people reported infected were traced to a seafood market."[70]

The term "novel coronavirus" emerged in AP news stories on January 9.[71] Identification of the novel coronavirus spurred expanded coverage of the emerging crisis. The *Record-Journal* in Meriden, Connecticut, *The Monitor* in McAllen, Texas, the Canadian *Whitehorse Daily Star*, the *Honolulu Star-Advertiser*, and other papers reprinted the AP information and stories from larger outlets. For example, the *Minneapolis Star Tribune* reprinted the *Washington Post* story "China Identifies New Strain of Coronavirus as Source of Pneumonia Outbreak."[72] Like most of the articles at this point, writers Gerry Shih and Lena H. Sun explained the crisis in Wuhan, defined coronaviruses, and distinguished the virus from SARS and MERS. "Symptoms of the new Wuhan pneumonia include fever and invasive lesions of the lungs when viewed under chest radiographs"—language repeated in other stories.[73]

Social media users circulated news stories, couched in their own comments. Posts at this time focused on distributing information, but also raised questions about China's credibility. For example, @DrAliSKhan retweeted a *BBC News* breaking story on the novel coronavirus identification, adding, "Days after rumors. Official that the #WuhanSARS Wuhan pneumonia outbreak is likely a novel coronavirus. But Coronaviruses span common cold to SARS. How do you trust #China to share the real epidemiology? Where is @WHO with PHEIC meeting? THIS is time." Tweeting from Madrid on January 8, @microRyC posted an image of a bat, paired with "WSJ Report Links Novel Coronavirus to Wuhan #Pneumonia Cluster. This virus seems to be quite similar to some previously described bat-borne Coronavirus. No official information was released yet." Heavy publicity surrounding the discovery of the novel coronavirus drew public attention. Boon-Itt, Sakun, and Yukolpat Skunkan's study of Twitter trends indicated that the keyword "outbreak" significantly spiked on January 9, 2020.[74]

Health agencies were already disseminating alerts on the outbreak. The CDC issued its first "CDC Health Advisory," titled, "Outbreak of Pneumonia of Unknown Etiology (PUE) in Wuhan, China" via the Health Alert Network on January 8, 2020.[75] The report confirmed, "Some of the patients were vendors at the Wuhan South China Seafood City (South China Seafood Wholesale Market) where, in addition to seafood, chickens, bats, marmots, and other wild animals are sold, suggesting a possible zoonotic origin to the outbreak."[76] This report advised health practitioners to "ask patients with severe respiratory disease about travel history to Wuhan City."[77]

The WHO tweeted further explanation on January 9, stating "Coronaviruses are a large family of viruses that are known to cause illness ranging from the common cold to more severe diseases, such as Middle East respiratory syndrome (MERS) and severe acute respiratory syndrome" (SARS). Part two read, "A novel #coronavirus is a new strain of the virus that has not been previously identified in humans." The tweets continued, "Some coronaviruses cause less-severe disease, some more severe. Some transmit easily from person to person, while others don't" (January 9, 2020).

WHO also produced its first tweet outlining precautions (with emojis for each tip), "Protect yourself & reduce risk from #coronavirus infection: Hand hygiene, Cover mouth & nose when coughing & sneezing. Thoroughly cook meat & eggs. Avoid close contact with anyone with respiratory illness. Avoid close contact with wild or live farm animals" (January 9, 2020). On January 10, Yanan Wang of the Associated Press, wrote a Q&A about the new coronavirus, explaining the type of virus, symptoms, and transmission, and distinguishing it from SARS.[78] WHO issued updated guidelines for travelers and trade, acknowledging the uncertainty of the moment: "Transmission potential and modes of transmission remain unclear. Therefore, it would be prudent to reduce the general risk of acute respiratory infections while traveling in or from affected areas (currently Wuhan City)," following the set of tips tweeted the previous day. Additionally, WHO offered advice for airline crew handling sick passengers and reiterated that trade and travel with China should not be restricted.[79]

On January 11, WHO provided guidelines for countries on preparing for the emerging crisis, tweeting (with emojis) about surveillance, treatment, infection control, supplies, and communication. WHO provided a slew of technical documents, including a "WHO tool for national authorities to review their capacity to detect and respond to a novel #coronavirus" (January 11, 2020), along with guidance on community preparation and necessary supplies.

In the midst of tweets about community preparedness, WHO announced online that it had "received the genetic sequences for the novel #coronavirus (2019-nCOV) from the Chinese authorities. We expect them to be made publicly available as soon as possible" (January 11, 2020). Following this tweet was an explanation of the significance, that these genetic sequences "will allow countries to develop specific diagnostic kits, quickly identify and then care for anyone infected, and ensure better health outcomes and containment of the virus" (January 11, 2020).

While WHO continued to instruct the global public on preparedness and caring for those with suspected respiratory infections, the organization continued to acknowledge its own uncertainty, "At this stage, there is no clear evidence of human-to-human transmission in the novel #coronavirus (2019-nCOV) outbreak in #Wuhan, #China. However, the Chinese authorities continue intensive surveillance and follow-up measures, including environmental investigations."

The first novel coronavirus death occurred in China on January 11, and was conveyed by WHO, news outlets, and others on January 12. At the same time, WHO's tweets also offered reassurance, "Currently, no case with infection of this novel #coronavirus (2019-nCOV) has been reported elsewhere other than #Wuhan, #China" (January 12, 2020).

THE VIRUS SPREADS: JANUARY 13–19

On January 12, the first coronavirus case outside of China had been confirmed—in Thailand. Chinese media outlets continued to downplay and ignore the rapidly expanding public health crisis.[80] *The People's Daily* website optimistically discussed the upcoming Spring Festival, boasted achievements in science, and offered feature stories on light topics. No headlines, links or images gave any indication that anything was out of the ordinary. For example, the homepage on January 14 featured an image of a woman prepping a train for the Spring Festival without a mask, gloves, or other health protection.

From January 6 through January 16, the *People's Daily* only offered two stories on the virus. An article linked at the bottom of the page on January 15 stated, "WHO Says No Clear Evidence of Human-to-Human Transmission of Novel Coronavirus."[81] Framed positively, the story downplayed the threat of the virus, repeating that it was limited to the market, and that "No additional cases have been detected since Jan. 3 in China."[82] The next day, the site included a link to the four-line article "Japan Confirms 1st Case of Pneumonia Linked to Coronavirus."[83] Instead, *The People's Daily* produced more content on upcoming festivals, Olympic hopefuls, and quirky tidbits, such as news of a water-skiing squirrel in Toronto.

But all was not well. Confirmed cases of the novel coronavirus had been identified in Thailand and Japan. Although no countries had yet to implement travel restrictions, public health agencies were preparing for the global crisis. WHO increased its public outreach, offering daily information and guidance through its website and on social media, including infographics on how to "Reduce your risk of coronavirus infection," instructing people to wash their hands, "cover nose and mouth when coughing," staying away from those with "cold or flu-like symptoms," fully cooking food, and "no unprotected contact with live wild or farm animals" (January 13, 2020). This and similar infographics continued to emphasize the risk of handling wild animals, reinforcing the possible connection to the Wuhan market. Along with educational materials, WHO's tweets linked detailed reports on significant developments and the implications for those developments.

With the spread of the virus to Thailand, other organizations, agencies, and individuals turned to social media to express concern about transmission to other countries. WHO warned, "Considering global travel patterns, additional cases in other countries are likely" (January 16, 2020). For example, officials in Spain, and Italy (writing in their native languages) explicitly acknowledged public fears. By the January 13, more tweets and stories about the current spread to Thailand and concerns about the transmission to other places had appeared. January 15 marked the CDC's first public communication about coronavirus, retweeting WHO content and adding, "CDC continues to monitor this ongoing investigation to learn more about this rapidly evolving outbreak #coronavirus. #2019-nCOV.[84]

At this point, breaking news about a confirmed case in Japan and a second death in China prompted the most comments on Twitter. Many were sympathetic, while others expressed alarm. Individuals also used the channel to educate fellow users. Columbian Infectious Disease Epidemiologist Dr. Zulma Cucunubá wrote, as @ZulmaCucunuba, (in Spanish), "Like many, I am fascinated and somewhat concerned that open science in just 17 days has allowed us to understand about a new virus with potential global implications. #coronavirus #2019nCov. As it is a relevant topic for everyone, I am going to tell you details," followed by seventeen informative tweets about the emerging virus. Her posts received over 10,000 retweets, 1,773 tweets with comments, and 14,700 likes—more than any other news or public health organization during that time period.

Still, some users made light of the rising crisis. For example, to the breaking news of a confirmed case in Japan by @spectatorindex, J@MixedTheKid replied with a GIF of a Corona Extra beer bottle dancing with an anthropomorphized lime wedge.[85] Along with other Corona beer references, users posted popular culture memes and GIFs of appalled reactions and clips from *Resident Evil* and *The Walking Dead* zombie scenes. A study of COVID tweets in mid-late January showed that humorous tweets were the most liked but were not as common as those that conveyed general information or expressed fear and other emotions.[86]

THE ESCALATING GLOBAL CRISIS: JANUARY 20–29

Following news stories in other countries that confirmed human-to-human transmission, on January 20, Chinese authorities publicly relayed the information that the virus could be transmitted from person to person.[87] WHO tweeted about the formation of the Emergency Committee on the novel #coronavirus (2019-nCOV), which would soon meet to "ascertain whether the outbreak constitutes a public health emergency of international concern, and what recommendations should be made to manage it" (WHO, January 20, 2020). This tweet grabbed the public's attention, with over 5,000 likes, 3,815 retweets, 854 quote tweets, and numerous comments, including,

> @LeslieHipp: "Eerily similar to the movie "Contagion" (linking a movie clip).
>
> @_cCaptainn_: "In the year 2016 alone, falling objects killed 4,693 U.S. construction workers. That's 29x more deaths than

> this "deadly virus" has caused. Why are trying to sow fear and panic?"
>
> @ElayneNahaman: "I guess you never heard of the Black Plague."[88]

Others made remarks about too little too late, advocated for Taiwan to be involved in the meeting, demanded travel restrictions, suggested the coverage overhyped the crisis, stated that China couldn't be trusted and may be spreading false information, or joked about Corona beer.

According to the US report, on January 20 the Chinese government became more transparent about its rising cases, demonstrated by the article on January 21, "All-out Efforts Ordered to Curb Spread of Virus," which appeared in multiple Chinese news sites including *The People's Daily*.[89] The lengthy article called for the need to "mobilize all available resources and take concrete and effective measures to contain further spread of the sickness," while at the same time, praising Chinese cities for their actions in "monitoring, prevention and control of infectious pulmonary diseases." Three other articles appeared on that day in *The People's Daily*, confirming human transmission, but also offering reassurance that the spread would be contained. Such stories continued to flood Chinese news sites, with notices about travel restrictions, businesses specifying their mitigation efforts, and demand for national unity to fight against disease spread.

The First US Case: January 21, 2020

In a media release on January 21, the CDC announced the first confirmed case in the United States in a man who had recently traveled from Wuhan.[90] The CDC released this information on Twitter, sparking emotional responses, debates about mitigation, and speculation.[91] Some users blamed the CDC for the lack of travel restrictions:

> @Galaxy48373323: "What about people exposed to him in his air travel[?]"

> @JKA2020_2030 replied to @CDCgov, "What are we doing about it? Just watching until it's too late? Seriously why haven't the airports been shut down? I mean completely shut down!"
>
> @aNorvsSomer: "Protect your people @TSA. The @CDCgov seems to think screening will control the situation. Give your employees all the protection gear, that they will need to protect themselves. Fellow #Americans protect yourself, especially in airports. Cause I don't ever count on #CDC."[92]

Other users blamed China, expressed disbelief at the rising crisis, or went so far as to suggest it was all a conspiracy. @justice4injured tweeted, "Just another illness for you to sell a vaccine for. You've created the panic. Now you have a vaccine to sell. Great job." @gyf728 replied, "How is QuestionVaccines still a thing in 2020?" While Twitter retroactively removed some of these early comments, speculation, misinformation, and conspiracy about coronavirus were not yet flagged or blocked by the platform.

Until this moment, the Trump administration had not publicly remarked on the burgeoning crisis. On January 22, 2020, then-President Trump commented in a *CNBC* interview, telling Joe Kernen, "It's one person coming in from China. We have it under control. It's going to be just fine."[93] This brief statement foreshadowed the Trump administration's overall coronavirus response and consideration.[94] Despite the US government's nonchalance, the rising transmission was already impacting economies. A brief article on January 22 listed the falling stock prices in the travel industry. Major airlines, hotels, cruise lines, resorts, and casinos' stock had already declined by 4–7 percent in anticipation of travel restrictions with China.[95]

WHO Director Dr. Tedros Ghebreyesus gave a speech on the global crisis on January 23, capturing the severity of the moment: "I am not declaring a public health emergency of international concern today . . . Make no mistake. This is an emergency in China, but it has not yet become a global health emergency. It may yet become one."[96] He went on to state that 575 out of the 584 known cases and all of the

17 deaths had occurred in China. Cases outside of China had appeared in Japan, the Republic of Korea, Singapore, Thailand, the United States, and Vietnam. He continued:

> Let me talk about what we know. We know that this virus can cause severe disease, and that it can kill, although for most people it causes milder symptoms. We know that among those infected, one quarter of patients have experienced severe disease. We know that most of those who have died had underlying health conditions such as hypertension, diabetes or cardiovascular disease that weakened their immune systems. We know that there is human-to-human transmission in China, but for now it appears limited to family groups and health workers caring for infected patients. At this time, there is no evidence of human-to-human transmission outside China, but that doesn't mean it won't happen.
>
> There is still a lot we don't know. We don't know the source of this virus, we don't understand how easily it spreads, and we don't fully understand its clinical features or severity.[97]

On January 24, as a second US coronavirus case was confirmed, Trump praised China in his first tweet[vi] about the crisis, "China has been working very hard to contain the Coronavirus. The United States greatly appreciates their efforts and transparency. It will all work out well. In particular, on behalf of the American People, I want to thank President Xi!"[98]

At this point, global public interest in the crisis was gaining momentum. Widespread television and print news coverage across countries speculated about the zoonotic origin of coronavirus, possibly from bats.[99] This fascination prompted Google and Wikipedia searches related to "bat virus," which reached 100 on Google Trends on January 25.[100] Repeated connections to the Wuhan market and to wet markets

---

vi Since Twitter permanently banned Trump, his tweets are no longer available on the social media platform. All of his tweets are available and cited through secondary news sources.

overall had also sparked a deluge of sinophobic public responses, in which news outlets and social media users ridiculed what they perceived as the eating habits in China, blaming them for the virus.[101] As will be further explored in chapter five, these early racist, false assumptions significantly set the tone for anti-Asian sentiment and hate crimes throughout the pandemic.

Cases were increasing significantly each day, up to 1,320, with 1,297 in China and 41 deaths reported by January 25.[102] WHO emphasized the need for global cooperation, announcing that major scientific journals would start sharing papers on coronavirus prior to publication, to "help us analyze the #coronavirus situation as it evolves, in real time. This helps us to provide the most informed advice and act more quickly" (shared on Twitter, January 26, 2020). Ten countries had identified cases by the January 26, with five in the United States.[103] The WHO situation report two days later showed up to 4,593 confirmed cases globally—56 outside of China, present in 14 countries.[104] WHO initiated a global platform for reporting clinical data and expanded guidance for health professionals on mitigation, stocking supplies, handling patients, and identifying potential coronavirus cases. Meanwhile, the CDC issued a media statement on helping 210 US citizens return home from Wuhan, China.[105]

Public health organizations focused on delivering up-to-date information to journalists and the general public, offering question and answer social media sessions, YouTube videos, briefs for health professionals, and abundant other materials. Cases continued to expand to new countries and US states. On January 30, the United States confirmed its first case of non-travel-related coronavirus, transmitted from human to human, as stated by the CDC, "The full picture of how easily and sustainably the 2019-nCOV spreads is still unclear." This press release concluded, "For the general public, no additional precautions are recommended at this time beyond the simple daily precautions that everyone should always take."[106]

On January 30, the WHO Emergency Committee determined that the coronavirus spread was officially a PHEIC.[107] Globally, 7,818 cases had been confirmed, with over 12,000 more cases suspected in

China. Eighty-two cases had been identified outside of China in eighteen countries and four continents.[108] By the next day, the confirmed numbers had risen to at least 9,709 cases in China, 213 deaths and 25 countries, with six cases in the United States.[109] Lockdowns were in place for Wuhan and other Chinese cities.[110] Hong Kong closed schools, libraries, and museums, canceled events, and facilitated remote work for government and other employees.[111] North Korea had closed borders to prevent transmission. However, at this point, most countries had just restricted travel to and from China and added airport screenings.[112]

Knowledge of the virus had become almost universal. At this point, 96 percent of US adults polled between Jan. 31 and Feb. 4 had heard about the virus.[113] Seventy percent of respondents said that they had "heard a great deal about coronavirus" and 66 percent perceived it as a threat.[114] Worldwide, "virus" steadily increased in Google search trends, reaching 100 on January 28 and 31.[115] In most parts of the world, though, life moved along as usual.

News Diffusion with the Global Crisis

The distribution and consumption of information set the foundation for how (what would become) the pandemic would unfold. Unlike other significant events (i.e., FDR's death or the *Challenger* explosion), news of the viral spread trickled before it exploded. Unlike epidemics and pandemics of a pre-digital age, most people found out about the virus long before it became an immediate threat. As such, it took weeks or even months before individuals outside of each rising Hot Zone paid attention to the crisis enough to share the information and modify their own behavior. Discussed in later chapters, this delay between learning about coronavirus and its presence in one's own community gave opportunities for preparation, but also contributed to "COVID fatigue" and resistance to mitigation later on.

What impacted the news diffusion of the "mystery pneumonia?" China's government/media structure shaped how and how much evolving information made it to the public within and outside the country. A US investigation into how China handled the initial crisis concluded that its government deliberately interfered with the delivery of timely, accurate information. The report titled "COVID-19 and China: A Chronology of Events (December 2019–January 2020)" provides evidence that the Chinese government downplayed the severity of the rising outbreak, delayed relaying genetic sequencing and other key information, and blocked news outlets from early reporting on the coronavirus.[116] The rising crisis was nearly invisible in state-affiliated media outlets. Individuals were discouraged and even punished for communicating information about the rising crisis. Dr. Li and others who publicly warned about the threat of disease faced questioning and even detainment.[117] Chinese authorities arrested citizen journalist Zhang Zan in May 2020 for uploading YouTube videos documenting the Wuhan lockdown.[118] Outside of China, it is difficult to ascertain the extent to which its media structure impacted the exterior channeling of information. And yet, even with censorship by the Chinese government, early action by Dr. Zhang Jixian, her hospital, the Wuhan Municipal Health Commission, and unnamed informants in China enabled information about the emerging virus to spread quickly, within minutes and hours of the updates.

Weeks before the novel coronavirus was identified, social media platforms provided global connections that relayed content instantaneously, jumping from Weibo posts to Twitter and other outlets in the first few days and then linking most of the world throughout. Local and national health departments and governments also distributed information and instruction through Facebook.[119] For example, Singapore's Ministry of Health produced 271 posts on coronavirus between January 1 and March 18, 2020. People turned to YouTube and TikTok as well to learn about coronavirus from public health agencies, news outlets, health professionals, and individuals.[120] Concerns about the spread of misinformation and conspiracy theories over social media platforms began early on. Even in January, some platforms took measures to cut down on false coronavirus content.[121]

Broadly speaking, news diffusion of the novel coronavirus was not simply about the release and distribution of new information through formal and informal channels. As social media platforms facilitated the spread of new knowledge, organizational and individual interest and perceived saliency also significantly impacted the rate at which other people found out about this new disease. News and public health agencies increasingly churned out content as cases spread in January (and beyond), yet the reach of those stories and messages depended on individual consumers to comment on and share the content.

What was not well understood was the ever-evolving nature of crisis messaging. WHO and other public health organizations issued numerous statements that were designed to be reassuring (i.e., the lack of evidence suggesting human transmission), but, in hindsight, were perceived as misleading. Combined with prevalent mis/disinformation, people struggled to discern between evolving facts, which changed with new evidence, and false information. Looking back, it is remarkable just how much information was garnered and what remained unknown in January 2020. In one month, scientists collectively genetically mapped the "mystery pneumonia," identified the source as a novel coronavirus, discovered how to diagnose the disease (initially with CT scans), learned that it could be spread through contact, observed its incubation period, and determined that healthy carriers could transmit the virus. News media around the world updated their publics on the ever-evolving information, but even after many breakthroughs, so much was still unknown. Would an effective test be developed and approved? Was the virus airborne? How contagious and lethal was it? Could it be transmitted on objects? For whom was it dangerous? It would take months before sound answers to these and many other questions could be provided and verified.

Early media also established the tone for global responses. The initial press statements set up the "mystery pneumonia" as a problem in Wuhan, for the people of Wuhan, with the focus on the seafood market. Speculation on the disease's potential to become epidemic or possibly pandemic was quickly squashed, particularly in the parallels to SARS in 2002–2003. Collectively, local, national, and international news outlets, briefings from public health agencies, and the comments and content of regular people (few of which were in Wuhan or even China) immediately and repeatedly dismissed the potential of this virus to impact the world. Google searches and social media posts reflected and perpetuated the focus on Wuhan at this time.[122] This shortsighted framework delayed travel restrictions and other mitigation efforts, blaming and stigmatizing China as "diseased," instead of developing cooperative efforts and public campaigns to prepare for (what we now know would be) the seemingly inevitable pandemic. On a related note, emphasis on bats as the possible origin could have long-lasting detrimental impact on conserving these mammals.[123] Although much of the focus was on the Huanan Seafood Market, the "Joint WHO China Study" final report concluded, "No firm conclusion therefore about the role of the Huanan market in the origin of the outbreak, or how the infection was introduced into the market, can currently be drawn."[124]

Overall, the initial media coverage set the path for how information would be produced and received throughout the pandemic. The perpetuation of stigma, early politicization, and distrust, couched in intensifying emotion emerged in content produced by governments, health agencies, news organizations, and individuals in January, before much of the action had even happened. Social media allowed for the quick sharing of content, public opinions to be expressed equally, and facilitated communication between experts, journalists, and lay people. At the same time, this digital landscape facilitated many of the troubling discourses of the "infodemic," significantly contributing to the deaths of more than 6.9 million people worldwide.[125]

CHAPTER THREE

"Like Sitting Ducks"

THE CRUISE SHIP CRISIS

We are now confined to the staterooms on the instructions of the Japanese health officials and that's all we've been told and we have to await further news. So it's not looking good . . All I can say is that every guest on board this ship is now confined to the stateroom.[1]

—David Abel, vlogging from the Diamond Princess cruise ship

On February 5, 2020, the *Diamond Princess* cruise ship abruptly shifted from a vacation vessel to a public health nightmare. Abel and other passengers documented their quarantine experiences online, connecting with news outlets internationally to tell their stories in real time. Despite the imposed quarantine and other mitigation efforts, over the next three weeks, 712 people tested positive for coronavirus. Fourteen of them died from the disease. The ship outbreak quickly became the largest cluster of cases outside of China.[2] Although the *Diamond Princess* certainly wasn't the only cruise ship quarantined with outbreaks, it produced the most cases and became the center of media attention.

February 2020—the month before WHO declared the pandemic—set the tone for much of how the next few years would unfold, both in the importance of citizen engagement and in the responses and debates that arose. Drawing from the history of disease at sea, this chapter traces the cruise ship crisis from before the first cases to the disembarkation of the last person on board on March 1, 2020 (the captain of the *Diamond Princess*). News coverage, cruise line press releases, social media posts, government communication with passengers, scholarly journal articles, documentaries, books, and other material produced about the quarantine were used to construct the narrative. To preserve the authenticity of the social media posts, all text has been repeated in its original form, including spelling and grammatical errors. Emojis have been removed.

Background: Ships and Infection

Long before disease causality was scientifically understood, people recognized that vessels could carry illness from one port to the next. Sailors often became ill at sea from poor nutrition, contaminated water, flea-carrying rats, unsanitary conditions, and infectious maladies.[3] In 1348, city-appointed public health guardians in Venice began inspecting arriving ships for signs of the Black Death and other disease.[4] The Republic of Ragusa on the Adriatic Sea, followed by Marseilles, Venice, Pisa, and Genoa first implemented quarantines in hopes of protecting against the Black Death, with 40 days becoming the standard in 1383.[5] In lieu of quarantine, ports also adopted the practice of issuing a *patente* (clean bill of health) for departing vessels, verifying that disease was not present.[6] Along with plague, smallpox, typhus, influenza, measles, and other contagious illness easily spread onboard.

As sea travel expanded over the next few centuries, illness continued to plague sailors—enough so that barber-surgeons and medical chests became standard onboard.[7] Quarantines and bills of health continued to be standard practice in Europe, effectively preventing at least some disease-ridden sailors from disembarking in established cities.[8] During this period, European ships regularly brought smallpox and other contagious diseases into the "New World," decimating Indigenous populations.[9]

By the twentieth century, vaccination, improved hygiene, antibiotics, and other medical discoveries rendered many of the past epidemiological threats irrelevant. As air travel replaced passenger ships as a mode of transportation by the late 1950s, leisure cruising became more common.[10] Sea travel nowadays obviously carries far less risk than its predecessors. A study of passenger and crew mortality found that from 2000 to 2019, 623 cruise ship deaths occurred across 78 ocean and river cruise lines.[11] Falls, suicide, and murder were among the top causes for the 557 passenger deaths, with 31 perishing from pneumonia, Norovirus, or another infectious illness.[12] For the sixty-six crew deaths, suicide, murder, and falls were most common, while only one was from disease.[13] In the year before COVID, twenty-seven passengers and ten crew members died on cruise ships out of the approximately thirty million people that sailed.[14] Even though disease is not usually fatal, people do get sick on board. Travelers' diarrhea, norovirus, and other gastrointestinal disease outbreaks have been attributed to contaminated fresh fruit, potato salad, swordfish, ice, and other contaminated food and water, as well as poor sanitation.[15] Respiratory illnesses are also common, although clusters of infection have been less documented.[16]

Since disease, injuries, and health emergencies do happen, contemporary cruise ships contain medical facilities and trained staff on board. Furthermore, every cruise line has extensive emergency plans for handling crises.[17] These procedures are largely hidden from cruise guests, aside from mandatory muster drills. WHO and the International Maritime Organization, working with other regulating bodies, shape health and safety on cruise ships.[18] Cruise ships that are part of the CDC's Vessel Sanitation Program must undergo sanitation inspections when arriving at domestic ports.[19] Individual governments also have their own inspection and regulatory processes that vary by country. Even with these structures in place, public health scholars before the COVID-19 pandemic noted a lack of crisis preparation for cruise ships to handle contagious disease.[20]

Pre-Crisis: January 2020

As addressed in the previous chapter, January 2020 marked the identification and rise of coronavirus as it quickly spread to twenty-five countries by the end of the month.[21] Despite its speedy transmission, much of the world continued to perceive the disease as a far-off threat.

Even with the WHO's declaration of coronavirus as a PHEIC on January 30, the United States and other countries outside of Asia had only restricted travel to and from China at this point.[22] The embarkation of cruise ships continued as normal.

The first news stories on coronavirus and travel did not mention transmission risk but focused on the looming financial impact. Stock prices in the travel industry had steeply declined, affecting airlines, hotels, resorts, casinos, and cruise ships.[23] On Twitter, @realwillmeade posted, "Can you imagine what will happen to cruise line stocks if and when SARS 2 Coronavirus breaks out $RCL $NCLH." Dan@optionscracker predicted, "Given the new items continue to compound as it relates to the coronavirus—expect this to take a toll over the next few days on $CCL and $RCL—cruise lines—as news spreads and the virus continues to spread." Those giving stock advice also warned of the decline. Stock Market Trading Money Making@stockMarketTrdg reflected on the day: "Hopefully you stayed away from banks, airlines, casinos, cruise lines and Chinese #coronavirus."

Shared on social media, *Seatrade Cruise News* tried to allay financial concerns with the story on January 21, "China's coronavirus outbreak will be something to closely monitor as it relates to the cruise industry but at present is not likely to be a material headwind, Wells Fargo Securities said in a note."[24] The shipping industry publication *Trade Winds* similarly stated, "China's coronavirus, an epidemic with flu-like symptoms that has alarmed the travel industry, should not have a major impact on cruise sector earnings, according to an analyst."[25] On January 23, Senior Editor of Empire Financial Research remarked, "Surprised there isn't more chatter about the coronavirus' impact on cruise lines. This is peak season for SE Asia cruises & Singapore is a HUGE port. If this continues it will cause havoc, not to mention cancellations of trips booked for NEXT year."

China continued to be the sole area of concern, even with cases spreading throughout the world. "China Virus Latest: Is It Safe to Travel to China?" asked by the UK-based *World of Cruising*. Despite the loaded (and stigmatizing) headline, the article's response was positive, noting that although Wuhan passengers were prohibited from cruising, other travelers should feel comfortable to do so as long as they feel healthy and practice good hygiene habits.[26] *Cruise Passenger* magazine offered prevention tips on January 25, including an infographic on the importance of washing hands, covering up while sneezing and coughing, avoiding ill people, cooking food thoroughly, and avoiding "unprotected contact with live wild or farm animals."[27]

On January 22, *Cruise Industry News* announced that Astro Ocean Cruises (out of China) and the Italian line Costa had begun to address passenger refunds to discourage sick people from coming on board.[28] Norwegian Cruise Lines (NCL) implemented touchless temperature screenings and denied entry to those who had visited Wuhan within the past thirty days.[29] Princess Cruises introduced temperature screenings and other measures. Royal Caribbean adding screenings for passengers and crews entering from China.[30] Soon after, other major cruise lines banned travelers from Wuhan and Hebei Province.[31] *The Maritime Executive* also covered the story, adding, "The virus is believed to have originated in a seafood market in Wuhan that was illegally selling wildlife, and the Chinese government has announced a temporary ban on the sale of wildlife in markets, restaurants and on e-commerce platforms."[32]

Trade publications, mainstream news outlets, fan blogs, and travel sites heavily covered suspension of Chinese cruise ship operations. *USA Today* reported on the story on January 26, conveying that MSC, Costa, and RCI had canceled departures from China "due to the deadly virus," citing the US Department of State's advisory not to travel to Hubei.[33] The UK tabloid *Daily Express* teased on social media: "Major #cruise lines cancel cruises as #coronavirus spreads—41 dead. A[r]e your holidays affected?"[34] *Fox Business* covered the story, weaving in the financial impact of the cancellations, along with specific measures taken by popular cruise lines, including the ban of passengers recently in Wuhan.[35] Across outlets, writers emphasized China as the source of disease, with port closure as the solution. Cruise lines implemented temperature screenings as precautions, yet reassured passengers that traveling continued to be safe.

On January 27, *Hindustan Times* reported that the Costa luxury ship Venezia had been quarantined at the southeastern Chinese port Shenzhen for a coronavirus outbreak, likely stemming from 148 people who had recently visited Hubei Province. Medical screenings of the 5,260 on board uncovered 13 symptomatic individuals.[36] Passengers on board that passed the medical inspection were then allowed to disembark at the port.[37] However, crew members were rumored to be stuck at sea for at least two weeks, according to this Facebook post circulated on social media:[38]

> I'm a crew members [*sic.*] from Costa Venezia Costa Crociere, we are from 26 of January around the sea From Cina and Japan, it's been almost 14 days that we are at sea without dock in any port, we are inside the ship CLOSED and for us it's not allowed to go out to buy sanitary products that we really need it. The company didn't give information to us and we don't know how the situation will involve. Our stress level is high and we need information about what to do, The Company has to know that is IMPOSSIBLE to keep us inside the ship closed for one month without working and at sea! Please share this message like this somebody Can help us to find a port and disembark crew members and stay safe in a future return at home. Thank you.[39]

The post received 930 shares and 1,100 responses, including the following:

> "Aimz Co": "Why are you complaining? You want to get off the ship and be infected? You are complaining because the local port authority and the company put first your safety? You should be thankful man."
>
> "Javier Gudiel Gamarra": "Costa cruises is taking care for all the crew onboard. . . . for the company first is the safety and help of each one onboard. . . . in my opinion they are doing the best and right decision. . . . .in 2010 when i was in new york to canada onboard in a american company the AH1N1 attack in 6 days more than 400 hundred people, passenger

> and crew because the company never stop the service. . . . now costa is taking cate first for the people onboard is time to be patient and understand the situation."
>
> 姜鑫蕊:"The company is protecting us and we're SAFE here!!!! It is hard to understand why the person has such strange ideas and complain about it . . . These days we even use free Internet,different shows only for crew every day, and we don't have too much work as the passengers onboard but we have the same salary . . . Please stop this untrue complaint . . . WE ARE SAFE AND GOOD IN COSTA VENEZIA!"

This story did not get a lot of attention—no social media tags, nor mentions in other cruise-related topics at this time.[40] Increasingly, cruise lines announced their immediate cancellations of ships in and out of China. *Cruise Industry News* reported on January 25 that Costa Crociere, Genting Cruise Lines, MSC, and Royal Caribbean had canceled all cruise operations in China.[41]

Online, people asked about their own upcoming reservations, especially for Southeast Asia. Marking one of the first social media posts linking coronavirus to cruises, Mo@Notts52 tweeted on January 21: "Re #coronavirus what is @VikingCruises position re upcoming Cruises in #china, starting 2 months time, especially as Wuhan is stopping point on Cruise." Viking Cruises immediately replied, "The safety of our guests is our top priority, @50sEKBOY, and we are monitoring the situation in China as it develops. Should there be any changes to scheduled sailings, guests will be notified directly. Thank you for reaching out."

Tagging Royal Caribbean (who did not respond), Serenity1@KurisutaBlue wondered, "What about #people going on #cruiseships in #Shanghai? I supposed to go on #SpectrumoftheSeas soon but with all these cases, I am not too sure now. Is anyone going to a #cruise #vacation soon in #China? #coronavirus #RoyalCaribbean." On January 23, Camille Denniss@camd8866 asked, @PrincessCruises, we're booked for an Asian cruise and we're extremely worried about the #coronavirus in China." Four days later, the corporation replied, "Thanks for asking,

Camille. Our medical experts are coordinating closely with the U.S. Centers for Disease Control and Prevention (CDC) and the WHO to implement recommended screening, prevention and control measures for our ships." Similar responses were generated to many potential passengers across cruise lines at this time.

People also shared safety protocols. On January 22nd, Seema Mody @seemacnbc tweeted about NCL's recent implementation of temperature checks to board their ships—information not shared on Twitter by the cruise line itself.

Those living in popular tourism destinations wondered online about the continued use of their cruise ports. Reporting from Trinidad and Tobago, *TTT News* commented on the latest government response: "Tourism Minister Randall Mitchell says the relevant authorities are taking all precautionary measures to prevent the coronavirus from entering the country. This, as thousands of cruise visitors are expected to arrive here tomorrow." Likewise, Trinidadian caffeinated tara @ TaraPersad commented, "OH LAWD a cruise with 5000 passengers/ foreigners arrive on Thursday and its raising fears and concerns regarding the coronavirus." On January 24, the *Philippine Daily Inquirer* briefly reported, "There is no hampering the arrival here of luxury cruise ships, some carrying Chinese tourists, despite a heightened alert raised by the Department of Health following the outbreak of the novel coronavirus in China, an official here said" and that no cruise itineraries had changed due to the virus.[42] Grp27@grp273 posted, "I sure hope Key West is paying close attention to this Coronavirus. Several Cruise Ships dock'n weekly 10K20K passengers get'n off & roaming around. I always worried about terrorist pull'n something there Backpacks & gym bags are a normal everyday item down there w/ Passengers."

Cruise Weekly addressed the cruise line responses in its January 24 newsletter: "Cruise ships are in a better position to minimize the risk of coronavirus infection than other forms of travel due to their stringent health procedures, Cruise Lines International Association (CLIA) claims."[43] The story reassured readers of the continued monitoring of the "status of the outbreak in Wuhan, China" and restated the new NCL protocols.[44] On January 26, China port calls were canceled, along with embarkation from the country.[45]

On *Cruise Critic* (a popular cruise fan site), user "Tee & Chilli" started what would become one of the lengthiest and most extensive coronavirus travel threads. "Corona virus RCI policy" initially posed the question, "Anyone changing plans due to the coronavirus? Has Royal issued a statement or offered a FCC? I'm not booked just wondering how cruise lines are handling this." Over the next few weeks, participants used this and other threads to speculate and debate the spreading virus's impact on the cruise industry. On January 24, "tybrkr17" wrote:

> I sail on the Spectrum of the Seas out of Shanghai on Feb 13th and haven't gotten any updates or emails about anything yet. I will let you know if I get anything before I go.
>
> I doubt anything will be affected. Shanghai isn't quarantined and I bet they will just screen for any sick people before you are allowed to board. And I also heard if you have been in in the Hubei area (like Wuhan) areas in the last 30 days, you will also not be allowed to board.

Two days later, "danv3" posted, including a news link:

> Read today (https://www.bbc.com/news/world-asia-china-51254523) that China believes that the virus spreads before symptoms are present and has an incubation period of up to 14 days. If that information is correct, it's reasonable to expect to see some much more aggressive countermeasures in the region, as the virus is going to be more difficult to contain than first thought.

"Joebucks" disagreed: "More people die from the flu than they have from Corona virus. How many of these "new virus" epidemics were anything to be concerned about?" Most responses were similarly dismissive, reassuring future cruise-takers that their bookings over the next few months would take place without issue.

The emphasis on China in this thread reflected news coverage of the rising crisis and press releases from cruise lines at that moment—all of which centered around viral containment in China, even with cases identified in twenty-six countries by the end of January.[46]

On January 30, WHO's declaration of the PHEIC rippled through the travel industry. Through social media, cruise line agents responded to customers asking about personal itineraries and the possibility of restrictions. @PrincessCruises tweeted on January 31: "Although the risk to our guests & crew is low, we're closely monitoring the evolving #Coronavirus response. Our medical experts are coordinating with @ CDCgov and @WHO to implement enhanced screening, prevention & control measures for our ships. Learn more" (attaching its updated travel advisory). Still, across cruise lines, most tweets at the end of January and early February were typical vacation promotions and passenger questions.

Meanwhile, the primary coronavirus *Cruise Critic* thread continued with an onboard observation. On January 30, "87turboii" wrote, "Im on Oasis right now and saw the crew steaming the hallway walls and handrails. Never seen that before. I asked the stateroom attendant and he said it was normal? Has anyone seen that before?" Biker19 replied: "During a noro outbreak, yes, other times not so much." Following suit, cruise lines began publicly communicating updated travel restrictions, refund policies, and improved sanitation practices.

THE DIAMOND PRINCESS: A QUARANTINE CASE STUDY

As public health authorities later chronicled,[47] a man from Hong Kong arrived in Japan on January 17, 2020, and developed a cough two days later. On January 20, he and thousands of other passengers began their sixteen-day Southeast Asia cruise on the *Diamond Princess* out of Yokohama, Japan, with stops scheduled in Japan, Vietnam, and Taiwan.[48] The man participated in a Kagoshima on-shore excursion with other passengers during his five-day ship stay before disembarking in Hong Kong on January 25. He developed a fever on January 30 and was officially diagnosed with coronavirus in a hospital that day.[49] On

Monday, February 3, Hong Kong authorities notified the Ministry of Health, Labor, and Welfare of Japan (MHLW) of the positive coronavirus case, prompting Japanese authorities to place the *Diamond Princess* under quarantine.[50] At this point, the ship had made six scheduled stops in three countries: Hong Kong, Vietnam, and Taiwan, before returning to its scheduled port in Japan.

Seatrade Cruise News was one of the first to report on the situation, explaining that the *Diamond Princess* would be held for "approximately 24 hours" to allow Japan public health authorities time to review the health status of all passengers and crew."[51] Other than the monitoring of guests' handwashing before dining, vacation life continued as normal that day. Guests dined at the buffet, enjoyed performances in the auditorium, and partied late into the night.[i]

At about midnight, guests were informed that "the Japanese medical health team would be boarding the ship and they would be coming to meet every single passenger in their cabins during the nighttime," as described by British passenger David Abel in his February 4 Facebook Live video. Japanese authorities conducted health screenings of the 2,645 guests and 1,068 crew members, while passengers continued to freely move around the ship.[52]

Confined to the Cabin

"We have been notified that amongst the second set of samples that have completed testing, 10 additional people have tested positive for Coronavirus."[53]

Guests woke up to this announcement from Captain Gennaro Arma on Wednesday, February 5th. The additional cases prompted Japanese health authorities to confine guests to their ship cabins for two weeks, expected to end on February 19.

Quarantine spaces varied significantly based on which of the five room classes guests had booked. On the *Diamond Princess*, the 377 interior staterooms ("our most affordable option," according to Princess

i As shown in the 2021 documentary of the Diamond Princess quarantine, *The Last Cruise*.

Cruises) contain 158–162 square feet without a window or balcony to access the outside.[54] Guests with oceanview staterooms, 146–217 square feet, can see outside, but not access fresh air.[55] Balcony stateroom cabins are a bit larger, at 214–279 square feet, including private outside spaces.[56] Mini, full, and grand suites have separate sitting rooms, outdoor spaces, and up to 932 square footage.[57] For the Southeast Asian January cruise, regular prices ranged from $2128 to $7,810 for the 16-day cruise.[58] Most of the 1,110 crew members shared rooms in the windowless lower decks. Doctors and nurses staffed the onboard seven-bed medical clinic.[59]

Out of the 2,666 guests, 50 countries were represented; 1,281 people were from Japan and 328 were Americans.[60] Filipinos made up over half of the crew, with other members representing Thailand, Indonesia, India, Ukraine, and Russia.[61] US citizens, residents, and their partners made up 109 of the crew on board.[62] Although more detailed demographics are not publicly available, data from the coronavirus testing suggests that the majority of the guests were at least age fifty. Crew members were younger and primarily came from the Philippines and other developing countries.[63]

Princess Cruises shared the quarantine update with the general public on social media and its website. News outlets around the globe exploded with the story, repeating the number of cases and the cabin restrictions for guests, saying little about the crew.[64] Many of the guests initiated their own regular web posts—primarily on Facebook and Twitter, but also on Instagram, YouTube, and TikTok—confirming that they were, indeed, stuck on the coronavirus ship. With the 13+ hour time difference, their posts on February 5 appeared on February 4.

> Sarah Arana: "Friends and family, I am getting so many messages that I cannot keep up. I want to be transparent and provide accurate information. I am indeed on this ship that is anchored off the coast of Yokohama . . ." (Facebook, Feb. 4)
>
> "だあ(On board the Diamond Princess / 乗船中乗客)@daxa_tw: "I'd like to share what it's like on board the Diamond Princess cruise. Please use this page to exchange info. #Dia-

mondPrincess #coronavirus." (Twitter, Feb. 4)

Hong Kong 97@Hong_Kong97: "14 days #Quarantine inside #diamondprincess near #yokohama begins. Still shocked and scared. But better precautions. Have faith in the crews and captain." (Twitter, Feb. 5)

Happy_girls_r_the_prettiest: "Yes, we are on THAT quarantined ship. But we are keeping calm and positive. We are safe. We are together. We are relatively comfortable with all the amenities we need. Food. Water. Internet. Power. #diamondprincesscruise #quarantine," paired with a photo of a woman and two teenagers in an interior cabin. (Instagram, Feb. 5)

British passenger David Abel also entered the spotlight early. After vlogging on the initial quarantine and the cabin confinement, on February 5, he pleaded via Facebook Live for Princess to deliver breakfast, posting videos at 8:00, 8:20, 10:12, and 11:50 a.m. Abel explained that they hadn't eaten since dinner on the previous night, putting him, as a diabetic, in severe danger: "So, all the media out there, please be aware of this situation for people such as me who are insulin-dependent and have to have a food intake to avoid going into a hypo. If this can be brought to the attention of Princess Cruises, I would be very grateful." This video was widely shared across platforms, prompting extensive media coverage and responses.

Abel updated at 2:05 p.m., stating that he had received food about an hour earlier: "I honestly believe this is a result from those of you who have really thankfully contacted Princess Cruise lines and made it known that I was in need of medical assistance . . ." Long after Princess had resolved the issue, people continued to post Abel's video clip. @PrincessCruises stated on Twitter, "Thank you for your concern for one of our passengers, we can confirm this situation has been resolved. While guests are quarantined to their cabins, food and beverage will be brought to their rooms via a daily menu."

Abel wasn't the only one using social media to connect to the cruise line. Panic and reassurance both dominated early social media posts as guests, along with family, friends, and internet strangers, tagged

@PrincessCruises to ask about food and dietary accommodations, water, fresh air, clean air, medication, and other issues. Some guests were exceptionally persistent. Canadian Nigel Finch-Cole @Nigel_Cole59 repeatedly tweeted @PrincessCruises, asking the cruise line for more English TV channels, more coffee and tea, cereal, and deodorant. Upon receiving the deodorant, he stated, "You sent secret . . . it's for women . . . we are two men," followed by "Please send old spice or something we can use." The cruise line frequently responded to Nigel and other individuals, either to their specific demands or by advising them to directly message them. Much of the public communication during this time consisted of such interactions.

Princess Cruises also issued broad updates online, reassuring the world of its humane guest and crew treatment. On February 6, the cruise line tweeted:

> "(1/3)#DiamondPrincess update: The well-being of our guests and crew remains our top priority, and we are working diligently to improve their experience during this challenging time. Food and beverages are being brought to their rooms via a daily menu."
>
> "(2/3)Guests in inside and non-balcony staterooms are now permitted to get fresh air on a rotating basis, as directed by Public Health authorities."
>
> "(3/3)We are also providing many in-room activities and additional entertainment options. This includes new TV channels, movies, audiobooks, exercise videos, arts and crafts, board and card games delivered to each stateroom, and more."

Over the next few days, Princess announced that guests would be able to receive their medications, interior cabin guests would have access to outdoor time, and that guests would receive a full refund for "all monies paid to Princess cruises," including the fare, money paid toward excursions, food and beverages, and travel expenses to go home.[65] Princess Cruise also promised a future cruise credit to each guest. In a four-minute YouTube video, Princess Cruise President Jan Swartz expressed justification for the quarantine and outlined resources for passengers and team members.[66]

Meanwhile, some individual governments also began contacting their citizens aboard the *Diamond Princess*. On February 6, the US Embassy Tokyo contacted all American guests, supporting the quarantine imposed by Japanese authorities.[67] The Centers for Disease Control and Prevention (CDC) distributed a similar message to passengers on February 8:

> Based on information CDC has at this time, remaining in your room on the ship is the safest option to minimize your risk of infection. Alternatives might increase the risk of spread of infection. We acknowledge that this situation is difficult. CDC is assisting Japanese health authorities and ship personnel to ensure precautions are being taken to prevent 2019-nCOV spread on the ship. We will continue to monitor the situation closely and take actions as necessary to safeguard your health. We will continue to provide you with information as it becomes available.[68]

The letter provided specific instructions for those on board, explaining and encouraging social distancing, mask-wearing, health monitoring, and what do to if symptoms begin. Government and health agency messages supported the actions of the Ministry of Health, Labor, and Welfare of Japan. Passengers needed to remain quarantined aboard the ship.

Life on the Boat

After the chaos of the first quarantine day, initial concerns were soon addressed. The majority of passengers did not publicly document their time on the ship, limiting communication to interpersonal means (calls and emails) or private social media groups. The dozen or so guests that did, however, flooded social media with updates, providing numerous posts and pictures each day. Through online platforms, these people described their individual experiences. Like David Abel and his wife, many of the guests were over 50 and traveling as couples or friends. Moreover, most of the regular social media posters and vloggers had balcony rooms.

Few social media users had interior cabins or were traveling with children, aside from Hong Kong citizen Yardley Wong and Australian Aun Na Tan. Wong (tweeting as Hong Kong 97@Hong_Kong97) was quarantined to an interior room with her husband and six-year-old son. Her elderly parents were in a cabin nearby, but she was not allowed to see them except during their sixty minutes of fresh air per day. Tan shared an interior cabin with her husband and two teenage children. Both Wong and Tan posted about their experiences multiple times per day, often including images and video.

They and other guests online most frequently addressed quarantine food. Although some guests criticized the menu options, overwhelmingly, guests praised the quarantine cuisine, including photos of their meals and snacks.

> Matthew Smith@mjswhitebread: "Princess stepping up its game with food service on #DiamondPrincess. Don't believe the honeymooners who would rather be in an American hospital. You might have to drag me off the ship when the quarantine ends." (Twitter, Feb. 7)
>
> Gay Coulter @GCourter: "Kudos to the magnificent pastry chefs on board the Diamond Princess. Delicious desserts twice a day chases the quarantine blues away. #diamondprincessquarantine." (Twitter, Feb. 11)
>
> happy_girls_r_the_prettiest (paired with an image of carefully packaged and labeled meals): "I haven't posted about food in a while—here's our lunch for today. We have dietary requirements (lactose free for me—no one would want to be stuck with me in a windowless room otherwise. Shellfish and nut allergy for my daughter) and the crew has been awesome in accommodating our needs. #diamondprincesscruise #quarantine #lunch #nomnomnom." (Feb. 10)

The Valentine's Day meal was highly regarded. Hong Kong 97@Hong_Kong97: "#day10 #HappyValentinesDay @PrincessCruises #coronavirus could you please forward my deep appreciation to the kitchen crew, Catering team and pastry team to make such a wonderful dinner tonight. No exception as always. bravo #HangintthereDiamondPrincess" (Twitter, Feb. 14). Other guests tweeted and posted about the special meal, complete with wine and dessert.

In addition to food, guests celebrated their time outside. Those with balconies expressed gratitude for their ongoing fresh air and used their vantage points to observe the dock area and ambulances. Matthew Smith@mjswhitebread tweeted a picture from his cabin on February 10, stating, "The captain just announced that we will be heading out to sea @ noon today (in about 2 and 1/2 hours) for normal marine operations. It's a lovely, bright day here Yokohama. Feeling very fortunate for our balcony." Balconies were also used as vantage points for information. To her public *Facebook* page, American Sarah Arana posted pictures and commented on the sights below from her balcony: "I can see a flurry of activity down below on the dock, ambulances and the ever-present "oompa loompas" all sealed up in their white hazmat suits. This is so surreal" (Feb. 13).

Guests in the interior cabins were less fortunate. On February 8, Australian Clare Hedger @clarehedger lamented from her interior cabin, "Now nearly 48 hours without fresh air or sunlight—even longer for some. @PrincessCruises, any chance the inside cabins can breath again? #DiamondPrincess #Quarantine." @PrincessCruises replied: "Hi Clare, all guests are now being scheduled for a 60 min fresh air walk, we appreciate your patience during this trying time." Later that day, she and other interior cabin guests were allowed time outside. Tweeting a picture of the ocean, she expressed, "We did!!! Feel alive again after 70 minutes of fresh air and sunshine." Yardley Wong (as Hong Kong 97@Hong_Kong97) tweeted short videos of her son and parents dancing during their daily deck visits, happy to be united and outside again.

Social media also helped to pass the time. American Karey Maniscalco as TikTok Karey Keys made a series of videos on silly ways to keep herself occupied. During her quarantine, she demonstrated "chin tightening" using a comb to flick herself in the neck, jumped on her bed, trimmed her bangs, dyed her hair, and showed off a bucket of beer. On Instagram, happy_girls_r_the_prettiest regularly posted pictures of different family members (as she was quarantined with her two teenagers and husband), playing games, exercising, and listening to music. She also documented her love of journaling with a photo of MUJI gel pens on February 8: "When your biggest worry is running out of ink in your favorite #mujipens from #muji and pages in your #leuchtturm1917 journal. Washi tape is getting low too! #daisojapan #daisoaustralia #delde #diamondprincesscruise #quarantine."

A sharp divide emerged between guests who supported the quarantine and those who resented their confinement. Abel's videoed concerns (which were later resolved) rapidly spread online. Maniscalco as Karey Keys on TikTok joked about being "held captive," pretended to escape using bedsheets, and called the ship "Corona Island." Her hashtags drive home these beliefs: "#trumpsaveus," "#getmeoffofhere," "#presidenttrumpsaveus," "#iwanttogohome," "#SaveMe," "#SaveUs," "#MisterPresidentIimwaiting," "#WhenWillThisEnd." On TikTok, another user asks if Kareykeys is being held hostage. She replies, "Locked in a room for 13 days by force, isnt freedom is it? But it's also a joke." Other social media users questioned those they perceived as too critical of the situation:

> Matthew Smith@mjswhitebread: "Be careful not to believe everything you read about conditions onboard the #DiamondPrincess. Some passengers appear to seeking media attention by exaggerations and outright falsehoods." (Twitter, Feb. 6)
>
> Matthew Smith@mjswhitebread "The truth is out there about conditions onboard #DiamondPrincess. Just be careful who you listen to." (Twitter, Feb. 6)
>
> Hong Kong 97@Hong_Kong97: "#day4 #coronavirus #CoronaOutbreak #quarantine on #DiamondPrincess I don't understand this. When someone make video w/criticism on crews, food, & the situation. Did they think of 3000+ ppl feeling who experience the same hardship?#complainisnot-

> productive #hanginthereprincess." (Twitter, Feb. 8)
>
> Hong Kong 97@Hong_Kong97: "#day5 #coronavirus #coronavirusoutbreak on #Quarantined one #diamondprincess whoever call the cruise is prison cell, prison food, oh gosh! I need to give them justice. We have more than ENOUGH! #hanginthereprincess." (Twitter, Feb. 8)
>
> happy_girls_r_the_prettiest: "We are ok. We are being well taken care of by the hardworking Captain, crew and company who have our best interests in mind. #diamondprincesscruise @princesscruise #princesscruise." (Instagram, Feb. 10)

Overall, selfie videos, pictures, and comments primarily conveyed the boredom of guests, a need to pass the time, and the uncertainty of the moment.

News Coverage of the Diamond Princess

To the outside world, the *Diamond Princess* quarantine was presented through limited frameworks. News outlets incorporated the ship quarantine into larger messages about what was quickly escalating to a global pandemic. Such stories featured photos of ambulances, people in protective gear, and cleaning supplies, with leads like "Large white sheets covering them head-to-knee, people infected with a new virus were led by gloved and masked officials today off a Japanese cruise ship, while the rest of the 3,700 people on board faced a two-week quarantine in their cabins."[69] Writers wove the ship's quarantine into broader news articles, exemplifying the growing reach of the virus, impacts on tourism, and mitigation measures implemented in various countries.[70] A story marking the first coronavirus death of a US citizen stated "Cruise ship passengers faced more woe as Japan reported three more cases for a total of 64 on one quarantined vessel and turned away another."[71] Offering a historical perspective, *Daily Oklahoman Sun* columnist Stephen Prescott wrote in support of the ship quarantine: "If the current quarantine of a cruise ship off the coast of Japan is going to work, every single passenger needs to stay on board for a full

14 days. Even the extremely wealthy, well-connected people who raise a ruckus."[72]

Even with coronavirus cases now identified in four continents,[73] media continued to focus on and blame China. Prescott used "Wuhan Coronavirus" in his title. Other outlets also incorporated the *Diamond Princess* quarantine into stigmatizing stories. "Chinese Leaders Face Public Anger Over Virus," "Virus Cases Surge in China," "China Mostly Closed Down as Virus Deaths Pass 1,000" all used the cruise outbreak to illustrate the magnitude of the problem, falsely framed as stemming from and perpetuated by China.[74] Likewise, *USA Today* printed a story attributing the epidemic to pangolins consumed in markets like the one in Wuhan (a widely shared theory early in the outbreak), referencing the ship to demonstrate its reach.[75] Such stories were less about global public health and more about protecting the world from China.

Smaller news outlets featured local people on board the *Diamond Princess*, personalizing the experience. *The Idaho Statesman* published "Buhl Man on Coronavirus Quarantined Cruise Ship in Tokyo," quoting passenger Tim Pond on his life in quarantine.[76] Similar articles appeared in many regional publications: "6 Hawaii Residents on Ship Quarantined" "Concern Grows for Canadians on Cruise Ship," "B.C. Couple Under 'Cabin Arrest,'" "Richland Couple Quarantined on Cruise Ship in Japan," "Olympia Woman Now Stuck on Quarantined Cruise Ship in Japan," "Citrus County Residents Quarantined in Japan," and "Coronavirus Quarantine Traps Paso Robles Woman."[77] These stories were all framed in the same way—guests were enjoying a wonderful vacation when it turned into a nightmare, with descriptions of their quarantine difficulties. For example, "Coronavirus Threat Strands B.C. Couple" explains that they "are confined to their room and doing their laundry in their bathroom with body wash."[78] Local TV news stations offered similar perspectives through Zoom and other video conferencing tools with the guests in their cabins.

Ethical questions about quarantine and civil liberties appeared in headlines and in quotes from guests and others, which included words like "confined," "trapped," and "prisoners." A story on February 7 in the *New York Times* cited UCLA professor Timothy Brewer: "Someone is going to have to weigh both the public health consequences of requiring hundreds of people to be in quarantine and the political consequences . . . Most people who end up in quarantine probably have not been exposed and do not have the disease—so you're restricting the civil liberties of a lot of people."[79] Regular people who were not on the ship also tweeted about it: BeachChik said, "Have you read articles where the people on the ship have been interviewed? They aren't allowed to leave their cabins. Imagine the people in interior rooms or the people with small kids. No thank you. Two weeks locked in a cruise ship room sounds horrible."

Videos and interviews with passengers who had tested positive reinforced this message, especially because they were either asymptomatic or had mild symptoms. *CNN* reporters interviewed Diamond guest Rebecca Frasure, who was restricted to a Tokyo hospital room after testing positive, while her husband remained on the ship. In her video exchange on February 18th, Frasure mentioned that she felt fine, except for the effects of solo quarantine and a lack of human interaction. The reporter responded, "It's like solitary confinement. I mean, you're describing that you are in solitary confinement, though you've done nothing wrong. What are doctors telling you about when you'll get out of this situation?" Other guests shared similar experiences—testing positive despite quarantine and then facing more confinement against their will, even while feeling healthy.

Across outlets and platforms, the *Diamond Princess* attracted attention. The Associated Press produced many stories, which were disseminated in both large and smaller markets in and outside of the United States. And yet, since those primarily affected were quarantined on the ship, hence difficult to reach, the content included in stories was generic, speculative, and drew from a small pool of interview subjects. Reporters begged *Diamond Princess* passengers for interviews, contacting them in DMs and in the comments of social media posts. In addition to passengers that agreed to tell their stories, writers quoted (and sometimes misquoted) social media posts, official statements from Japanese health authorities, Princess Cruise Line news releases, and infectious disease and other public health experts (speculating on the situation) to construct the unfolding story. Crew members rarely gave interviews and, when they did, the interviews were usually anonymous. The story was far-reaching, but with little content. News outlets also encouraged readers to check out social media for passenger updates, noting how guests were tweeting and posting about their time on the ship.[80]

For selected guests, media interviews became a regular part of the day. Passengers received and gave numerous interviews to outlets all over the world. For example, *BuzzFeed*, *CNN*, *NBC*, *Beijing News*, a Russian TV station, and other outlets contacted Australian Aun Na Tan[ii] in the comments' section of her Instagram posts. Reporters also drew from social media entries to write their stories. A lengthy Associated Press article on February 14 summarized passengers' experiences and varying tones: "Fear. Surprising moments of levity. Soul-crushing boredom," citing both interviews and "a growing stream of tweets and YouTube videos."[81] While still on the ship, author Gay Coulter wrote the first of four articles on her quarantine experiences, publishing in the *Washington Post*.[82] Student Spencer Fehrenbacher wrote an op-ed for *USA Today* about the importance of staying optimistic during quarantine.[83] Journalists from all over had rushed to interview Abel after his urgent video went viral. By Thursday, February 6, Abel announced that due to time and exhaustion, "I will not be talking to any more news stations unless they are based in the UK." Yet, he continued posting his own content until he left the ship.

Some guests declined all interviews, even stating such on their social media profiles. Guests also objected to media framing of the quarantine, especially later on. Hong Kong 97@Hong_Kong97 criticized the *New York Times* for describing the *Diamond Princess* as a "Cruel experiment," tweeting, "That's why I hate mainstream media,

---

ii Family featured in this *BuzzFeed* story: Jamieson, Amber. "Here's how Two Teens are Dealing with Being Trapped on a Cruise Ship Quarantined for Coronavirus." *BuzzFeed News*. February 8, 2020, https://www.buzzfeednews.com/article/amberjamieson/diamond-princess-coronavirus-quarantine-cruise.

the writer just so ignorance and self interested by making up fact to get famous! NEW YORK TIME is disappointing. Captain said so million times the air system is fresh air #Quarantined #COVID19 #diamondprinces" (Twitter, Feb. 24).

Crew members were nearly invisible to those not on the ship. They were not creating content for social media. News outlets and guests talked about the crew, but they were scarcely shown or heard from. The *New York Times* primarily focused on guests, but featured crew in a February 10 article:

> "Down below, more than 1,000 crew members live and work elbow-to-elbow, preparing the passengers' dishes and eating simple buffet-style together, with as many as four sharing a bathroom—and sharing the risk of possible infection from the coronavirus."[84]

The story explained how the crew, mostly from developing nations, declined interviews. Those that gave them primarily remained anonymous "for fear of losing their jobs."[85] While more details of their challenging conditions came out later, in the moment, little space or airtime was given.

Rising Cases: The Plan Shifts

Despite the quarantine and other mitigation measures, coronavirus continued to spread on the *Diamond Princess*. News of the rising cases punctuated the day's monotony, causing worry and uncertainty for those on board. Testing was slow and selective, especially at first, with only symptomatic passengers and close contacts swabbed for the virus. Groups tested expanded to include guests with medical conditions, or eighty years and older, along with those in interior cabins.[86] All remaining guests were not evaluated until they prepared for evacuation.

Results took several days and, at least sometimes, passengers were only notified of positive tests, with others left wondering. Social media users documented the uncertainty, noting that passengers were sometimes taken away with only minutes to vacate the cabin. Captain Arma's February 13 announcement explained, "Guests who test positive will be disembarked to a medical facility ashore to continue their quarantine," while close contacts remained on the ship.[87] Rumors circulating among passengers suggested this process was not always followed. What happened after passengers tested positive was somewhat of a mystery.

Hospital experiences were not documented with the same detail as the mundane life of quarantine. *Diamond Princess* passengers Renee and Clyde Smith relayed their experiences of testing positive and hospitalization through their adult son in *The Atlanta Constitution*.[88] Even heavy social media users slowed down or stopped posting once they became ill. On February 18, Abel posted on Facebook, "There is going to be a time of quiet. We have been proved positive and leaving for hospital soon. Blessings all xxx." He and his wife updated a few days later to let viewers know they were doing well in the hospital.

Uncertainty also stemmed from the slow and sometimes inaccurate dissemination of information on the ship. Through TV[iii] and free Wi-Fi, guests could access outside sources. News media regularly updated the case count faster than what was communicated to passengers on board. Throughout Abel's updates, he repeatedly noted that he learned the accurate number of cases from the *Washington Post* and other outlets, not from the captain's announcements. On Friday, February 7, Abel stated in his Facebook Live video (shared on YouTube):

> We as passengers, we want to be informed of what's going on. We don't want secondhand news. We don't want rumors. We want to hear precisely what is happening to passengers on this ship. Now we are on a 14-day quarantine. That's what we were told when we came back to Yokohama to disembark, but of course, everything changed. 14-day quarantine, but the couple of days later it was then discovered, well, we've now got 22 infected people. They've been taken off the ship or at least 20 of them, but does that 14-day quarantine start all over again? We don't know. We haven't been informed . . .

In the first two days of quarantine, identified coronavirus cases doubled. The US Embassy in Tokyo noted the case count at twenty on February

iii Cabins contained television sets with access to news and other channels.

6. On February 7, the Associated Press reported, "Japan Finds 41 More Cases on Ship," bringing the positive number to 61.[89] Two days later, the case count rose to 64 and then 70 by February 10.[90] From February 3 through February 9, 490 out of 3,713 individuals were tested, with 172 positive cases.[91] As of Wednesday, February 12, 174 people on the ship had tested positive. Forty-four additional passengers tested positive the next day.[92]

As was conveyed by the US Embassy's message to guests, more than 100 pharmacists, physicians, nurses and other health professionals boarded the *Diamond Princess* to help with medication, coronavirus testing, and patient care.[93] In *The Miami Herald*, journalist Taylor Dolven detailed the process of providing all passengers with their necessary medication throughout the quarantine, calling it "nothing short of herculean," as 45 Japanese pharmacists helped to acquire 2,000 prescriptions for guests.[94]

Across outlets, news coverage highlighted concern for the passengers about the escalating viral spread. On February 10, 2020, the *New York Times* referred to the ship "a floating, mini-version of Wuhan," stating, "passengers have grown increasingly fearful that the quarantine—meant to protect people in Japan and contain the virus's spread—could be putting them in jeopardy."[95] In another *New York Times* article, passenger John Montgomery referred to the *Diamond Princess* as a "petri dish of a ship."[96] On February 13, *The Gazette* (Montreal) quoted guest Bryan Doyle, "The virus is now infecting the crew . . Once this thing gets into the crew, it's just going to blow completely apart. Although we're isolated, we're eating the food that they prepare. So we feel like we're sitting ducks here."[97] The story addressed the overall spread of the virus, calling the *Diamond Princess* "a virtual prison."[98]

Some crew members broke their media silence in hopes of getting off the ship. Crew member Binay Kumar Sarkar posted a public Facebook video of himself and four crew members, begging their government (India) to evacuate them.[iv] Featured in *The Last Crew* docu-

iv See this video, https://www.facebook.com/100003617015316/videos/1780986532031897/.

mentary, a group of Indonesian crew members made a similar video on February 24: "We are afraid we are being killed slowly. We work here to support our families in Indonesia. Please don't let us catch the virus and die slowly because we got evacuated too late."

As cases continued to rise, public health experts increasingly blamed Japan and Japanese health authorities for their handling of the cases, channeled through news outlets. Others weighed in on what to do about the *Diamond Princess* guests. On February 11, the editorial board of *USA Today* advocated for the evacuation of the Americans on the ship. After laying out the passenger quarantine situations and rising cases, the board argued, "The Japanese and U.S. governments are effectively gambling with the health of all the passengers who haven't fallen ill. It's possible that the crew, which lives and works in close quarters, could be spreading the virus among themselves."[99] The board concluded, "There is a prudent step here for the State Department. Offer the Americans aboard a chance to come home. Now."[100] This essay, under title variations, appeared in papers across the United States and in Guam.

USA Today published a response statement from the State Department's Bureau of Consular Affairs on February 12, explaining, "We have consulted with the CDC, and current medical consensus and protocols state that the safest and most reliable way to prevent further spread of viral infections on cruise ships is for passengers to shelter in place, as the passengers of the Diamond Princess are doing."[101] On February 12, an AP article on an emergency WHO meeting about coronavirus stated that the case count had reached 174 on the ship, demonstrating the need for global action.[102]

Leaving the Diamond Princess

On February 12, the CDC issued its second letter to passengers and crew, explaining the Japanese health officials' tiered voluntary disembarkation plan, noting that "medically vulnerable" passengers would leave first. Testing would then determine the next steps, with positive cases transferred to a nearby hospital and those testing negative would move to "a quarantine housing facility."[103] The escalating case count accelerated the evacuation strategy. On February 15, the US Department of Health and Human Services announced the plan to support American passengers in their return journey.[104] News outlets reported the evacuation plan. Following testing and health screenings, Americans that elected to leave the ship would fly to the US and do a two-week quarantine at either Travis Air Force Base or Joint Base San Antonio-Lackland.[105]

The mass evacuation of 328 Americans received heavy media attention, especially since the process did not go as smoothly as planned. Guests shared their experiences through social media and news outlets. Online videos and TV stations showed the difficult, crowded journey in which passengers were forced to sit on a bus for hours and then ride home in a cargo plane with fourteen people who had tested positive for coronavirus.[106] Once back in the United States, cruise passengers expressed frustration at having to undergo a second two-week quarantine period in the United States, once again becoming "prisoners." American Matthew Smith@mjswhitebread chose to finish out his time on the ship, stating, "My health is fine. And my 2-week quarantine is almost over. Why would I want to be put on a bus and a plane with other people they think may be infected when I have spent nearly 2 weeks isolated from those people?" (Twitter, February 15).

Australia and Hong Kong soon evacuated their citizens from the ship. Next, Matthew Smith and the remaining guests were permitted to leave with the end of the quarantine, cheered on by masked Princess Cruises President Jan Swartz. Over the next week, crew members were evacuated, with the last ones leaving by March 1. Princess Cruises@PrincessCruises tweeted: "Captain Arma was last to leave #DiamondPrincess. He is a hero in our eyes. We thank him & our exceptional onboard team. We offer our sincere gratitude to all the agencies in Japan & around the world who worked with us to support our guests & crew through this extraordinary time."

Even before the ship had emptied, the quarantine had already been deemed a failure. In a *USA Today* article on February 18, 2020. Dr. Anthony Fauci stated that the quarantine, social distancing during outside time, and masks were "very ineffective in preventing spread on the ship."[107] Indeed, they were. Out of the 3,711 passengers on the ship, 712 tested positive for the coronavirus, many of whom were asymptomatic.[108] Fourteen people died from the virus—all older guests, yet their names were never released.[109] The *Diamond Princess* coronavirus outbreak contained the largest number of cases outside of China at that time, demonstrating the transmission potential of the virus. On March 12, Princess Cruises voluntarily ceased global operations for sixty days, halting cruises for its eighteen ships.[110] The pause was later extended into summer and Fall 2020.

In the time that followed, additional information and documented experiences helped to shed light on what happened aboard the *Diamond Princess*. Author Gay Coulter wrote more newspaper articles in 2020, created a blog, and eventually published a book, *Quarantine!*, about her time on the ship. In March 2021, HBO released *The Last Cruise*, documenting the *Diamond Princess* quarantine. Unlike most of the fragmented narratives captured earlier, this film coherently constructed the story of the *Diamond Princess*, incorporating pictures and video from guests and employees. Some crew members' perspectives were incorporated through interviews with Dede Samsul Fuad, Maruja Daya, Luke Hefner, Dr. Franco Swart, and Sonali Thakkar.[111] The documentary showed much of what was unknown and unseen at the time—the crew's tiny, windowless shared quarters and dining area, their overburdening workload, and the lack of measures taken to protect the employees. Still, only a fraction of their experiences were captured and shared. The majority of the film featured experiences of the American guests.

Impressions from the Diamond Princess Quarantine

The public's lasting impressions of what happened to the *Diamond Princess* set the tone for the rest of the pandemic. The mundane tweets of good food and silly dances didn't receive nearly the attention of temporary cries for help and hashtags that implied imprisonment. At the same time, messages that could have profoundly shaped this moment as the public health crisis were nearly non-existent, as people who were actually sick did not have the same large blocks of time, consistent Wi-Fi, and motivation, compared to the healthy "trapped" guests on the ship.

Extensive media content was both consumed and produced by guests upon the *Diamond Princess*. News outlets emphasized the difficult living quarters, documented the rising cases, and spread criticism of Japan's handling of the crisis. What people on and off the ship did not see were the effects and experiences of being sick. News outlets around the world documented the boredom of quarantine living. But, once sick passengers left the ship, we seldom got to view their experiences.

Lack of time, stable Wi-Fi, and the willingness to show these experiences or to be interviewed meant that the reasons for the quarantine remained largely unseen. As such, questions with no answers arose: Why quarantine if you will just get sick anyway? Why wear a mask if it seems to do nothing? Moreover, discourses that framed passengers as "captives" or "victims" on a "floating petri dish" undermined the need for quarantine, especially when only asymptomatic or mild-case coronavirus patients were interviewed.

News and social media framed the *Diamond Princess* as a problem of Japan and China, amplifying already existing stigma and xenophobia. It should be noted that this messaging did not stem from guests (some of whom were Asian) but appeared in threads and comments from those not on the ship. As with the initial news and social media about coronavirus in January, prevalent discourse across news outlets that linked disease to geography (Wuhan then China then Asia as a whole), encouraged racist denigration about Asian food, culture, "appearance," way of life, and existence. From a public health stance, media framing of the *Diamond Princess* and coronavirus in February as an "Asian scourge" diminished the perceived threat of the virus, despite its reach at that moment.

What was also lost in communication was the lack of diversity in perspectives and voice during the *Diamond Princess* quarantine. To have the time, knowledge, and access to post on social media was a privilege onboard. Around the world, in spots with technology, the public heard from this narrow pool of voices. We did not get the perspectives of guests who couldn't or chose not to capture their experiences in words, images, and videos. Crew members could not/would not document their (much longer) quarantined stays, for lack of time and fear of retaliation. An economic and, for the most part, ethnic disparity existed between guests and crew. In not telling the stories of those stuck below, they become further marginalized, as would later occur with sectors of the "essential workers" and others invisibly impacted by the pandemic.

Public health authorities never pinpointed the specific cause of transmission after the quarantining of guests. This lack of identification manifested in media constructions as a lack of transparency and speculations of a cover-up. Additionally, media attention was not given equally to effective quarantines, like that of the MS Artania off the coast of Australia in 2020.[112] On that cruise ship, careful mitigation measures and the use of an outside catering company enabled the crew to also quarantine.[113] Instead, the spread and media framing of the *Diamond Princess* fueled misperceptions that the quarantine created the outbreak, not prevented it. As will be addressed throughout this book, misinformed people and groups repeatedly put forth that mitigation measures (like masking and vaccination) caused disease. The roots of this inaccurate messaging stem from this moment.

Even though the production of social media content and news media enabled people on shore around the world to learn of the *Diamond Princess*, this live presentation offered raw, unchecked, emotional moments left uncontextualized. For example, Abel's diabetic cry for help continued to circulate after the problem had been solved, unbeknownst to those consuming the content. Similarly, guests were blamed on social media for embarking during coronavirus. Yet, as background information is lost on Twitter and other platforms, this attribution of responsibility fails to account for the length of the cruise, which left Yokohama on January 20—before even the lockdown of Wuhan. Little was known about the virus in January. Knowledge about coronavirus greatly increased in February (much of which was from the ship outbreak). The expanding body of information was often perceived as contradictory or false, instead of connected to a particular moment in time.

Last, the *Diamond Princess* outbreak signified a contemporary arrogance toward disease that undermined public knowledge and willingness to modify behavior throughout the pandemic. Given the history of disease at sea, the coronavirus outbreak should not have taken the world by surprise. And yet, like the pandemic as a whole, people ignored the rising threat and criticized mitigation measures under the guise that a true crisis could not happen. This minimalizing assumption delayed both the quarantine on the *Diamond Princess* and global public health actions.

CHAPTER FOUR

"Essential" or Sheltered in Place?

MEDIA IN SPRING 2020

Stay home for everyone who can't.[1]

By the time the WHO declared COVID-19 a pandemic, the crisis had been building for more than two months. From a global perspective, January made people aware of the novel coronavirus. Early February brought the cruise quarantines and a new name: COVID-19. In the United States and many other countries, the new virus still seemed like a far-off threat, falsely constructed as solely an Asian crisis. Then, in the last week of February, an explosion of cases in northern Italy and its subsequent lockdown started to shift public perception.[2] For the first time, people outside of the epicenter could see the impact of the virus on particular regions, as news and social media from Italy showed the world what the virus could do in a way that the heavily regulated Chinese media had not. Unlike Chinese citizens, Italians could freely access Twitter and other social media platforms. Thus, people locked down in Italy could and did produce content consumed by the rest of the world.

Cases outside of China and Italy also continued to rise. The United States had 52 cases on February 19 and 83 cases one week later.[3] The epidemic in Italy, paired with escalating cases elsewhere, fueled global news coverage about the virus. Behind the scenes, public health departments around the world began to prepare for the worst.

At the end of February, people in the United States and other countries began panic buying supplies, leading to a shortage of household goods. Stock prices surged for masks, hand sanitizer, disinfectant sprays, and thermometers.[4] Sales for pet medicine, and bottled water, and pantry items also spiked as people prepared for the looming crisis.[5] News and social media messages exacerbated frenzied purchasing through images of empty grocery shelves and headlines like "Coronavirus Fears Empty Store Shelves of Toilet Paper, Bottled Water, Masks as Shoppers Stock Up."[6] Local newspapers mentioned shortages in specific stores, quoting individuals as they searched for increasingly scarce products.[7] Online searches for toilet paper peaked in mid-March, as individuals struggled to find products in stores.[8] Meanwhile, the virus continued to spread.

March 11, 2020, marked a pivotal moment. WHO Director Ghebreyesus gave a media briefing, listing the global case number at 118,000 across 114 countries, with 4,291 deaths.[9] He continued, "WHO has been assessing this outbreak around the clock and we are deeply concerned both by the alarming levels of spread and severity, and by the alarming levels of inaction. We have therefore made the assessment that COVID-19 can be characterized as a pandemic."[10] That same day, actor Tom Hanks shared the following message on Instagram:

> Hello, folks. @ritawilson and I are down here in Australia. We felt a bit tired, like we had colds, and some body aches. Rita had some chills that came and went. Slight fevers too. To play things right, as is needed in the world right now, we were tested for the Coronavirus, and were found to be positive. Well, now. What to do next? The Medical Officials have protocols that must be followed. We Hanks' will be tested, observed, and isolated for as long as public health and safety requires. Not much more to it than a one-day-at-a-time approach, no? We'll keep the world posted and updated.
>
> Take care of yourselves!
>
> Hanx![11]

The post received widespread in news outlets and on social media.[12] Later that night, the National Basketball Association suspended its season after a player tested positive and the National Collegiate Athletic Association also announced the cancellation of the season for all spring college sports.[13]

At this point, US cases had reached 1,437 and school closings had already impacted more than 850,000 K-12 students.[14] Some colleges and universities had already announced their plans to move classes online. The pandemic declaration, Hanks's announcement (which received more than 2.8 million likes) and the suspension of professional and collegiate sports greatly heightened public concern about COVID-19. On March 12, 2020, #CoronavirusPandemic reached number one on Twitter. By the end of the week, the rising crisis had initiated more school closings, stay-at-home orders, and lockdowns across the country. Restrictions varied somewhat regionally, yet almost every US town, city, and state implemented some measures at this point. By March 15, every state in the United States had declared a state of emergency.[15] #StayTheFHome topped Twitter as "Coronavirus tips" was the most searched phrase on Google.[16] By March 18, 2020, the US had 9,918 cases and 149 deaths, which exploded to 70,602 cases and 1,306 deaths by the next week.[17]

Over the next few weeks, the world was sent home, or at least it seemed like it. Nearly every country in the world implemented some COVID restrictions in the spring of 2020: banning international travel, closing borders, and implementing additional mitigation efforts. Most countries in Asia, Europe, and South America imposed national lockdowns.[18] Some parts of South America and Africa, Finland, Norway, North Macedonia, Ukraine, Bosnia, Malta, and Canada used localized restrictions.[19]

The United States did as well. Even though all states temporarily closed schools, the level of restriction on businesses and individuals varied significantly.[20] Five states—Arkansas, Iowa, Nebraska, North Dakota, and South Dakota—did not issue stay-at-home orders. Utah, Wyoming, and Oklahoma varied by county and city. The remaining forty-two had statewide orders, but ranged in the name, timeframe, definition, and implementation of COVID restrictions.[21] For example, the statewide stay-at-home order in Alabama stated "every person is ordered to stay at his or her place of residence except as necessary to perform any of the following 'essential activities'," specifying a lengthy list of exceptions that included acquiring "necessary supplies," "essential services," outside time, caregiving, and attending worship services with capacities and social distancing implemented.[22] On the other hand, California's order did not include exceptions for individuals unless they were part of the "16 critical infrastructure sectors whose assets, systems, and networks, whether physical or virtual, are considered so vital to the United States that their incapacitation or destruction would have a debilitating effect on security, economic security, public health or safety, or any combination thereof."[23]

States also differed in the enforcement of stay-at-home orders. Eleven states mentioned specific consequences in their orders, running the gamut on severity. Wisconsin had the most minimal, with up to 30 days in jail and a $250 fine for violating the "Safer-At-Home" order.[24] In Alaska, offenders could face up to a year in prison and a $25,000 fine.[25] Overall, 316 million people in the United States and Puerto Rico were under some form of a stay-at-home order in April 2020.[26]

This chapter addresses the mediated story of Spring 2020, articulating the often-conflicting discourses of essential workers and those forced to stay at home. In this isolating time period, news, entertainment, and social media became even more important, as face-to-face, in-person interpersonal communication was largely severed by the circumstances. The production and consumption of news, entertainment, and social media captured and defined this unique time, as COVID cases exploded to 1,329,799 by May 2020—many of whom were healthcare providers and other "essential" workers.[27]

REDEFINING WORK

Outbreaks of disease redefine the hierarchy of what is considered important in the workforce. Who needs to perform their duties in order for society to function? What jobs become in-demand? Who bears the brunt of the work to be done? It is not surprising that caregivers and medical workers are needed during epidemics. The "plague doctor" is one of the most iconic images in the history of medicine, signified by its ominous beaked mask and black cloak. Other types of caregivers, postal workers, gravediggers, florists, and coffin makers have also been sought after in past epidemics.[28] And yet, this work has not been equally valued. Dr. Benjamin Rush, Dr. Curtis Welch, and other physicians became famous for leading their respective towns through disease outbreaks.[29] Missing in the historical narratives are the names of nurses and other caregivers, gravediggers, and other people vital to a community in crisis—many of which were women and workers of color, who were not allotted newspaper or other mediated public spaces[i] to capture their experiences.[30]

The closure of schools and public spaces frequently occurred during past epidemics, with the understanding that those critical to the functioning of society would continue working. For the COVID-19 pandemic, "shelter in place" and other similarly named orders used the term "essential worker" as those with permission to continue working in person. The US federal government's Cybersecurity and Infrastructure Security Agency listed 16 critical infrastructure sectors "considered so vital to the United States that their incapacitation or destruction would have a debilitating effect on security, national economic security, national public health or safety, or any combination thereof."[31] These sectors include public health and health care, law enforcement and emergency services, critical retail businesses (grocery stores, pharmacies, hardware stores), manufacturing, construction, food and agriculture production, government, and other sectors.[32] The April 2020 Gallup Polls

---

i One exception is the pamphlet written by Richard Allen and Absalom Jones about the Free African Society's many contributions during the 1793 yellow fever epidemic in Philadelphia. See Absalom Jones and Richard Allen, *A Narrative of the Proceedings of the Black People during the Late Awful Calamity in Philadelphia in the Year 1793 and a Refutation of Some Censures Thrown upon Them in Some Late Publications* (Philadelphia: William W. Woodward, 1794), 18.

showed that 57–59 percent of those employed were in jobs considered "essential," exempting them from stay-at-home orders, however, even with federal guidelines, this definition varied significantly by state.[33]

Because of racial disparities by occupation, non-Hispanic Black people disproportionately held essential worker positions (i.e., transportation, health care support, food preparation, and cleaning and maintenance) and were therefore put at a higher risk of contracting COVID-19. As such, deaths among non-Hispanic Black people were disproportionately high.[34] In comparison, the ability to work from home was more common for occupational categories dominated by white or Asian workers.[35] Remote working protected people both from the virus and from unemployment for those fortunate enough to have the option.

Although many people were able to shift to remote work, Spring 2020 brought massive unemployment. Globally, an estimated 114 million people became unemployed in 2020, totaling lost income of approximately $3.7 trillion.[36] In the US, unemployment jumped from 3.5 percent in February to 14.8 percent in April.[37] People of color and those with lower levels of education faced higher rates of unemployment, while older, Caucasian, educated groups fared better.[38] Some businesses began recovery as early as May 2020, while other industries lagged behind for months.

The Burden of Care

In addition to the reconfiguration of work in society, care for others without additional support contributed to the difficulty of Spring 2020. The closing of schools and daycares created hardships for parents and guardians. Only selected facilities remained open for essential workers. Caregivers, who were disproportionately female, had to shoulder the responsibility of working from home and caring for children.[39] The suspension of therapies and care for children and adults with disabilities caused further hardship.[40] This moment also changed household dynamics, as universities closed dormitories, ousting college students to return home with parents or figure out their own housing situations, with little notice given.[41] Moreover, senior citizens and others in long-term care facilities were at high-risk for COVID, leading to a ban on visitors and prompting some people to remove residents from these places.[42] In other words, household dynamics had changed dramatically at this time, with experiences far from universal.

MEDIA CONSUMPTION IN SPRING 2020

With no in-person work, school, activities, sports, events, or travel, or other face-to-face interactions, media channels served as the primary connections to the outside world. As such, people viewed and produced content in new ways. Consumption of news, entertainment, and social media surged during March and April 2020. They consumed more news, read more books, watched more videos, played more video games, posted to social media platforms, and interacted using digital technology more than ever before.[43] Individuals spent an average of twelve hours and twenty minutes interacting with content.[44] Nearly half of that time was spent on watching videos.[45]

Desperate for information in March 2020, Americans more than doubled the amount of time they devoted to consuming content on global news and current events, compared to the previous year.[46] News became much more part of daily media diets, with 66 percent of participants in an April 2020 survey by Digital Third Coast reporting that they had increased their news consumption.[47] Approximately 22 percent of respondents took in one to two hours of news per day, compared to 14 percent before the pandemic.[48] Fifteen percent consumed more than two hours.[49] Web traffic for the *Washington Post*, the *New York Times*, and *CNBC* experienced more than a 50 percent increase.[50] Web visits to local news sites also soared, with more than 50–150 percent growth.[51] Consumers sought real-time numbers of COVID cases and deaths, turning to the Johns Hopkins University "COVID-19 Dashboard" and other online data sets.[52] Online Google searches for "coronavirus" and "COVID-19" spiked in mid-late March, both globally and in the United States.[53] "Handwashing," "social distance," "quarantine," "stay at home," and other terms related to the pandemic also dominated internet searches.

Unprecedented was the rise in visitors to the WHO and CDC websites, as people sought information and guidance on preventing, identifying, and treating COVID-19.[54] In addition to regularly updating their websites and producing special news briefs on COVID, WHO and CDC used Twitter and Facebook to disseminate infographics on COVID prevention and other information. Through these outlets, the public health organizations interacted with the public, responding to comments and questions in real time. People tuned in to the numerous news conferences, webinars, and interviews with leading public health authorities: WHO Director Dr. Ghebreyesus and members of the White House Coronavirus Task Force, including then Vice President Mike Pence, Dr. Deborah Birx (response coordinator), Dr. Anthony Fauci, director of the National Institute of Allergy and Infectious Disease, Surgeon General Vice Admiral Jerome Adams, and others.[ii] Digital platforms offered a global connection, at least to those who had access. YouTube, TikTok, and other platforms enabled users to see glimpses of experiences in other places. Pandemic-themed content dominated platforms. Consumers could view signs of what was to come through scenes of the coronavirus epicenter in New York: lengthy testing lines, overflowing hospitals, and makeshift triage areas.[55]

Media content, across platform, type, and political affiliation, overwhelming pushed for people to stay home. Countries and local governments launched formal campaigns.[56] California, Hawaii, Tennessee, Washington, and many other US states encouraged people to social distance and stay home.[57] Op-eds in *USA Today*, Fox News, NPR, and numerous other outlets pleaded with readers to avoid public spaces and gatherings to reduce the spread of coronavirus.[58] Instagram added a "Stay Home" sticker, enabling users to become part of a shared story on the importance of sheltering-in-place.[59] The platform also launched a "co-watching feature," through which people could consume content online together.[60] TikTok added #HappyAtHome—a daily series of

---

ii This task force and the overall politicization of the pandemic is discussed in more depth in chapter 6.

livestreamed comedians, actors, and musicians to provide entertainment during the lockdown.[61]

Sports leagues chimed in with their own messaging. US Soccer initiated "Bend the Curve, Stay at Home."[62] Tom Brady and other NFL players participated in the "Stay Home, Stay Strong" public service announcement distributed on YouTube and other social media channels.[63] Celebrities led their own informal campaigns. On March 18, 2020, actor Kevin Bacon posted this message on Twitter:

> Hey everybody, now it's so important to STAY HOME and keep our distance from others. Join me and post a video or photo with a sign like this, with #IStayHomeFor, telling who you are staying home for, & tag 6 friends. Let's work together to stay home and keep each other safe.

He included a video of himself talking about the importance of staying home.[64] Bacon's challenge was widely popular. Carrie Underwood, New Mexico Governor Michelle Lujan Grisham, Demi Lovato, DePaul Women's Basketball, Cleveland State Volleyball, Cancer Research UK, various reality show stars of The Learning Channel, Boston Public Schools, and numerous organizations, health professionals, and individuals participated. Bacon later won the Webby People's Voice Award for Best Viral PR Campaign for #IStayHomeFor.[65]

Corporations contributed their own messages on the importance of staying home, using much of the same types of content, with sappy music paired with photos and videos of empty public spaces and at-home scenes.[66] For its COVID ad, Heineken featured a compilation of at-home frustrations, highlighting poor internet connections, pet interruptions, and charger difficulties, as Frank Sinatra's "That's Life" played in the background. The ad concluded, "It's not the best get-together, but it's the best way to get together." Honda produced a commercial using a toy car, with the phrase, "Until we drive again." Other companies used similar messaging: "Stay home. Go forridge" (Quaker Oats), "Stay home of the Whopper" (Burger King), and "We're never lost if we can find each other" (Facebook). Dove and Clorox offered instruction on effective handwashing and surface disinfecting. Heinz Ketchup created a puzzle, consisting of 570 identical pieces and an invitation: "Tell us who you'd finish this with" on social media. Actor Ryan Reynolds, owner of Mint Mobile, instructed his customers to leave voicemails with their least favorite one of his movies. Oscar Meyer encouraged a "Front-Yard Cookout" on May 2, promising to donate a meal to Feed America for each #FrontYardCookout posted.

People who did not stay home were heavily criticized on social media platforms. One of the most widely viewed tweets of March 2020 showed an aerial news footage of a packed Florida beach with the teaser, "Clearwater Beach, Florida is PACKED today despite 'social distancing' recommendations." In a similar vein, a *CBS News* interview of young adults partying on spring break received 41.7 million views (Twitter, March 18, 2020). In the clip, a student identified as Brady Sluder stated:

> If I get corona, I get corona. At the end of the day, I'm not going to let it stop me from partying. You know, I've been waiting, we've been waiting, for Miami spring break for a while, about two months, we've had this trip planned, two, three months, and we're just out here having a good time. Whatever happens, happens.

Another young adult, Brianna Leeder, added, "It's really messing up with my spring break. What is there to do here other than go to the bars or to the beach? And they're closing. I think they're blowing it way out of proportion. I think it's doing way too much." Similarly, Atlantis Walker said, "What they're doing is bad. We need a refund. This virus ain't that serious. There's more serious things out there like hunger and poverty and we need to address that." Tweeted clips like these extended the reach of the news station, while also shedding light on resistance to social distancing orders and other mitigation.

Stay-at-home messaging frequently was intertwined with reminders of those risking their lives in the pandemic. On social media, health professionals reminded users, "We stay here for you, please stay home for us."[67] Images of wearied frontline workers showing their faces raw and red from Personal Protective Equipment (PPE) circulated online. Other videos depicted a lighter side, as masked nurses, doctors, respiratory therapists, and other health professionals performed short dances or formed lines to celebrate COVID patients' recoveries.

Spring 2020 celebrated health professionals as the frontline workers of the pandemic. The governor of Alabama led "Ribbons of Hope," encouraging people to display ribbons as prayer reminders for medical personnel, first responders, and others.[68] WHO initiated #ThanksHealthHeroes, as a means to show appreciation for frontline health workers.[69] On March 29, 2020, the Fox channel aired "iHeartRadio's Living Room Concerts for America," an hour filled with artists performing from their homes.[70] The event raised $10 million for COVID victims and first responders, as more than 8.7 million people tuned in.[71] Brands celebrated frontline workers as well. Dove showed photos of mask-chafed faces and the tagline "Courage is beautiful. As a thank you, Dove is donating care products to front-line healthcare workers in Canada." A McDonald's ad featured a sign, stating, "First Responders & Healthcare Workers Enjoy a Thank You Meal For Free." In its "couch-patriot" commercial, Burger King mentioned donating Whoppers to nurses and supporting the American Nurses Foundation. Frontline healthcare workers received visibility in other ways.

In addition to campaigns and praise for frontline workers, people became fascinated with crisis entertainment content. Interest in the epidemic-themed films *Outbreak* (1995) and *Contagion* (2011) first increased in late January and reached peak public interest in mid-March.[72] Films, podcasts, and books on epidemics were also heavily consumed.[73] Numerous popular media and scholarly journals published comparisons between the 1918 influenza pandemic ("Spanish Flu") and COVID—a trend that would continue over the next year.[74] Zombie and dystopic narratives also ranked high on fictional consumption as people struggled to make sense of their new reality.[75]

Overall, the various COVID restrictions, social pressure to stay at home, and fear of the virus had already shaped public perception and behavior by the end of March. Of the 11,537 adults surveyed between March 19 and 24, 88 percent said their lives had been changed by the coronavirus outbreak.[76] Over 90 percent of participants indicated that they would feel uncomfortable attending a crowded party and 77 percent reported discomfort with eating at a restaurant.[77] Besides the pandemic's social impact, economic effects had already started to take a toll. One-third of respondents had personally experienced or had someone in their household experience losing jobs or taking pay cuts.[78]

Entertainment and Social Media in Spring 2020

Pandemic-themed entertainment dominated in popularity. March and April 2020 impacted other forms of media consumption as well. Games in all forms surged in popularity. On March 20, the social simulation game *Animal Crossing* reached the fifth spot on Twitter. Twitch and other online platforms for video-gaming engagement also achieved record participation.[79]

With the halting of sports events and television shows (see chapter 9), only programs that had previously been completed were released at this time. And yet, never had people binge-watched so much entertainment programming. On Netflix, a docu-series about big cat owners, *Tiger King*, became the most-watched program shortly after its release on March 20, 2020.[80] The show sparked fervent discussions and memes to Facebook and other social media platforms and became Twitter's most talked about topic on March 28, 2020.[81]

Not surprisingly, in the absence of interpersonal interaction, social media platform use jumped, with a 27 percent increase in Facebook.com activity, 15.3 percent for YouTube, and 15.4 percent for TikTok.[82] Social media platforms released special features to aid people during the shelter-in-place orders. Snapchat moved up its mental health resource center and added a COVID-specific section.[83] While specific social media trends evolved over the course of the stay-at-home orders, patterns in the type of content consumed emerged.

In Spring 2020, media users wanted content that reflected their time in isolation. Gifs created and shared online captured the moment, featuring hand washing, hand sanitizer, and the toilet paper shortage.[84] Simple and mundane posts and videos became popular. One of the most retweeted posts of 2020 was Jamie@gnuman1979's nine-second video of a sock puppet pretending to eat passing cars through the window, titled "Quarantine day 6." Posted on March 16, 2020, this video received more than 2.7 million likes and 21,800 replies.[85] Pets playing Tic Tac Toe also ranked among the most viewed videos on Instagram and Twitter. And, at a time in which many could not go out in public, digitally skilled content creators artificially placed themselves in fun places, exemplified by ant-honey@aanthonyy07's video of himself pretending to be in a speed boat, which garnered nearly 27 million views (Twitter, March 20, 2020).

Challenges on social media addressed the absurdity of the moment. #pillowchallenge involved making an outfit from a pillow and then posting a picture of it. Celebrities (also stuck at home) participated in the home creation of media content. In an at-home interview on the *Today Show*, late-night host Jimmy Fallon started banging a bell, declaring, "It's the cowbell challenge. I want everyone to get out your cowbell, get out a pot and pan, 3:00 p.m. Open a window. Open a door. If you have a balcony, good for you. Let's go. Let's make some noise."[86] Numerous groups and people participated, posting videos of themselves on Twitter, Instagram, and Tik-Tok.

In March 2020, *Wonder Woman* actor Gal Gadot shared to social media a video of herself singing "Imagine," collaborating with other celebrities at home. Her video immediately faced mockery on social media. Among the numerous posts, Ray Reynolds @RayReynoldsNMS tweeted, "It's really nice that all those celebrities singing imagine with Gal Gadot donated a million of their many millions of dollars to buy vital masks and medical equipment for struggling health workers and hospitals. Oh, they didn't? They just sang out of tune? Oh Oh OK." (Twitter, March 20, 2020). Musicians parodied the random key changes among the singers. Celebrities not in the video also created their own parodies. The backlash was great enough that news media addressed the response. *New York Times* Pop Music Critic Jon Caramanica summed up the response, stating, "The actress Gal Gadot assembled celebrities singing John Lennon's anthem on social media. The result is far from inspiring."[87] The *Washington Post* ran the headline "Gal Gadot, Mark Ruffalo and other celebrities asked us to 'Imagine' in a viral video. It did not go well."[88] Heather Schwedel wrote in *Slate*, "Gal Gadot's video of self-isolated celebrities singing 'Imagine' is one of the worst things to have ever happened."[89] The *Jerusalem Post* similarly captured public sentiment: "Labeling the video 'cringe' and 'tone deaf,' many were not charmed by celebrities who can retreat to their mansions when they 'self-isolate' singing about imagining no possessions."[90] Reflections on 2020 cultural trends list this moment as one of the most cringeworthy in the pandemic.[91] Gadot herself later called the video "in poor taste."[92]

On the other hand, actor John Krasinski's *Some Good News*—segments filmed from his home that highlighted uplifting moments and people—became widely popular.[93] Krasinski's fifteen-minute quarantine show debuted on March 29, 2020, bringing together uplifting regular people and celebrities through video clips and Zoom interviews. Featuring a logo drawn by his daughters, Krasinski began the series:

> For years now I've been wondering why there is not a news show entirely dedicated to good news. Well, desperately seeking my fix somewhere else, I reached out to all of you this week, asking, nay begging, for some good news. And boy did you deliver. After reading those replies and the incredibly heartwarming stories that came with them, I thought, 'Alright, enough is enough world. Why not us? Why not now? So ladies and gentlemen, this is your fault, and this is SGN.

The first episode featured a cancer survivor receiving her last treatment and a reunion from the sitcom *The Office*, in which Krasinski had had his breakout role. Over its eight episodes, *Some Good News* reunited the original *Hamilton* cast, praised essential workers, facilitated a real-life wedding, and held a virtual prom for high school students missing out due to the pandemic. In eight weeks, the show received more than 72 million views and 2.58 million subscribers.[94] Krasinski sold the series to ViacomCBS at the end of May 2020, explaining that it "wasn't sustainable" past the stay-at-home period.[95]

Singer Mariah Carey's YouTube performance of her song "Hero" on April 10, 2020 was also well-received. In the introduction to her video, she stated:

> Quite the unique time in history. A time that doesn't allow us to be together in person and to be festive, and worship with one another, but I'm grateful that so many of us are staying home, staying safe, and in doing so, keeping each other safe. We're united in this effort and in this moment. I want to take this time to acknowledge and honor the sacrifices of those who work everyday taking care of their communities in this time of need and uncertainty. The heroes who are making our daily lives possible. Let's continue to support them and each other.[96]

The video description included links to Feeding America, The First Responders Children's Foundation, Direct Relief, World Central Kitchen, and National Domestic Workers.[97] Carey's performance received over three million views.

Across platforms, celebrities' content consistently ranked among popular social media posts. On Instagram, more than half of the top-viewed posts for March 2020 featured celebrities. Singer Cardi B's rant about the coronavirus received more than twenty-seven million views, topping the list. She produced four other videos in the top ten, including her post on March 24 about the need for widespread access to COVID testing. Selena Gomez, Dwayne Johnson, Jennifer Lopez, Kim Kardashian, LeBron James, and Justin Bieber also had top-viewed videos, featuring throwbacks to past events and clips of themselves dancing or chatting with their kids at home.[98] On Twitter, Idris Elba's announcement that he had tested positive for COVID received 34 million views between March 16 and March 30.[99]

People looked for ways to create structure in their stay-at-home days, as video titles with "quarantine" and "routine" received 10.5 million views.[100] With gyms closed in the second half of March, average daily views with "home workout" in YouTube video titles rose 515 percent compared to viewership in January through March 14, 2020.[101] Videos on dance workouts, ab challenges, handstands, jump rope activities, and other fitness activities exploded in viewership.[102] Searches for yoga, guided meditation, and other "self-care" content increased in views by 215 percent.[103]

As stay-at-home orders extended into April, online consumption expanded to include more content to replace public activities. YouTube videos on "how to cut hair" received over 2.5 million views.[104] Videos on cooking, gardening, raising chickens, playing guitar, and journaling were among the new skills people sought to develop at this time. Sourdough bread instructions and recipes for Dalgona trended on social media, reflecting the time at home. Nostalgic videos also gained traction. For example, for the "I'm Just a Kid" challenge in April 2020, TikTok users recreated old photos and posted them, accompanied by the Simple Plan song.[105] The challenge grew in popularity, especially as JoJo Siwa, Ed Sheeran, Usher, and other celebrities participated. Since then, recreations have included famous scenes from TV and movies, featuring the original actors, including Will Smith and the cast of *The Fresh Prince of Bel-Air*, and Patrick Renna's reprise of his role in the 1993 film *The Sandlot*.

Social media production and consumption also reflected the shift to working from home. The use of Zoom, Google Classrooms, and other virtual meeting spaces skyrocketed.[106] People made numerous videos about their home offices, as global production of video content with "home office" grew 700 percent.[107] A widely circulated GIF showed a dog reclining on a couch using a laptop with the phrase "Working from home" on it.[108] From March 15 through March 31, YouTube videos with "home office" in the title received a 210 percent spike in views.[109] More than five million people viewed YouTuber HotandFlashy's "How To Look Good on Video Calls. Zoom FaceTime Skype. Blogger Secrets," posted on March 31, 2020.[110] In this twelve-minute video, the fifty-seven-year-old woman offered straightforward tips on creating flattering Zoom calls, addressing optimal lighting, camera angles, other practice advice, paired with shopping links to purchase equipment to improve video sessions. Videos that spoofed working from home also became popular, like Caitlin Reilly's "The co-worker you hate during a Zoom meeting" (1.1 million likes on TikTok).[111]

Spring 2020 brought a spirit of altruistic education online, especially since many school districts offered little or no instruction. Community organizations, gyms, and recreation centers offered abundant virtual programming without geographic restraint. Online became the place for people to connect, even locally. With houses of worship closed in most places, members tuned in online to stream services for their regular churches, mosques, temples, and other faith homes.[112] Only 3 percent of participants in an April 2020 Pew Research Poll said that their houses of worship had continued to hold in-person services.[113] City and school board meetings moved to virtual spaces, with political leaders checking in on their communities.

At home, people could participate in (often free) classes for yoga, martial arts, dance, and other fitness, art, poetry, cooking, and other activities. Individuals and organizations provided digital experiences for places all over the world. Visitors could see the cherry blossoms in Washington, DC, or Greenland's Northern Lights, sail through webcams in the British Virgin Islands, watch pandas in China or gorillas in Uganda, learn about Egypt's great pyramids, India's Mehrangarh Fort, and other historic sites, or check out conservation efforts in Brazil.[114] Virtual museums also became popular, with exhibits featured online. Many cities also created virtual tours, enabling tourists from home to "wander" around destinations ranging from Antakya, Turkey to Austin, Texas.[115] Webinars offered additional insights and education for different audiences. The NBA produced "Jr. NBA at Home," offering basketball drills for kids, and "NBA Math Hoops"—virtual educational content.[116]

REOPENING SOCIETY

The March 2020 shutdown happened abruptly and somewhat uniformly, as most US states and countries implemented shelter-in-place orders about the same time. At the peak of the shelter-in-place orders,

81 percent of Americans surveyed were interacting with 0–5 people outside their homes within a 24-hour period.[117] A Gallup poll from March 2020 indicated that over 80 percent of participants believed the COVID disruption would only last a few weeks or months.[118] Very few people anticipated that it would be months or even years before life returned to "normal."

In May, governors and public health authorities communicated and implemented their plans for reopening. These ranged significantly, based on population density, COVID cases, and political affiliation, with Democrat-led states much more likely to continue moderate or major mitigation. California remained the most restrictive, with all businesses closed. Beaches reopened with mask requirements. East Coast and Democrat-led states had moderate restrictions. Most Midwest and Southern states greatly eased restrictions, reopening retail shops, salons, barber shops, restaurants, bars, gyms, movie theaters, and other spaces, with capacity rules in place. North Dakota and West Virginia reopened all businesses, only placing restrictions on nightclubs, sporting venues, and large events.[119]

From March 30 to April 5, 75 percent of people surveyed were completely isolated, compared to 43 percent during the first week of June 2020.[120] Over the next few months, mask mandates (or no mandate at all) replaced shelter-at-home orders. In the strictest states, mitigation ebbed and flowed depending on COVID cases.

IMPLICATIONS OF THIS MOMENT

This global pause was unprecedented in world history. Never before had countries implemented disease restrictions at the same time in so many places. Towns, cities, and broader geographic regions had closed businesses or even locked down before, but not simultaneously on this scale, and with the ability for people to easily connect and share their experiences on a global level. Despite the ubiquitous mantra of "all in this together," experiences differed dramatically, depending on geography, food and housing security, household structure, caregiving, relationship status, personality, and intersectional positions of race, gender, gender identity, disability, socioeconomic class, and other characteristics. Of course, experience was profoundly impacted by occupation and employment—whether or not people got to keep their jobs during the pandemic and the extent to which work could be done remotely. The majority of media production and consumption, then, was done by those sheltering-in-place. With vacant streets due to sheltering-in-place and journalists primarily working remotely, traditional interviewing of people on the streets halted during the pandemic.[121]

The surge in consumption of news, entertainment, and social media obviously reflects a time when so many people were at home. This rise only tells part of the story, as does an analysis of the popular content. A look at the number of views, time on devices, trending tweets/posts, memes and so forth ignores significant perspectives that need to be contextualized. Consumers varied by platform and type of content. Older consumers watched more television and were much less likely to participate in social media, especially on Instagram or TikTok.[122] In other words, those tuning in to cable news were not the same as the majority of TikTok viewers.[123] Moreover, who produced content during Spring 2020 depended then on digital knowledge, access, personal preferences, and the desire to put material online for others to consume. With much of the popular content featuring wealthy celebrities or mundane activities at home, the stories of those facing food scarcity and other hardships of unemployment were largely rendered invisible.

Themes of staying-at-home dominated all forms of media, ignoring the experiences of "essential" workers still in the field. Moreover, the overwhelming praise for health professionals, though deserving, overlooked those in other "essential" positions directly and indirectly related to the care of COVID patients and survival of society as a whole. Those in health care support, environmental health, social work, janitorial and housekeeping, transportation, food service, and other sectors, disproportionately people of color, risked their lives to perform vital duties, and were infected and succumbed to COVID-19 at higher rates.[124] Their stories and sacrifices largely went unrecognized.

To many, the shutdown without visibility of the pandemic itself spurred disbelief about the necessity of sheltering-in-place. An overabundance of content on life in the lockdown was produced, as individuals made song parodies, baked bread, invented new driveway sports, and connected with others online. In this sea of leisure production, however, was a dearth of crisis messaging. Most of the content did not reflect the tragedy, as those at home only received glimpses of what was happening in the pandemic. Put bluntly, not enough coverage of sickness and death was produced, distributed, and consumed. The public—assuming they happened to consume the right video at the right time—saw a few refrigerated trucks to hold COVID victims, rows of respirators ready for use, and occasional images of patients on ventilators. Very little footage of COVID wards became accessible to the public, as journalists were not allowed in hospitals and health professionals were discouraged from sharing online.[125] Stay-at-home orders, plus the prohibition of visitors in hospitals, clinics, and long-term care facilities, blocked firsthand views of COVID's true impact. Most of the horror of this pandemic went unseen. This was especially the case in Spring 2020, as patients died without friends or family members at their side.[126]

From a public health perspective, the isolation of the very ill and dying was necessary. However, the lack of documented experiences of those hospitalized in news (as journalists were not allowed in hospitals) or on social media further removed those at-home from the rationale of staying home. This moment, which was highly politicized, defined the course of the pandemic, especially as many believed sheltering-in-place to be unfounded. Messages of the initial COVID shutdown largely conveyed *what did not happen*, rather than the tragedy of *what could happen*, especially in regions that faced delayed outbreaks of the virus.

This was a unique moment, as people were cut off from their communities, while, at the same time, consuming more news, entertainment, and social media messaging than ever. Adding to this isolation was the tension over perceptions of the pandemic. From the April 2020 Digital Third Coast survey results, a quarter of participants reported arguing over COVID-19 on social media and 20 percent had already "unfriended" at least one person over divided beliefs.[127] This time frame also produced other negative effects, including heightened anxiety, depression, and suicidal ideation, loneliness, learning loss, poverty, and food scarcity.[128]

Overall, Spring 2020 profoundly impacted how people consumed and produced media. This moment redefined how work, school, and leisure could be carried out, with life events, proms and graduations, book clubs, worship services, fitness classes, and just about any activity one could dream of taking place online. Never before had the world been so linked, at least in superficial ways. This isolation brought Zoom and Teams into homes, skyrocketed the purchasing of puzzles and board games, and changed how individuals interacted with each other. From January to March 2020, media played an integral role in the growing global acceptance of the impending crisis, setting the stage for shelter-in-place and lockdown orders. In Spring 2020, media served as the means of entertainment and connection. And, as discussed in the upcoming chapters of this book, media in many forms continued to significantly impact public function, perception, and behavior.

CHAPTER FIVE

Not In It Together

STIGMA, INJUSTICE, AND DISPARITY IN THE PANDEMIC

In Spring 2020, business owners, politicians, celebrities, media producers, and individuals declared solidarity in the lockdown, with false proclamations about shared equal perspectives and hardships. And yet, life in the global crisis was anything but homogeneous, as geography, socioeconomic class, occupation, digital access, and other factors significantly shaped perspectives and experiences. Adding to existing disparities, the pandemic magnified difference, stigmatizing communities unified by race, ethnicity, immigrant status, disability, and gender identity.

People who were Asian or perceived as Asian were especially targeted, facing unjustifiable prejudice that persisted throughout the pandemic. From March 19, 2020, through March 31, 2022, almost 11,500 hate incidents[1] were reported to Stop Asian American and Pacific Islander (AAPI) Hate.[i] Crimes included "verbal hate speech and/or harassment," workplace discrimination, "avoidance or shunning," physical attacks, "online misconduct," being "coughed or spat on," "refusal of service," and other

i AAPI Equity Alliance, Chinese for Affirmative Action, and San Francisco State University's Asian American Studies Department initiated the "Stop AAPI Hate Coalition" to document and combat "incidents of hate, violence, harassment, discrimination, shunning, and child bullying against Asian Americans and Pacific Islanders in the United States." "About." *Stop AAPI Hate*, https://stopaapihate.org/about/.

types of discrimination in public spaces, businesses, private residences, schools, universities, hospitals, and other locations.[2]

This chapter specifically examines the construction of anti-Asian sentiments and actions in the pandemic, contextualizing this time in the stigmatized history of this group. From the early news out of China, organizations, policies, news, and social media perpetuated unjustified attributions of blame, with profound effects on public perception, mitigation strategies, and other aspects. Certain pivotal moments escalated existing racist-driven beliefs and actions that continued to gain momentum throughout the pandemic. Although this chapter focuses on anti-Asian discrimination, it also addresses violence, discrimination, and stigma against African Americans, Indigenous populations, other communities of color, immigrants, people with disabilities, LGBTQIA+, and their respective intersectional positions during the pandemic, examining the roles of media content and resulting implications. All social media posts are presented in their original form, including spelling and grammatical errors.

BACKGROUND

The discrimination and stigma that occurred during COVID-19 obviously didn't originate in 2020 but have been deeply rooted in the history in the US and other places. Those in power (i.e., white, privileged cis-men) have repeatedly used the threat of disease to blame and punish the "other"–marginalized due to race, ethnicity, religion, gender/gender identity, nationality, sexuality, socioeconomic class, and their cross-positions. Media tend to reproduce ideologies from those in authority, which then can become common sense—stigmatizing and marginalizing "othered" groups.[3] Conversely, media content can also challenge hegemonic structures, eventually leading to change in power dynamics, perceptions, policies, laws, and culture.[4]

Discriminatory acts related to (or in the name of) health have generally been derived from three false assumptions. The first is "medicalizing nativism," in which people believe immigrants or other "foreigners" to be diseased.[5] In the 1793 yellow fever epidemic in Philadelphia, the refugees from Santo Domingo were blamed for the scourge upon the city.[6] Under the guise of protecting public health, entire groups have been generalized to be considered diseased, typically drawing from racist "dirty" or "unclean" stereotypes.[7] Certain groups have been perceived as less likely to be diseased (different ethnicity, socioeconomic class, or religion), even when they shared risk factors with a stigmatized group (i.e., arrived on the same ship). For example, in the nineteenth century, Irish immigrants were believed to spread cholera, yet German immigrants were not.[8] Such generalizations also occurred with the quarantining of Russian Jewish immigrants in 1892 due to false assumptions that they carried cholera.[9] Stereotypes of Asian immigrants as "rat eaters" or as harborers of disease were used to justify the 1882 Chinese Exclusion Act, the quarantine of Chinatown in San Francisco in 1902, and other racist actions, as newspapers at the time perpetuated stigma.[10] This excuse underscored the tightened medical evaluations of immigrants at Ellis Island, in which 69 percent of immigrants were turned away for disability or disease in 1915, correlating with the amplification of anti-immigrant sentiment.[11] "Medicalizing nativism" has also been also used to justify quarantine or removal even when an individual of the group or the group has had no actual exposure or connection, such as the discrimination against Asian Americans in New York City's Chinatown during SARS.[12]

A second manner of health discrimination occurs when those in power do not value the lives of "the othered," therefore are not concerned about infecting them with disease. As mentioned in the "cruise ship" chapter, while quarantines were regularly practiced in fifteenth and sixteenth century Europe, explorers of the "New World" gave no thought to how their diseases might impact Indigenous people.[13] Related to this apathy are false assumptions that communities of color cannot get infected by a particular disease. Enslaved and free Black people were regularly forced to care for and clean up after white patients in various epidemics. In the 1793 yellow fever outbreak, the Free African Society—an organization of Black Philadelphians—rescued much of the town, as (white) doctors claimed that Black people could not get the disease.[14] The false assumption that darker skin protected against disease was also used to deny health care. In 1903, Dr. Thomas D. Coleman wrote a lengthy essay arguing that Black people only became susceptible to tuberculosis after emancipation, arguing that slavery helped to protect their health.[15] Similarly, Black polio survivors were undercounted and struggled to received rehabilitation in the 1930s and 1940s, compared to their white counterparts.[16]

Last, the othering of disease itself perpetuates stigma. Naming disease after people or places carries negative connotations, as evident with "Spanish Flu," Gay-Related Immune Deficiency (AIDS), Ebola, and Middle East respiratory syndrome."[17] Regarding the use of stigmatizing labels or phrases, scholars Wenshan Jia and Fangzhu Lu explained that the choice of labels or names "designating or ascribing someone as something negative, inferior, or undesirable" perpetuates stereotypes and biases conveying "untruthful, unfair, and unjust judgments and attitudes."[18] Media messages can perpetuate these stereotypes, stigmatizing marginalized groups as "the other." At the same time, news framing defines what is considered salient by the content creators, establishing what is perceived as having value, while rending other topics, individuals, and groups invisible. In the United States, stigma that flourished during the pandemic came from earlier sentiments spread by Trump and his administration even before the 2016 election.[19] His labeling of China as "a revisionist power" in a 2017 National Security Report, attempts to ban the Chinese-owned WeChat and TikTok, and repeated ridicule of the country led to an already-strained relationship in 2019.[20] Moreover, Trump's open endorsement of white supremacists, anti-immigrant policies, and his statements against many already marginalized groups set the stage for the explosion of stigma and discrimination that would take place in the pandemic.[21]

BUILDING TO THE PANDEMIC

Stigmatizing COVID messages initially stemmed from early theories connecting the outbreak to a wet market in China. The Wuhan

Municipal Health Commission's first briefing on December 31, 2019, mentioned Huanan Seafood City three times as possibly connected to the outbreak of pneumonia.[22] At least four Chinese news outlets that day referred to a seafood market as a potential source.[23] On January 1, 2020, the story broke internationally, repeating a limited pool of information: Wuhan had "27 cases" of unexplained illness, likely linked to a Huanan market. These few facts were couched in speculation, with many references to SARS and its impact.

As discussed in chapter 2, for the first part of January, coronavirus had yet to grab the attention of the mainstream public outside of China. Aside from a few social media users that passed along news stories, little was said about the growing crisis. Posts mentioning the virus did not get many shares, likes, or retweets. Still, opinions voiced foreshadowing discourses that would later dominate media. On January 3, Nate Klingenstein@GlenwoodNate tweeted, "It is still weird that only Hong Kong has seen cases outside Wuhan. Do they plan to look like heroes saving HK? Are they trying to win Hong Kong's love by infecting you with a deadly disease? Or did 1 HK'er and hundreds of Wuhan people eat bats? The rumor rings of possibility. ." This post received no likes or retweets. Similarly, on January 9, replying to a Chinese news outlet, Unfrozen@alive_unfrozen stated, "Why has the authorities allowed the wildlife market to flourish? When ordinary citizens can buy and eat bats, civet cats, bears and other wild creatures easily, one can be sure the risks of them catching diseases like the unidentifiable pneumonia will increase manifold and spread" (15 likes, 2 retweets, January 9, 2020).

News reports across international outlets continued to focus on Wuhan and mention seafood markets. And, despite no concrete evidence tracing the virus to exotic animals, WHO emphasized this possible link in its first of many public infographics addressing the virus. Starting on January 15, WHO posted infographics on preventing sickness, advising people to avoid "unprotected contact with sick people (including spitting in public, touching one's eyes, nose or mouth) and with live farm or wild animals."[24] Numerous similar social media posts from WHO repeated this warning about "handling animals," especially as part of coronavirus prevention.

Growing coverage of coronavirus information and cases emerging in Thailand (January 13), Japan (January 15), and the United States (January 20) heightened awareness of the escalating crisis. On January 21, *South China Morning Post* published, "Coronavirus Weaker Than SARS But May Share Link to Bats, Chinese Scientists Say," with a Shutterstock image of a bat hanging in a tree.[25] The article stated that the virus "shares a common ancestor" with SARS in "a virus found in fruit bats."[26] It did not refer to transmission of the virus or mention consuming bats.[27] Later that day, the paper published, "Why Wild Animals Are a Key Ingredient in China's Coronavirus Outbreak," teasing:

> Civets and wolf cubs were just some of the exotic items advertised for sale at the Wuhan market at the epicentre of the infections. Novel dishes are part of identity for some people in China but diners just need to say no to eating such food, researcher says.[28]

Accompanying this text was a large image showing vendors crouching next to plastic tubs of bloody, unidentifiable meat, with a graphic labeling the issues ("improvised table for cutting meat," "live frogs for sale," "unwashed buckets," "dirty scale"). The story listed various exotic animals sold at the market, "which experts believe is the source of the outbreak, with the virus jumping from wild animals on sale there."[29] Although bats were not mentioned as a market item, Twitter responses suggested that readers made their own conclusions. For example, Alex Spring @AlexSpring 17 replied, "OMG, please don't tell me they eat bats too! Bats are so ugly" (January 21, 2020).

In social media spaces, the possible link to seafood markets jumped to broader assumptions and criticism about Chinese diets. On January 22, to nearly half a million followers, citizen journalist and lawyer 陈秋实 Chen Qiushi@chenqiushi404 tweeted an eleven-second video of a dead bat floating in a bowl of soup, commenting (translated from Chinese), "Does this thing look like death lying in your bowl? I watched a documentary before. Bats live in caves and excrete on the spot. There is a thick layer of feces in the caves, and all kinds of disgusting bugs live in the feces . . . Will the experience of this incident make Chinese people give up eating game completely?"[30] It received 2,195 retweets, 2,748 quote tweets, and 4,680 likes. This tweet coincided with the WHO's confirmation of human-to-human transmission and Hong Kong's first case.

The brief video of the dead bat and a second one, an Asian woman happily eating a bowl of soup with a bat in it, went viral. Through social media, people expressed their disgust, connecting the image and video to China and coronavirus.

> alpнacenтaυrι@alphacentauriii: "Bats: "The flying mammals are reservoirs for more than 60 viruses that can infect humans, and host more viruses per species than even rodents do, new research shows." Chinese people eat them! #WuhanPneumonia #WuhanVirus" (with "bat soup" video, January 22, 2020, 247 comments, 5,361 retweets, 2,678 likes)
>
> woppa 🎗😌@WopparWoppa (Hong Kong): "When you eat bats and bamboo rats and shit and call it a 'Chinese delicacy,' why y'all be acting surprised when diseases like #coronavirus appear?" (500 comments, 11.1K retweets, 10.2K likes, January 22, 2020)
>
> Catturd@catturd2 tweeted, "Dear China . . . Stop eating bat soup. Signed, America." (January 23, 2020, 925 retweets, 127 quote tweets, 4,797 likes)

Myths about Chinese culture and food causing coronavirus went viral. The "bat soup" videos spread on YouTube, Facebook, and other platforms, as "bat" memes also emerged, fueling misinformation and stereotypes about Chinese culture and the origin of coronavirus.

Tabloids were quick to publish the story, failing to identify the woman or location of the photo.[31] The *New York Post* circulated two of the videos, leading with, "The first gag-inducing clip features an unidentified woman at an undisclosed restaurant in the Wuhan province clutching what appears to be a fruit bat with chopsticks while nibbling its wing like chicken."[32] *The Daily Mail* declared in a lengthy headline, "Revolting Footage Shows Chinese Woman Eating a Whole Bat at a Fancy Restaurant as Scientists Link the Deadly Coronavirus to the Flying Mammals."[33] "'Coronavirus Could be Linked to Fruit Bats': Scientists as Bat Soup Videos Emerge Online," "Is This Objectively Disgusting Soup What's Causing China's Disease Outbreak?" "Stomach-churning Recipe for Bat Soup as Animals Named as Possible Coronavirus Host."[34] ABS-CBN News@ABSCBNNews shared the "bat soup" video, "The snake or bat eaten by the people of Wuhan, China is said to be the source of the new strain of #coronavirus #nCoV." (January 23, 2020, translated from Tagalog, 6,491 retweets, 5,337 quote tweets, 15.3K likes). "Bat soup" rose worldwide as a Google search on January 23, peaking on January 25.[35] Related terms to the human consumption of bats and coronavirus also increased in popularity at this time.[36] Rumors about Chinese food carrying the virus also spread on WhatsApp and other social media platforms.[37]

While the majority of comments on these tweets were disparaging, perpetuating stereotypes about Chinese culture, a few social media users tried to correct these myths.

> June@June69851711 (replying to @alphacentauriii's post quoted above): "Only a tiny tiny amount of people in China will ever eat that! Don't confuse people by including all Chinese!" (0 comments, 0 retweets, 1 like, January 22, 2020)
>
> Wuhan专注@lannyone (a Twitter user from Wuhan) tweeted, "Although the epidemic was caused by eating wild animals, let me tell you that most people in China don't eat bats or mice. I think that less than one in 10, 000 people eat them. I hoped that after this incident, the government must severely ban the consumption of wild animals." (January 25, 2020)
>
> Shut down the devil sound@JerpaDerpa (New York, replying in a thread): "The vast majority of Chinese people don't eat bats though, so yeah you are a bigot for making it seem like they do" (No comments, retweets, or likes, January 25, 2020).

> @sunshinesdae (California): "Bruh Chinese people don't eat bats. It's a small minority jsut like I can't just say white people eat snails?? Like who do you actually know that eats snails on the daily? My entire family is in China and no one has ever or known anyone that has ever eaten BAT." (1 comment, no retweets, 3 likes, January 30, 2020)

Even in the midst of a popular thread, these types of posts did not receive much attention.

On January 26, "bat soup" video creator and influencer Wang Mengyun apologized on her microblog for the video, explaining that it had been filmed in Palau, not China, back in 2016. Her intent (in 2016) had been to "to introduce the life of local people" to fans of her vlog.[38] *Foreign Policy*, Fox News, the *Toronto Sun*, and other outlets covered Mengyun's apology, confirming that the videos were not from Wuhan or even China.[39] It wasn't just Mengyun's content that was misleading. Five of the most widely shared videos about bat soup were actually made in Palau and Indonesia, with no connection to the pandemic.[40] On January 30, the *BBC* included "bat soup" as an example of coronavirus misinformation.[41] Online searches for "bat soup" peaked on January 25, declined in February, and then rose again in March.[42] Despite the debunked myth, the "bat soup" racist trope prevailed throughout the pandemic—its effects lingering.

The effects of early stigmatizing content and Sinophobia were noted by the end of January. On social media, individuals and groups described bigoted acts that they experienced or witnessed tied to the coronavirus. On January 27, 2020, French filmmaker Amandine Gay@ OrpheoNegra shared a friend's message on Twitter: her photo with the words #JeNeSuisPasUnVirus on a poster held in front of her face.[43] The hashtag went viral, spreading in different languages, as Asian people documented their experiences online:

> Adam Rugnetta@Rugnettanews (Italy): "Thinking all Asians have #coronavirus is like thinking all Italians are mafiosi. Act don't overreact to #Pandemics. #IamNotAVirus" with a drawing to illustrate his point." (January 30, 2020)

RickyOishi@iromiudo211: "Even in Japan, I saw a few people who used language that meant to avoid Chinese because of this. They're hiding "racism" under the pretext of "prevention", but of course, it was language that went beyond the "prevention." (January 30, 2020)

Jason Oliver Chang@chinotronic (Connecticut): "Started by our brothers and sisters in France #JeSuisPasUnVirus. Consider using #IAmNotAVirus in solidarity with them and to reject the racism prompted by the coronavirus." (January 30, 2020)

CGTN (China state-affiliated media): "As a Chinese official said, "It is the virus that is our common enemy, not people from Wuhan." People across the world have been showing their support for those in Wuhan #IamNotAVirus #StandWithWuhan." (January 30, 2020)

chong zhang@zhangchongzc (Durham, England): "#JeNeSuisPasUnVirus #IamNotAVirus Hey! Xenophobia and racism towards Asians have come! A ten-year-old alike kid on a school bus yelled 'Get out ' at me today! @Chinese4Labour." (January 31, 2020)

News stories relayed harassment and discrimination of Asian-looking people in England, the Netherlands, Italy, and other countries.[44] In Berlin, two German women attacked a young Chinese woman. Yelling racist remarks, they spit on her, yanked her hair, and knocked her down, then kicked and hit her.[45] A food sample distributor at a Washington Costco turned away an 8 year-old boy wearing a mask because she worried that he was from China and "might infect her."[46] An event at a Melbourne night club promoted a "Corona Chinese New Year Special" online, featuring with a racist illustration of a Chinese stereotype holding a beer (canceled due to backlash).[47] Incidents like these were becoming more common across countries.

Additionally, news and social media's emphasis on China as the source of transmission fueled public fears of contracting the virus from Asian people, even when they had not recently ventured abroad.

Customers raised questions about ingredients imported from China. As such, Asian restaurant owners reported business declines in London, New York, Boston, San Francisco, Seattle, Arizona, Toronto, India, Australia, and other cities around the world.[48] Moreover, some of the newly implemented travel restrictions at the end of January targeted all citizens with Chinese passports, even those who had lived abroad for months or years.[49] This perceived culpability expanded to Japan with the February quarantine of the *Diamond Princess*.

On February 24, WHO publicly recognized the growing problem of stereotyping and stigmatization in language about the escalating crisis in its latest situation report.[50] The supplemental public guide stated, "The current COVID-19 outbreak has provoked social stigma and discriminatory behaviors against people of certain ethnic backgrounds as well as anyone perceived to have been in contact with the virus" and cautioned against using location-specific names, including "Wuhan Virus," "Chinese Virus," and "Asian Virus."[51] WHO produced a series of social media posts on stigma, parceling out components of the guide.

Despite this guidance, anti-Asian messaging and bigotry continued. A study of news articles from February 9, 2020, through March 7, 2020, found a 50 percent increase in stories on discrimination.[52] In this time period, 471 discriminatory and xenophobic incidents were identified. Individuals continued to share their concerns and experiences on social media. aiMEEEE@chivolute stated, "Every time I look, I see another story on a violent and vicious attack against Asians. Every time I go outside, I feel more and more afraid of being the next. Just this evening, people would move away or stare or cover their mouths when I walk by. I am terrified. #IAmNotAVirus" (March 4, 2020). In this time period, Asian and Chinese American businesses continued to face hardship, experiencing an 18 percent decline due to public fear of catching coronavirus in these establishments.[53] Ethnic clumping also continued to occur frequently, in which anyone who was perceived to be Asian was assumed to be Chinese, and thus, targeted.[54] For example, on March 5, a London art fair excluded a Vietnamese curator for fear that she would be "'seen as carrying the virus,'" as stated in an email to her.[55]

At the same time, movement against anti-Asian racism started to gain momentum.[56] The California-based Asian Pacific Policy and Planning Council (A3PCON, now called the AAPI Equity Alliance) and the Chinese for Affirmative Action civil rights organization issued "News Accounts of COVID-19 Discrimination 2/9–3/7/20." This ten-page report documented news articles that promoted xenophobia and noted coverage of harassment, bullying, event cancellation, travel bans, and other incidents of racism. Statements against discrimination and Asian American resistance were also included in the document.[57] Individuals also challenged racist media messaging. For example, Diana M. Kwon@diana-m-kwon (Washington State) called out NPR for reinforcing stereotypes, tweeting, "News sources need to stop using stock images of Asians for their headlines on COVID-19. They are perpetuating the xenophobia and racism. Standing strong with my Asian community #IAmNotAVirus #WeAreNotAVirus" (March 8, 2020).

FUELING THE FIRE: POLITICIZING STIGMA

Patterns of stigmatizing language spiked again in March 2020, when Trump and other GOP leaders began introducing phrases in interviews and social media posts, significantly escalating existing sinophobic and xenophobic beliefs. This turn was foreshadowed one month earlier in the *Wall Street Journal* when Walter Russell Mead[ii] wrote, "The mighty Chinese juggernaut has been humbled this week, apparently by a species-hopping bat virus."[58] He blamed China, stating, "Chinese authorities are still trying to conceal the true scale of the problem," called the Wuhan government "secretive and self-serving," and speculated on the economic fallout.[59] According to Jia and Lu, this article marked a critical moment: "Mead and the *WSJ* successfully set the stage on which Trump daringly picked it up and elevated this smear campaign against China onto the podium of the White House."[60] On March 2, The Five on Fox News TV show further stigmatized and blamed China.

ii Mead held a position in a right-wing think tank that aided Trump with policymaking.

JESSE WATTERS (co-host of *The Five*): "I'd like to just ask the Chinese for a formal apology. This coronavirus originated in China and I have not heard one word from the Chinese. A simple 'I'm sorry' would do. It would go a long way. I expect a formal apology tomorrow. Doesn't matter if it comes from Qi or the Embassy and I think all of my colleagues around this table will join arm and arm with me, also demanding a formal apology."

DANA: "What if the outbreak had started here?"

JESSE: "It didn't start here, Dana."

DANA: "But what if it had?"

JESSE: "It didn't start here, Dana, and I'll tell you why it started in China. 'Cause they have these markets where they're eating raw bats and snakes and they are very hungry people. The Chinese communist government cannot feed the people. And they are desperate. This food is uncooked. It is unsafe. And that is why scientists believe that's where it originated from."[61] (The other hosts of the show laughed.)

On March 6, then Secretary of State Mike Pompeo called the disease "Wuhan coronavirus" and "Wuhan virus" in a CNBC interview and press briefing.[62] He continued to use these terms as part of an overarching discourse blaming China. Two days later, Republican Paul Gosar tweeted that he was in quarantine because of "the Wuhan Virus."[63] Within an hour, this phrase was retweeted 24,049 times.[64] Retweets with "Chinese virus" included increased 650 percent.[65] The next day, GOP House Leader Kevin McCarthy included the phrase "Chinese coronavirus" in a tweet.[66] Conservative radio host and Trump supporter, Charlie Kirk, teased his latest episode on March 10 (retweeted by Trump): "Now, more than ever, we need the wall. With China Virus spreading across the globe, the US stands a chance if we can control of our borders. President Trump is making it happen. I explain why this matters & SO MUCH MORE!"[67] Trump also started referencing both "China virus" and "the Chinese virus" on social media and in press conferences, greatly amplifying others' publicly sharing these beliefs as well.[68] For example, Senior White House Correspondent for CBS News Weijia Jiang@weijia shared, "This morning a White House official referred to #Coronavirus as the "Kung-Flu" to my face. Makes me wonder what they're calling it behind my back" (March 17, 2020, retweeted over 87,000 times, 19.7 quote tweets, 412,000 likes).

Mainstream media outlets, organizations, and individuals quickly denounced this use of stigmatizing statements.[69] Like many social media users, Anna Spain Bradley (she/her)@ASpainBradley (Los Angeles, CA) objected, "Just say no to President Trump's #xenophobic and #racist labeling of COVID-19. Only massive global solidarity and cooperation will get us to the other side of this. #IamNotAVirus" (March 18, 2020). Similarly, HuffPost@*HuffPost* stated, "Tucker Carlson praised President Donald Trump's racism against the Chinese community at a time when Asian Americans are being attacked in response to the coronavirus," tweeting a *Huff Post* video documenting Fox News host Carlson's pattern of supporting Trump's racist comments.[70]

Despite criticism, Trump and his political allies continued to repeat stigmatizing labels and fan racist stereotyping. "Chinese virus" usage in conservative news articles quickly rose by 800 percent.[71] #ChineseVirus" had become the top trending hashtag on Twitter.[72] Over the next two weeks, Trump spoke the words "Chinese virus" over 20 times, choosing this phrase for social media, press conferences, and TV interviews on Fox News.[73]

The GOP's endorsement and spread of racist statement profoundly impacted public opinion. Sinophobic racial slurs on the anonymous political discussion board */pol/* and Twitter surged higher than ever before in mid-March.[74]A study of implicit bias against Asian Americans showed a significant increase in bias after March 8th, which was much higher in extreme conservatives, reflecting the use of stigmatizing language by Republican political leaders and news outlets.[75]

At the end of March, the *New York Times* and other news outlets documented the surge in hateful and discriminatory moments experienced by Asian Americans, describing how they'd been publicly harassed, spit on, and assaulted.[76] Stories captured the rising hate crimes, such as a New York City attack in which a woman yelled racial slurs and punched an Asian American woman.[77] Stop AAPI Hate received over 650 reports of bigoted acts within one week of opening its online reporting system on March 18.[78] In addition to verbal and physical assaults, Asian Americans also experienced discrimination from ride-share drivers and store employees.[79] People continued to share their experiences with prejudice and bigotry online:

> Tiffanie Chan@tiffaniechan (Richmond, VA): "Went to my neighborhood Kroger today and scared some old white ladies just by being in the aisle as they turned the corner. It was not a good feeling. #IamNotAVirus." (March 9, 2020)
>
> Kim newmoney@kimnewmoney (Los Angeles, CA): To be an Asian American right now . . . it's tiring. I have so many words . . . I'm going to try to spit them out to prevent an outburst or mental break in a few months from now. On January 30th, I went to a hospital in Burbank, California to have eight vials of blood drawn to have . . . some things checked. In the full hour I was at this hospital, everyone was staring at me and couldn't figure out why. Then it dawned on me, this is when everyone was first whispering about #covid. I am familiar with racist stares. I grew up in a small town in Southern Georgia." (March 11, 2020)
>
> Greg Lee@GregLeeKTVU (CA): "Walked by a couple. Lady says to her husband "doesn't he know he's like the plague right now?" Let's go ahead and take a deep breath from that xenophobia folks. We'll get through this." (March 14, 2020)
>
> Internet=Immortal@InternetImmort (Pacific Northwest): "How do I explain to my 8 year old that because she is Asian that she has to be careful of racist acts against her? She is correlating what she is seeing & hearing to the racism towards African Americans/MLK. Anyone feeding this hate. @POTUS, WTH are you doing? #IamNotAVirus." (March 19, 2020)
>
> Jiayang Fan@JiayangFan (staff writer at *The New Yorker*, New York): "Went to take out trash.Was talking on phone in Chinese. Man walked by on sidewalk & in interest of social dis-

> tancing, I said,"sorry, go ahead." "FUCKING CHINESE," he yelled loud enough I could hear him over aide's voice on phone. I turned to look at him to make sure I heard right . . . For the longest time,Ive been telling friends in China that altho racism against Chinese exists in this country, that's NOT what I feel in a pandemic. I've never felt like this in my 27 yrs in this country. I've never felt afraid to leave my home to take out the trash bc of my face." (March 17, 2020)

Although Trump's usage of stigmatizing phrases briefly declined in April, his statements soon returned as he continued to promote anti-Asian sentiment throughout the pandemic.[80] In 2020, Trump referred to "Chinese virus" 27 times and "China Virus" approximately 365 times on social media and in press conferences, political rallies, TV interviews, and other public events.[81] This number doesn't include similar derogatory remarks that Trump made, such as "kung flu," which he stated at a June 20, 2020, political rally in Tulsa, Oklahoma, prompting the crowd to wildly cheer.[82]

Other Republican political leaders also repeatedly made false and pejorative statements about China, including many that tied in the pandemic.[83] In May 2020, Senators Marsha Blackburn, Martha McSally, and Steve Daines proposed the "Stop China-Originated Viral Infectious Disease (Stop COVID Act)," encouraging Americans to file lawsuits against the Chinese Communist Party, claiming "they sent us the virus this year." Blackburn tweeted a promotional video on the Act. As ominous music played in the background, the video montage featured Blackburn (juxtaposed with clips from Fox News) accusing China of covering up the virus, "stealing our jobs," and "stealing our intellectual property," and declaring that China needed to be "held accountable."[84] Even though the Act never passed, Blackburn's messaging contributed to public fear and blame of China, along with anyone perceived as associated with China (i.e., Asian Americans). Blackburn reintroduced the Act in June 2021, to "empower Americans to sue China in US court and seek compensation for the devastating harm the deadly virus has caused to the economy and human life."[85]

Publicly captured anti-Asian sentiment wasn't limited to political leaders. People sold "Chinese bat-eating" t-shirts and other racist merchandise online.[86] "Bat soup," "China Virus," and "yellow peril" memes circulated on TikTok, Instagram, and other platforms.[87] Designed to be humorous, this content perpetuated racist stereotypes of Chinese/Asians, othering them as "diseased," blaming them for the pandemic, and ridiculing their accents and culture.[88] "Kung Flu Fighting" parody video went viral, containing numerous racist references (i.e., "China men," a Chinese cover-up, bat-eating, and China as the source of COVID).[89] Even scholars were called out for using stigmatizing labels ("Wuhan virus," "China virus," "Chinese virus") in academic publications.[90] By August 2020, over 2,000 scholarly manuscripts about COVID on PubMed included a reference to Wuhan, perpetuating stigma and prejudice.[91]

DISCUSSION AND IMPLICATIONS

Why did this happen? The stigma and blame attached to China (and broadened to people perceived as Asian) was deeply entrenched in a history of Sinophobia that existed long before 2019. The initial messaging put forth about the "mystery pneumonia" contained little information—a place (Wuhan), a disease that might be SARS, and speculation about connections to a wet market and to SARS. Trump and his political allies didn't create the situation but exploited it for their own agenda. As some scholars have noted, Trump's racist statements intensified Sinophobia, serving as a "call" to his supporters "to take up racist action against the members of the target group."[92] The Trump administration also shifted blame to China, using stigmatizing language to make the pandemic seem like a far-off threat, which contributed to downplaying the impending pandemic.

Despite WHO guidance on stopping stigmatizing COVID language, it was too little, too late, as the association between COVID and China and Chinese people had long been established. WHO and the CDC contributed with messaging about handling exotic animals. Public health organizations also delayed in emphasizing the importance of using a non-stigmatizing name for the virus. What many people missed or chose to ignore was that its origin was unknown and that the disease has no ethnicity. News and social media repeatedly stigmatized COVID as a "Chinese" or Asian disease, inciting discrimination against people who "looked Asian" and against Asian food online.[93] The racism and stigma against Asian people and Asian Americans extended beyond the parameters of the pandemic.

In the summer of 2020, 73 percent of US adults held unfavorable views of China—an increase of 26 percent from 2018 and 7 percent just from March 2020.[94] Approximately 78 percent overall blamed China for the global pandemic because of the country's initial handling of the crisis.[95] A partisan disparity existed in perceptions, with significantly more Republicans/Leaning Republican than Democrats holding unfavorable views of China and believing the country was responsible for the pandemic.[96] It also became more socially acceptable to voice bigoted opinions. In a survey of nearly 10,000 Americans, approximately 40 percent believed it had become "more common for people to express racist views about people who are Asian" than before the pandemic.[97] Many Asian Americans experienced the impact of escalating Sinophobia. Approximately 39 percent reported that "people acted as if they were uncomfortable around them," compared to 13 percent of white respondents.[98] Nearly a third of Asian Americans had been subjected to "slurs or jokes and 26 percent "feared someone might threaten or physically attack them."[99] Chinese American college students experienced increased perceived discrimination and anxiety.[100]

This fear was unfortunately justified as violence against Asian Americans/those perceived as Asian Americans continued to skyrocket, with 164 percent increase in anti-Asian hate crimes reported to police from the first quarter of 2020 to the same time period in 2021.[101] From March 19, 2020 through March 31, 2022, almost 11,500 hate incidents were reported to Stop AAPI Hate.[102] Crimes included "verbal hate speech and/or harassment," workplace discrimination, "avoidance or shunning," physical attacks, "online misconduct," being "coughed or spat on," "refusal of service," and other types of discrimination in public spaces, businesses, private residences, schools, universities, hospitals and other locations.[103] This number does not encompass, of course, unreported hate crimes, discrimination, casual racism, and microaggressions.

PANDEMIC STIGMA AND INEQUITY FOR OTHER GROUPS

In addition to people of Asian descent, the pandemic also fueled stigma, hate, and inequity for other marginalized groups as well. Immigrants were frequently (falsely) blamed for COVID cases, as initiated by Senator Ted Cruz and other Republican leaders in summer 2021.[104] According to a September 2021 survey, 55 percent of Republicans believed that the 2021 "third wave" of COVID occurred because "immigrants and tourists" carried the virus into the United States.[105] Migrants and refugees were not only more susceptible to COVID infections, but also faced additional pandemic challenges.[106]

Black and brown people succumbed to COVID at a much higher rate than other ethnic groups.[107] By population, people of multiple races, American Indian and Alaska Native, followed by Native Hawaiian and Pacific Islander, and Black or African American, disproportionately died from COVID.[108] Structural racism contributed to a heightened risk, including positions as essential workers, their disproportionate representation in prison, poverty, lack of health care access, and incidence of comorbidities.[109] Moreover, people of color were less likely to receive equitable, quality care when they became infected.[110] Frontline health care providers observed that other health professionals gave BIPOC and disabled patients less interaction and not as much explanation.[111] Patients of marginalized communities also experienced more barriers to quality care, including difficulty in accessing telehealth services and making appointments for health conditions unrelated to COVID.[112] Delayed care was also observed as more prevalent for individuals from underrepresented groups, especially for those with language barriers.[113] Hispanic women struggled more than women of other ethnicities to get medical appointments or to fill prescriptions.[114]

Adding to the difficulty of the pandemic was the continuation of police brutality against people of color. On May 31, 2020, former Minneapolis white police officer Derek Chauvin murdered a Black Minneapolis man, George Floyd.[115] A call to end such violence sparked protests for social justice all over the world.[116] With approximately fifteen to twenty-six million people participating in the United States alone, Black Lives Matter became one of the largest mass demonstrations in history.[117] Although media coverage of the protests helped to highlight systematic racism and inequality in the pandemic, backlash in the forms of memes and other media discourse perpetuated stereotypes.[118]

COVID profoundly impacted LGBTQIA+ communities, who experienced a higher percentage of job loss, as well as negative impact on stress and mental health, compared to the general population.[119] Shelter-in-place orders meant that many LGBTQIA+ adolescents and young adults lost their in-person affirming spaces. Over 80 percent of LGBTQIA+ youth surveyed indicated that the pandemic heightened the stress in their living situations, which was even higher for Native/Indigenous adolescents.[120] Furthermore, LGBTQIA+ youth of color reported experiencing multiple forms of discrimination and found that COVID hindered their abilities to express their gender identities and sexual orientation.[121]

Older people faced negative stereotypes and higher risks for contracting disease, especially those living in nursing homes and other congregated settings.[122] Those in homes with domestic violence experienced heightened incidence during lockdown with the need for restraining/protective orders up 40 percent.[123] People with disabilities experienced accessibility issues and other obstacles.[124] The reliance on technology for school and work amplified the digital divide and knowledge gap, especially among low-income households.[125]

Overall, this was a pandemic of inequality. COVID's effects were devastating for a privileged public. They were catastrophic for already marginalized communities, confounded by systematic inequalities. Stigma and discrimination didn't originate in January 2020, but were amplified, resulting in much more difficult experiences for the under-represented. The long-term implications of COVID's inequalities are not yet known.

CHAPTER SIX

A Pivotal Moment

MEDIA AND THE COVID VACCINES

Pfizer's Early Data Shows Vaccine Is More Than 90 Percent Effective.[1]

On November 9, 2020, the pharmaceutical company Pfizer released their coronavirus vaccine trial results, declaring high rates of effectiveness.[2] Five days later, Moderna announced similarly successful vaccine trial results.[3] Within just over a month, both had received Emergency Use Authorization from the US Food & Drug Administration, permitting the vaccines to be given to the general public, ages eighteen and over.[4] Vaccine administration began with health care workers on December 14, 2020.[5] Over the next two months, health professionals, essential workers, long-term care residents, and senior citizens received their COVID-19 doses. Vaccine eligibility varied by state, slowly expanding to include more groups considered high-priority.[6]

In March 2021, adults that did not fit a pre-approved category desperately awaited their turn for the COVID vaccination, checking health department websites for the tiered rollout of Moderna, Pfizer-BioNTech (mRNA), and the one-dose vaccine Johnson & Johnson (approved February 27, 2021).[7] Talk of driving hours for the chance at a shot buzzed in certain circles.[8] Online, people shared tips for getting immunized as soon as possible. Some volunteered as traffic control, entry screeners, and monitors at vaccine clinics, hoping to receive their first dose.[9] For many, COVID vaccination came with tears of joy and celebration, optimism about returning to "normal life," and the dissipation of fear from a disease that had disrupted the world. Among those vaccinated, hospitalizations and deaths plummeted, paling in comparison to the high rates experienced in unvaccinated individuals.[10]

Two years later, the eligible population had expanded to age six months and older, and over 230 million people had completed a primary series (69.5 percent of the US population).[11] More than 92 percent of adults eventually received at least one dose and nearly 80 percent completed the primary series.[12] Yet, reaching these numbers took time. And the significant fluctuation in vaccine rates by demographics, partisan affiliation, and geographic region cannot be overlooked. For example, the percentage of adults fully vaccinated with the primary series ranged from 63.3 percent in Wyoming to over 95 percent in Rhode Island.[13] Some individuals were so ardently opposed that they elected to lose their jobs rather than receive the vaccine.[14] Worse, vocal anti-vax leaders crafted and spread conspiracies and disinformation about the vaccines, persuading those who were uncertain to wait or decline immunization altogether.[15]

The COVID vaccine rollout marked a unique moment, both in the pandemic and in history. Never before had a successful vaccine been developed in the midst of the crisis, before cases had subsided. And, just as important (and unfortunate), never before had the introduction of an effective vaccine been so publicly scrutinized. This chapter explores media constructions leading up to the vaccine rollout, from the first references to the initial distribution. Although each country faced its own challenges (ideological and practical) in vaccine dissemination, this chapter specifically focuses on the United States. Three key contextual factors dramatically shaped how the approved vaccines would be received: Rise of vaccine opposition in the digital landscape, a lack of media interest in coronavirus vaccines pre-2020, and the framing of vaccines and science as a whole early in the global crisis.

VACCINES, VACCINE OPPOSITION, AND MEDIA

As David Heath eloquently articulated in *Longshot: The Inside Story of the Race for a COVID-19 Vaccine*, the development and implementation of COVID vaccines was made possible because of centuries of scientific work and progress.[16] The practice of inoculation or variolation (intentionally infecting one with smallpox to reduce the disease's potency) dates back to at least tenth century China, and saved numerous lives in colonial America after it was introduced in 1721.[17] Edward Jenner improved upon inoculation practice by replacing smallpox matter with cowpox, significantly reducing risks while providing immunity. which he called "vaccine inoculation."[18] Within only of a few years of Jenner's initial publication, programs emerged to provide public immunization.[19] Smallpox vaccination campaigns gained momentum and continued throughout the nineteenth century.[20] In the 1880s, Louis Pasteur developed an effective vaccine against rabies, marking the first laboratory vaccine to be used on humans.[21] By the 1930s, scientists had created effective vaccines against tetanus, cholera, typhoid fever, bubonic plague, tuberculosis, diphtheria, scarlet fever, pertussis, yellow fever, typhus, and influenza.[22] In 1954, Jonas Salk's polio vaccine was tested in the largest trial in history, with 623,972 children receiving a placebo or the vaccine.[23] Its approval in 1955 signified a triumph over the dreaded disease.[24] Vaccines against measles, mumps, rubella, and other diseases were developed in the 1960s and 1970s.[25] Meanwhile extensive global vaccination programs, surveillance, and preventative measures successfully eradicated smallpox and once-common childhood diseases became nearly unheard of in developed countries.[26]

Pockets of opposition first emerged with the practice of inoculation. Anti-vaccination groups have existed since the first vaccines. Yet, for the most part, their positions received little coverage in mainstream news.[27] As Martin Kaufman wrote about nineteenth century opponents, "Many anti-vaccinationists were lone wolves, doing their best to convince others of the danger of vaccination."[28] With the mainstream acceptance of the germ theory, by the twentieth century, anti-vaccination groups began embracing anti-science rhetoric as a primary justification for not immunizing.[29] Editorial gatekeeping reduced unsubstantiated claims from being published. At the same time, people had firsthand experience of the devastation of what these diseases could do, having witnessed "the strangler" (diphtheria) attack school classmates or "the crippler" (polio) paralyze neighbors, making them more willing to vaccinate. Outbreaks and epidemics regularly shut down towns, sometimes causing so many deaths that funeral bells ceased to toll and coffins ran out.[30] Fear and experience prompted nearly everyone to get whatever vaccines scientists could create and try out. By the time that WHO declared the eradication of smallpox on May 8, 1980, the prevalence of most contagious childhood diseases had declined significantly due to effective vaccines.[31]

Fast-forward nearly forty years to COVID, and much of the developed world took health and herd immunity for granted, with generations separated by memories of iron lung imagery and sugar cube vaccines. Routine immunization continues to save approximately four million lives each year, rendering vaccine-preventable illnesses nearly invisible in developed countries.[32] In the absence of collective memory of disease, the digital landscape amplified the once-outlier groups of anti-vaxxers. This mediated revolution started to occur at the same time as Andrew Wakefield's quickly retracted *Lancet* article that, without any evidence, linked the MMR vaccine to autism.[33] Even back in 2000, anti-vaccination websites spread myths that vaccines caused illness, hindered immunity, helped pharmaceutical companies profit, offered content on opting out of vaccine requirements, and provided links to other disinformation-filled sites.[34] Searches on "vaccines" were much more likely to produce anti-vaccine sites than scientific information supporting immunization.[35]

An anti-vaccination movement further gained momentum with the advent of social media platforms, enabling regular people to distribute their opinions online, oftentimes presenting them as factual and science based.[36] Ideas that never would have passed through the chains of editors and news producers can appear instantly on blogs and social media channels. Adding to this, bots can produce and reproduce content.[37] Loopholes in state mandates have also enabled parents to avoid vaccinating their children.[38]

The twenty-first century digital climate expanded opportunities for unchecked content about vaccines. Trump's wavering position on vaccines brought outliers into the mainstream. A 2017 *JAMA* article highlighted Trump's anti-vaccination messaging, explaining how he had publicly repeated false claims that vaccines cause autism and supported Wakefield and others known for anti-vaccination messaging.[39] Pockets of unvaccinated kids increased, leading to measles outbreaks in the United States.[40] Overall, though, most people continued with recommended vaccines. In 2019, a survey of US adolescents showed that over 90 percent of US children had received two doses or more of the measles, mumps, and rubella (MMR) vaccine and Tdap (tetanus-diphtheria-pertussis).[41] Yet, the simmering distrust of science and vaccines among various groups, especially far-right extremists, set the foundation for how COVID vaccines would later be received.

Outside of epidemics (SARS, H1N1, Ebola, Zika), twenty-first century news outlets did not prioritize vaccine innovation. Scientists made significant progress toward successful messenger RNA (mRNA) vaccines in a series of developments stretching back to 2005 but received very little media recognition for their work.[42] For example, from 2000 to 2019, only 31 news articles addressed coronavirus vaccines. The *New York Times* only produced one article, focusing on Middle Eastern respiratory syndrome, published in 2013.[43] Writer Donald G. McNeil, Jr. commented on this disinterest, "While flu vaccines have been produced around the world for 60 years, the passion for a coronavirus vaccine has faded since the SARS epidemic."[44] Scientists occasionally tweeted that they were working on coronavirus vaccines—mostly for cats and dogs—with little engagement (receiving almost no likes, retweets, or comments). In other words, progress toward effective coronavirus vaccines had already begun, yet no one was paying attention.[i] Media framing and agenda setting leading up to the pandemic set the stage for how COVID vaccines would be received.

VACCINATING AGAINST COVID-19

Early news coverage of the emerging crisis set the foundation for much of what would come later on in the pandemic. References to a vaccine appeared even before the virus had been identified. On January 5, 2020, *Channel News Asia's* website posted "As Singapore's first suspected case of the Wuhan pneumonia virus turned out to be a false alarm, an infectious diseases expert tells CNA there is currently no vaccine against the little-known strain and that it would take at least three to four years to develop one."[45]

On January 10, 2020, the *Washington Post* published, "China Identifies New Strain of Coronavirus as Source of Pneumonia Outbreak," quoting Chinese researcher Xu Jianguo: "Developing specific drugs and vaccines against a new pathogen could take years."[46] A week later, ScienceNews@ScienceNews posted, "It's been 17 years since SARS, and we still don't have any coronavirus vaccine. We don't have any coronavirus antivirals," linking to a lengthy article about coronavirus.[47] The few articles on coronavirus that trickled out over the next week took a similar approach, repeating statements like, "There are no vaccines to prevent it or specific treatments" (*Daily Record*, January 18, 2020), "There is no vaccine and efforts are being accelerated to develop treatments" (*Evening Standard*, January 22, 2020), and from the Associated Press: "There are no specific medicines for the illness and no vaccine to prevent it" (*Democrat and Chronicle* and other outlets, January 23, 2020).[48]

Unbeknownst to the public, the release of the genetic sequencing of the novel coronavirus instigated the development of the vaccine. As Heath chronicled, the work to quickly create a new coronavirus vaccine

i For a detailed history on scientific developments that paved the way for COVID vaccine success, see David Heath's *The Inside Story of the Race for a COVID-19 Vaccine* (2022).

had been done in the decades leading up to 2020. Jesper Pallesen, Nianshuang Wang, Kizzmekia Corbett, and their team had published a road map on using a spike protein to fight coronaviruses in a 2017 publication.[49] Yet, this progress existed outside of media content, receiving almost no attention for the initial article or in its critical application in developing a COVID-19 vaccine.

From January 20 through January 25, social media mentioning coronavirus vaccines primarily involved sharing news articles about competing companies and the vaccine quest, with almost no engagement. An Associated Press story on January 21 stated, "There is no vaccine yet, although nine studies are examining coronavirus vaccine development."[50] Biotech company Moderna circulated its press release on social media two days later: "We just announced a funding award from @CEPIvaccines to accelerate development of an #mRNA vaccine against novel coronavirus."[51] Coverage appeared speculative and distant, promising vaccines in the hopefully not-too-distant future.

As cases expanded to new countries, including the United States, news coverage of coronavirus also increased. On January 24, headlines about vaccine developments appeared in a barrage of news outlets: "U of S Scientists Working on Vaccine for Coronavirus," "$9M Grant to Develop Coronavirus Vaccine," and "Virus Vaccine Plans Boost Drugmakers, But Time is Short"[52] Such articles were common on social media, yet still received few likes, shares, comments, or other engagement. Urgency and speed were repeatedly emphasized in headlines. For example, *ABC News Australia* announced, "The University of Queensland (UQ) is confident it can develop a vaccine for the potentially deadly coronavirus in as few as 16 weeks as four people in NSW and two people in Brisbane are monitored for the virus."[53] *The Guardian* published "Lessons From Sars Outbreak Help in Race for Coronavirus Vaccine," on January 24: "Companies aim to have vaccine in production within 16 weeks before entering testing stage."[54] Announcements from the pharmaceutical companies also took place, including "Different Outbreak, Same Strategy: Inside Novavax's Plans for a Coronavirus Vaccine" and "Cambridge's Moderna Therapeutics Ramps Up Search For Coronavirus Vaccine."[55]

That day, a *CNBC* interview with Dr. Anthony Fauci aired (shared on YouTube and on Twitter). When asked about the timeline, Fauci first spoke about the possibility of mRNA vaccines:

> A phase one trial to determine safety of a vaccine, we think we'll be able to put material into a human and a safety trial within the next three months. And I think that's a pretty good number. I don't think that's an exaggeration or too optimistic. And then after that, it takes a few months to get enough data to know at least whether you're dealing with a compound that's safe. So three months from now to get into a human. Another three months to get some data. But then the real problem is when you want to develop something to use for people, if you have to use it even on an emergency basis, that's going to take several months more, but the process is already started in developing vaccines.[56]

On January 28, the *New York Times* published a lengthy article about coronavirus with a section on potential vaccines, stating, "The hunt began Jan. 10, when Chinese scientists posted the genetic makeup of the virus on a public database. The next morning, researchers at the National Institutes of Health's Vaccine Research Center in Maryland went to work. Within hours, they had pinpointed the letters of the genetic code that could be used to make a vaccine."[57] Another story unveiled that Australian scientists had figured out how to grow the coronavirus in a lab—progress toward developing tests and possible vaccines.[58]

As the virus continued to appear in more countries, media content about vaccine development exploded, with questions about the timeline dominating headlines and social media teasers:

> "'We Thought We Had Three Years': UQ Team To Fast-Track Coronavirus Vaccine." (*Brisbane Times*, January 24, 2020)[59]
>
> "Novavax Exec: Making a Coronavirus Vaccine Could Take a Long Time." (*Yahoo!Finance*, January 24, 2020)[60]

> One News Page@One_News_Page tweeted: "Wuhan Coronavirus Vaccine Could Take Years," paired with a story.[61]
>
> "Drugmakers are rushing to create and test a coronavirus vaccine. Here's how they're doing it." (*USA Today*, January 24, 2020)[62]
>
> "Coronavirus Vaccine May Be Ready in Months." (*Financial Express*, January 24, 2020)[63]
>
> "Australia's Been Asked to Make a Coronavirus Vaccine at 'Unprecedented Speed. We're not prepared." (ScienceAlert@ScienceAlert, January 24, 2020)[64]
>
> "J&J Scientific Officer 'Pretty Confident' They Can Create Coronavirus Vaccine As Outbreak Widens." (*CNBC*, January 27, 2020)[65]

Carolyn Johnson's article in the *Washington Post* "Coronavirus vaccine research is moving at record speed. The science is fast, but the virus is faster" outlined the unprecedented pace of the vaccine, mentioning how it had not occurred successfully with SARS and other epidemics due to limited resources and technology in the past.[66] Similarly, *The Conversation* explored the timeline more in-depth in "When Will There be a Coronavirus Vaccine? Five Questions Answered." Authors Aubree Gordon and Florian Krammer emphasized that vaccine "work was ongoing for other closely related coronaviruses that have caused severe disease in humans, namely MERS and SARS."[67]

News of companies working on vaccine development correlated with surging stock prices and speculation on profit. According to a January 24 *Atlanta Constitution* article, Novavax stock shares had increased by 71 percent and Moderna had received an 11 percent boost due to both companies' "news of their plans for coronavirus vaccines."[68] Twitter user Bagsy@Bagsy posted a meme of a frog holding up a stack of cash, with "Which company has the patent to the coronavirus vaccine?"[69] News told of Bill and Melinda Gates' $100 million donation to vaccine development.[70] Actor Jackie Chan pledged a reward for a successful vaccine.[71] Around the world, money and resources flowed into swift vaccine development.

Toward the end of January, regular people started producing random comments on the crisis (as also discussed in both the news diffusion and stigma chapters). As news stories became increasingly concerned about the crisis, individuals joked through beer-themed tweets. Don't Lie@passfirstmafia: "Drank a Corona as a coronavirus vaccine. Decided I would rather contract the virus than drink a second Corona." (Twitter, January 25, 2020). Comments about and from anti-vaxxers also entered at this point, scarcely receiving attention.

> Tiffany Berry, MD@DocMom_TX: "Bet if there was a coronavirus vaccine, there would suddenly be a line of die hard #antivaxxers lining their kids up." (1 retweet, 7 likes, January 24, 2020).[72]
>
> Lina@agirlcalledlina, "Am sure the anti vaccine brigade will refuse to have the coronavirus vaccine? if they end up coming up with one." (13 likes, January 24, 2020).[73]
>
> Phillip Mcilwain@dendrades: "Breaking! A massive anti-vaccination protest has assembled outside the laboratory working on the coronavirus vaccine at the Queensland University." (No engagement, January 25, 2020).[74]
>
> Juugman Laflare@ThaSouth: "So are they gonna blow this coronavirus shxt outta proportion and then tell everyone you need the coronavirus vaccine, that has.......... wait for it............ keep waiting. . . . the RFID chip in it???" (4 retweets, 5 likes, January 25, 2020).[75]

As the virus spread to new countries and locked down cruise ships, scientists around the world worked diligently to create effective coronavirus vaccines. News outlets reported increments of progress, sharing stories on social media. Sky News@SkyNews tweeted, "The scientist leading the UK's research into a #coronavirus vaccine says he is now at the stage to start testing the vaccine on animals as early as next week" (February 5, 2020).[76] The linked news story mentioned that this step indicated a reduction "of the normal development time from 'two to three years to just 14 days.'" *Hindustan Times* in India celebrated, "Indian scientist in Australia helps grow first batch of #coronavirus for preclinical studies" with a news article.[77] KVUE News@KVUE posted, "San Diego lab discovers #coronavirus vaccine in 3 hours" discussing the company Inovio and vaccine development.[78] On February 24, Moderna Inc. produced a press release declaring that "vials of mRNA-1273 have been shipped to the National Institute of Allergy and Infectious Diseases (NIAID), a part of the National Institutes of Health (NIH) to be used in the planned Phase 1 study in the U.S."[79] Its announcement on Twitter received 27 comments, 645 retweets, and 591 likes. The *Washington Post* summed up the need for urgency: "This sounds like great news: Drugmakers are starting to develop a coronavirus vaccine. The downside: That's because they believe the virus is so deadly that developing a vaccine is worth risking a lot of money."[80]

As scientists moved forward, the Trump administration continued communication politicizing the rising crisis and muddling questions about vaccine development. Trump repeatedly downplayed the imminent threat, assuring the public that it would "go away in April."[81] At the end of February, Donald J. Trump@realDonaldTrump tweeted,

> The Coronavirus is very much under control in the USA. We are in contact with everyone and all relevant countries. CDC & World Health have been working hard and very smart. Stock Market starting to look very good to me! (February 24, 2020).[82]

Among many of those who commented, Eugene Gu@eugenegu replied, tagging Trump, "Republicans have been waging a war on science, women's reproductive freedom, and fetal tissue research for so long that we have no vaccine for the coronavirus despite having more than 17 years to prepare since the SARS outbreak first alerted us to the dangers of coronavirus." (February 24, 2020)[83]

During the February 25, 2020, press conference, Trump repeatedly diminished the threat of COVID-19, stating, "Because of all we've done, the risk to the American people remains very low," promising that a vaccine could be developed "fairly rapidly."[84] Online, Quoth the

Raven@QTRResearch responded: "TRUMP SAYS CORONAVIRUS VACCINE IS 'VERY CLOSE' The fuck is he talking about—clinical trials take at least 3–6 months." (February 25, 2020).[85] Meanwhile, Dr. Fauci appeared much more cautious during the same briefing:

> It's probably going to be closer to two months. That would then take about three months to determine if it's safe and immunogenic, which gives us six months. Then you graduate from a trial—which is phase one—of 45 people, to a trial that involves hundreds if not low thousands of people to determine efficacy. At the earliest, an efficacy trial would take an additional six to eight months. So although this is the fastest we have ever gone from a sequence of a virus to a trial, it still would not be any applicable to the epidemic unless we really wait about a year to a year and a half.[86]

In addition to continued questions about timeline, vaccine cost became politicized after Health and Human Services Secretary Alex Azar stated in a budget hearing to Congress, "We would want to ensure that we work to make it affordable, but we can't control that price, because we need the private sector to invest" (February 26, 2020). Congressional Reporter Michael McAuliff shared the clip on social media. Fearing that emerging vaccines might be cost-prohibitive, members of Congress rallied on and off-line. Senator Chuck Schumer@SenSchumer directly responded to the clip: "Any emergency Coronavirus funding supplemental Congress approves must include provisions ensuring: 1—Pres. Trump can't transfer the funds to anything other than Coronavirus 2—Vaccines are affordable & available to all who need it 3—State & local governments are reimbursed" (February 26, 2020).[87] Democratic US Representative Jan Schakowsky@janschakowsky declared, "Today I led 45 of my colleagues to demand that @realDonaldTrump ensures any #coronavirus vaccine or treatment developed with U.S. taxpayer $ is accessible & affordable. That goal can't be met if #BigPharma sets prices & determines distribution, putting profits over public health" (February 20, 2020).[88] Other US Representative Democrats made similar posts.

PREVENTING COVID IN SPRING 2020

As the now-pandemic virus shut down much of the world, trials for three potential COVID vaccines ensued, and seventy potential vaccines globally were being developed.[89] The NIH, partnering with Moderna, launched the first human clinical testing phase for their potential vaccine, mRNA-1273, on March 16, 2020.[90] Pfizer-BioNTech initiated its first round of vaccine testing on twelve participants in Germany on April 29, expanding to the United States on May 5.[91] CanSino Biologics and the Beijing Institute of Biotechnology had also reached phase two with their vaccine at this point.[92] The Oxford COVID-19 (using adenovirus vaccine vector) vaccine trial, consisting of approximately 1,110 people, started on April 23, 2020.[93] Online, people were talking about vaccines, sharing information about the vaccine trials, offering advice on protection against COVID, and speculating on the costs of vaccines.[94] A relatively small percentage of social media posts spread conspiracies, primarily about government and the companies producing the vaccines.[95]

Trump retweeted stories documenting the trials, however, his messages to the public more often touted untested treatments.[96] He brought up the possibility of using hydroxychloroquine to treat or prevent COVID, drawing from the unsubstantiated claims of its effectiveness by Phillipe Gautret, Didier Raoult, and others.[97] In a March 19 press briefing, Trump stated:

> Now, a drug called chloroquine—and some people would add to it "hydroxy-." Hydroxychloroquine. So chloroquine or hydroxychloroquine. Now, this is a common malaria drug. It is also a drug used for strong arthritis. If somebody has pretty serious arthritis, also uses this in a somewhat different form. But it is known as a malaria drug, and it's been around for a long time and it's very powerful. But the nice part is, it's been around for a long time, so we know that if it—if things don't go as planned, it's not going to kill anybody.

> When you go with a brand-new drug, you don't know that that's going to happen. You have to see and you have to go—long test. But this has been used in different forms—very powerful drug—in different forms. And it's shown very encouraging—very, very encouraging early results. And we're going to be able to make that drug available almost immediately. And that's where the FDA has been so great. They—they've gone through the approval process; it's been approved. And they did it—they took it down from many, many months to immediate. So we're going to be able to make that drug available by prescription or states.[98]

Following Trump's briefing, Google searches for "hydroxychloroquine" spiked on March 19 and surged repeatedly in the following months, paralleling further endorsement by Trump and other prominent figures.[99] Despite no scientific confirmation that the drug was effective in treating COVID, Trump continued to promote hydroxychloroquine and an array of other untested treatments much more than approved treatments (the drug Remdesivir) through social media, television, and press briefings.[100] His frequent tweets and remarks endorsing chloroquine, hydroxychloroquine, and azithromycin, conveyed and confirmed in conservative media outlets, produced surges in Google searches for the drugs and in Amazon purchases.[101] Hydroxychloroquine prescriptions were especially sought-after in geographic areas with high numbers of Trump supporters, indicating a correlation between political affiliation and use of the untested medication.[102]

In an April 23, 2020, televised press briefing, Trump proposed yet another "treatment" for coronavirus. Acting Undersecretary William Bryan discussed the effects of direct sunlight and disinfectants on the virus. The following dialogue ensued without interruption:

TRUMP: Thank you very much. So I asked Bill a question that probably some of you are thinking of, if you're totally into that world, which I find to be very interesting. So, supposing we hit the body with a tremendous—whether it's ultraviolet or just very powerful light—and I think you said that that hasn't been checked, but you're going to test it. And then I said, supposing you brought the light inside the body, which you can do either through the skin or in some other way, and I think you said you're going to test that too. It sounds interesting.

BRYAN: We'll get to the right folks who could.

TRUMP: Right. And then I see the disinfectant, where it knocks it out in a minute. One minute. And is there a way we can do something like that, by injection inside or almost a cleaning. Because you see it gets in the lungs and it does a tremendous number on the lungs. So it would be interesting to check that. So, that, you're going to have to use medical doctors with. But it sounds—it sounds interesting to me.[103]

Trump's unsubstantiated speculation that "injecting bleach" could prevent the virus spurred immediate, detrimental responses. Various organizations promptly issued warnings:

> Harvard Toxicology@Harvard_Tox: "Please don't inject bleach or drink disinfectant. Bleach injections cause hemolysis (where your red blood cells that carry OXYGEN break apart) and cause liver damage, and many disinfectants can cause dangerous burns or bleeding in your stomach. This tweet IS medical advice." (April 24, 2020)

The message included evidence that bleach injection could cause black urine and kidney injury, blood clots, and esophageal perforation. It received 10.8K Retweets, 1,121 Quote Tweets, and 30.2K likes.

> Lysol US@Lysol (the leading disinfectant manufacturer) replied to individual tweets related to Trump's dangerous suggestion: "Hi, under no circumstance should our disinfectant products be administered into the human body (through injection, ingestion or any other route). For More Info, please visit our website: https://bit.ly/2Vz8TVh. (April 25, 2020).

This press release was heavily covered in news.[104] Much of the content emphasized the dangers of heeding Trump's advice, like *Rolling Stone*'s article "What Would Actually Happen to Your Body If You Actually Injected Bleach?"[105] Despite the warnings, calls to poison control centers doubled in NYC and increased so much in Maryland that an emergency alert had to be issued.[106] More liberal-leaning media framed this moment as another demonstration of Trump's "general mismanagement of the government's response to the COVID-19 pandemic and his tendency to spread misinformation, whether by mistake or as an intentional distraction tactic."[107] On the other hand, conservative outlets repeated the content of the press conference, defended Trump for his statements, and accused other media outlets of distorting what the president had said.[108] Trump's repeated declarations of untested treatments would later complicate the successful vaccine rollout.

Trump regularly flip-flopped between boasting of vaccine development to mainstream media while downplaying the severity of the pandemic to his followers. On April 29, 2020, *Bloomberg News* published "Trump's 'Operation Warp Speed' Aims to Rush Coronavirus Vaccine."[109] This article introduced Trump administration's vaccine development plan and explained, "the program will pull together pharmaceutical companies, government agencies and the military to try to cut the development time for a vaccine by as much as eight months.[110] News coverage of "Operation Warp Speed" focused on the short timeline. *The Hill* reported, "Trump administration launches 'Operation Warp Speed' to accelerate vaccine development."[111] Similarly, the *New York Times* printed, "Trump Seeks Push to Speed Vaccine, Despite Safety Concerns."[112] Author David E. Sanger wrote:

> President Trump is pressing his health officials to pursue a crash development program for a coronavirus vaccine that could be widely distributed by the beginning of next year, despite widespread skepticism that such an effort could succeed and considerable concern about the implications for safety.[113]

Backlash to both the name "Operation Warp Speed" and its plan appeared that day on social media, much of which highlighted Trump's move from downplaying the crisis to rushing for a vaccine:

> Shawn@ShawnRockk: Trump is initiating operation Warp speed on a vaccine. Where was this operation when we Needed PPE? Or Ventilators? Or a plan back In December and January when he knew about the coming Pandemic? (April 29, 2020)

> Dastardly Democrat @LifeLongWanderR (Replying to @axios): "Operation Warp Speed" Trump admin pushing for a vaccine by end of year at the cost of billions, pass or fail. I'm as anxious as many, but would prefer it be SAFE and EFFECTIVE rather then rapid. (April 29, 2020)

> ®øbę®†@NotyalcTrebor, Apr 29, 2020: Operation Warp Speed would be a lot cooler if it had something to do with Star Trek. Unfortunately it's some dumbass name the current admin came up with for accelerating vaccine research/production. (April 29, 2020)

> Lafayette@Freedomstrasse: Too late for that and the @GOP. Trump is now in full reopen mode, Operation Warp Speed. He fears an ongoing tanked economy more than any number of deaths. He doesn't get it. The consumer decides when and if it wants to play. No stop-gap therapies, no vaccine? Forget about it. (April 29, 2020)

Star Wars memes accompanied many of the posts, parodying the film franchise's reference. Republican legislators referred to "Operation Warp Speed" and praised Trump for the vaccine success on Twitter.[114] Democratic legislators were more likely to relay public health messaging, along with a broader range of topics.[115] According to some public health officials and academic scholars, the name (Operation Warp Speed) and mission appeared vague and reinforced a misperception that the vaccines had been developed too quickly.[116]

SUMMER 2020: MASKS & VACCINE TRIALS

As trials were underway for Moderna, Pfizer, and other potential vaccines, journalists, public health officials, and others continued to speculate about the timeline and effectiveness. At this point in time, politicians across party lines spoke in favor of the vaccine. On July 27, 2020: Donald J. Trump posted a video of his briefing to *Facebook*. "And we're here actually today to discuss the exciting progress that we've achieved under the Operation Warp Speed, our historic initiative to develop tests, manufacture and deliver a vaccine in record time and that's what it is, in record time . . . This morning, the Moderna has officially entered phase 3 already and that's phase 3 clinical trials, the final stage before approval." Even with these intermittent briefings, the clinical trials for potential vaccines did not yet receive much media attention, likely because it took months to immunize participants and then wait to see on the results.

Disinformation about the vaccines in development continued to circle. For example, Twitter user Doug Alexander (a layperson) shared a video titled, "Dr. Claims New COVID-19 Vaccines will alter your DNA," along with this diatribe on July 24, 2020:

> #OperationWarpSpeed = Operation Stupid Speed. VACCINE DESCRIPTION BY EXPERT: "It is recombinant DNA . . . This is what is proposed for COVID vaccine . . . to make genetically modified organisms" (comparable to the genetically modified Monsanto vegetable seed strains) with financial backing from the Bill and Melinda Gates Foundation. These vaccines have never been used before and the fast tracking without normal clinical trials is VERY DANGEROUS. The producers of these vaccines will be exempt from any liability.—According to Dr. Carrie Madej, Internal Medicine Specialist—with Doug Alexander MDew.

Such content went unchecked, even with social media platforms' policies and screening for misinformation.

Meanwhile, mask-wearing became the temporary measure for

preventing COVID-19. Months earlier, in April 2020, the CDC had officially recommended that individuals wear face masks.[117] Summer and the reopening of many public spaces prompted mask ordinances. The CDC strengthened its position in a July 14 press release, citing two studies that demonstrated the protection of masks against COVID transmission.[118] Over the summer, governors in thirty-three states implemented mask requirements.[119] Fourteen states varied by county or municipality and two had no mandates.[120]

Yet, Trump continued to downplay the severity of COVID, criticizing public health authorities and mask-wearing, especially to his constituents.[121] He was photographed unmasked and mocked those who donned face coverings.[122] Presidential candidate Joe Biden and other prominent Democrats consistently spoke in favor of public health and mitigation and were seen practicing social distancing and wearing masks in public spaces. Mask-wearing became highly politicized, with right-wing conservatives much more likely to resist masks and ordinances enforcing them.[123] This tension escalated over the following year, particularly in regard to mask requirements in schools.[124] This politicization of mask-wearing laid the foundation for the strong partisan division later on with COVID vaccination.

NOVEMBER/DECEMBER 2020: EFFECTIVE VACCINES!

The events of November 2020 significantly impacted the vaccine rollout. As scientists concluded data analysis for the vaccine trials and prepared to announce the results, the 2020 election further divided the nation. After media outlets confirmed Joe Biden as the winner of the presidential election, Trump contested the results, refusing to concede.[125] Despite numerous ballot recounts and no evidence of election fraud, Trump insisted, especially to his followers, that the election had been stolen from him—a lie that incited the 2021 Capitol insurrection.[126] After mainstream platforms censored "Stop the Steal" rhetoric, a surge of Trump supporters began using the right-wing, gatekeeper-free social media platform *Parler*.[127] It is outside the focus of this book to deconstruct the media messages surrounding Trump's election myth. That said, it should be noted that this moment dramatically influenced public reception of the vaccine, especially among Republicans.

A little more than a week after media outlets confirmed Biden's presidential victory, the same outlets aired Pfizer's vaccine trial results: the vaccine was 95 percent effective with no serious side effects.[128] The initial Pfizer trials consisted of 21,720 out of 43,548 participants, ages 16 and older, who had received the two-dose vaccine.[129] Coverage of the Pfizer announcement was surprisingly positive and optimistic. Front page news expressed joy and amazement at both the high levels of efficacy and the absence of alarming effects. Vaccine news dominated media on November 10, 2020, with numerous stories on COVID appearing that day. Banners reiterated the Pfizer press release, while other articles spoke of COVID cases surging, speculated on the vaccine rollout, and contextualized the vaccine within the post-election turmoil.[130] Even tabloids and right-wing conservative outlets favorably reported on the vaccine trials, repeating Pfizer's results, but stating that Trump should have been credited.[131]

Twelve days later, Moderna released similar results on its trials of 30,251 participants and applied for FDA emergency approval.[132] On December 2, 2020, the United Kingdom authorized Pfizer for mass vaccination, becoming the first country to do so.[133] Due to the urgent need for effective vaccines, the initial FDA meetings and review took less than a month. The FDA issued Emergency Use Authorization for the Pfizer vaccine on December 11 and for Moderna on December 18.[134] Both the Pfizer and Moderna vaccines use messenger RNA and require two doses to be administered, two weeks apart. The Pfizer vaccine was approved for ages sixteen and older, while Moderna was eighteen and older. A third COVID vaccine, Johnson & Johnson achieved EUA approval on February 27, 2021.[135] At 71 percent effective against hospitalizations, it was not quite as effective initially as the mRNA vaccines, yet the J&J vaccine appealed to many people because of the type (the more established viral vector) and dosage (only one dose, not two).[136]

The J&J vaccine offered little protection against COVID-19 variants and its recipients were later advised to get mRNA boosters. As such, this vaccine went off the market in the United States by 2023.[137]

THE VACCINE ROLLOUT

On December 14, 2020, Long Island Nurse Sandra Lindsay received the first vaccine administered outside of trials.[138] Health professionals and long-term care facility residents were the first groups to be eligible for COVID vaccines, followed by adults aged 65 and older.[139] At the time of the rollout, approximately 71 percent of Americans surveyed indicated a willingness to get vaccinated.[140] On the other hand, 27 percent said that they probably or definitely would not get vaccinated. Republicans, people under 50, and those in rural areas had higher rates of vaccine hesitancy. Concerns about side effects and vaccine safety, distrust in the government, and the influence of politics in the vaccine development were cited as the most common justifications for vaccine hesitancy. For many, receiving a vaccine was both a privilege and a reason to celebrate, as newly immunized people posted vaccine selfies to social media platforms.[141] These public acknowledgments did more than captured elated Pfizer and Moderna recipients. Since many of the early vaccine recipients were health professionals, their endorsements of the vaccines spurred online questions and conversations, encouraging others to get immunized as well.[142]

Over the next few months, vaccine eligibility opened up to new groups, which varied by state—nonessential health care workers, law enforcement officials, people with high-risk medical conditions, incarcerated and homeless populations, and others.[143] As more people became eligible for vaccination, they too announced their immunization online. By April 19, 2021, all states had expanded vaccine eligibility to include all adults.[144] At this point, over 131 million American adults had already had at least one COVID vaccine dose and 84.3 were considered fully vaccinated.[145]

Individuals, media outlets, and other entities widely promoted vaccination. *Good Housekeeping*, *Elite Daily*, and other sites offered playful caption suggestions for vaccine selfies, including "Oops, I did it again #fullyvaccinated" and "Maybe she's born with it . . . maybe she's fully vaccinated."[146] Working with the Department of Health and Human Services and the CDC, Facebook added a "I got my COVID-19 vaccine" profile frame to highlight such photos.[147] Instagram and WhatsApp users could choose "I Got Vaccinated" stickers for their stories.[148]

On May 12, kids twelve and older became eligible for the Pfizer vaccine series.[149] Once vaccine eligibility opened up, public health authorities, counties, and various nonprofits launched massive campaigns to encourage even more people to get vaccinated. Some counties hired youth-focused vaccine ambassadors to encourage younger people and members of disproportionately affected populations to get their vaccines.[150] The US Department of Health and Human Services produced a plethora of informative materials to be used in various campaigns, from countering vaccine myths to reasons for vaccinating children.[151] Cambria County, Pennsylvania launched #CAMBRIACRUSHESCOVID, calling for individuals to submit their selfies and reasons for getting vaccinated.[152] The Alabama Public Health Department launched the "Vaccinate Alabama TikTok contest," inviting teens and young adults to submit videos about getting vaccinated, awarding four $250 Visa gift cards to winners.[153] Targeting young people, the US government partnered with influencers to spread positive messages about vaccines, called "Gen Z for Change."[154] Celebrities reached out to persuade people to get vaccinated. Most notably, to encourage more people of color to get vaccinated, Tyler Perry interviewed medical experts and then received the vaccine himself in a thirty-minute TV special airing on BET.[155]

Vaccines drastically reduced the number of hospitalizations and deaths for those immunized.[156] On August 23, 2021, the FDA upgraded the EUA for the Pfizer and Moderna vaccines to full approval.[157] Requirements and mandates became more common, determined by cities, states, and places of employment (as opposed to the national mandates in other countries). New York City implemented vaccination requirements for indoor dining and activities, requiring patrons to show proof to enter.[158] Many colleges and universities also required vaccination for students to return to campus.[159] Amtrak, McDonald's and other large corporations mandated vaccines, as did rideshare companies, airlines, and health care industries.[160] Many tech and media corporations also required vaccination, including NBC Universal, Facebook, Google, Twitter, the *New York Times*, and the *Washington Post*.[161] Even Fox Corp. employees had to get vaccinated, despite the Fox News network's content that had contributed to vaccine misinformation.[162] An April 2022 survey indicated that 40 percent of workers had been required to get vaccinated by their employers.[163]

Eligibility expanded to include children aged five through eleven on October 29, 2021, and then six months to four years old on June 15, 2022.[164] Yet, vaccination rates among children were significantly lower than for adults at 32 percent of 5–11 year-olds receiving two doses and only 13 percent of those under 5.[165] Parents' perceptions that kids were not as susceptible to COVID and concerns about side effects impacted decisions to vaccinate.[166] Vaccines and boosters protected people against severe COVID cases and death, but did not stop them from getting infected.[167] COVID variants caused spikes in rates over the next two years, as first Delta than Omicron surged.

In the early months of the rollout, celebration overshadowed skepticism. As the vaccine selfie craze illustrated, many people were overwhelmingly grateful for their vaccine doses. By the end of 2020, at least 385,676 people in the United States had died from COVID.[168] A desire to protect vulnerable family and friends and a fear of catching and spreading COVID were among the top reasons for getting vaccinated.[169] Others were ready to resume "normal" life after experiencing months of social distancing, mask-wearing, distance learning, canceled activities, and other pandemic effects. COVID vaccines became synonymous with freedom.[170] Demographics strongly impacted willingness to get vaccinated. Age, partisan affiliation, and education were the greatest predictors of vaccination, with those sixty-five and older, Democrats, and college graduates most likely to get vaccinated.[171]

Two very different types of people defined those initially hesitant to receive COVID vaccines. Some communities of color expressed reluctance at getting immunized yet were more likely to wear masks and take COVID precautions. A history of medical atrocities against people of color, racism in care, and other complex factors created deep-seated distrust toward health professionals and medical establishments as a whole.[172] Extensive media and interpersonal campaigns and community outreach with prominent Black and Hispanic leaders helped to significantly increase vaccine rates among Black and Hispanic adults up to the level of other populations.[173]

Vaccine hesitancy also appeared among Republicans, who were significantly less likely to trust the CDC, FDA, and Dr. Fauci for vaccine information, compared to Democrats.[174] Partisanship impacted people's perceptions of their state's COVID policies, especially for Republicans.[175] They were also less concerned about COVID and were less willing to wear masks and adhere to social distancing and other mitigation measures.[176] Instead, Trump voters were more apt to use alternative "treatments," as hydroxychloroquine and ivermectin prescriptions were significantly higher in Republican-dominant counties.[177]

DISCUSSION: MEDIA & THE ROLLOUT

Media consumption and engagement profoundly shaped the COVID vaccine uptake. The absence of news coverage of coronavirus vaccines prior to 2020 likely hindered confidence in the vaccine.[178] While the trials were concluding, 78 percent of participants in a Pew Research Center poll believed that the vaccine approval process was happening "too fast, before safety and effectiveness [was] fully understood"—a perception that ignored decades of research in developing models for the successful mRNA approach used with Pfizer and Moderna.[179] Speculation about the vaccine development process early on, paired with the name "Operation Warp Speed," reinforced this misperception that the vaccines had been developed too quickly.

Most mainstream American print and cable news coverage was fairly consistent in tone about vaccines.[180] Similarly, most tweets early in the rollout were positive and contained accurate information, according to a study of 419,495 tweets from December 9, 2020, to January 12, 2021.[181] However, conservative and fringe media outlets produced significantly more negative vaccine coverage and spread conspiracy theories and other disinformation, especially after Biden took office in January 2021.[182] The Fox News Network aired false claims and undermined vaccinations in other ways on almost a daily basis during the first six months of Biden's administration.[183] In 2021, Fox News personality Tucker Carlson spread false claims about COVID vaccines in 113 out of 114 episodes with vaccine segments: exaggerating vaccine-related complications, lying about government cover-ups of vaccine deaths, challenging efficacy rates, equating mandates to forced sterilization, apartheid, and Jim Crow laws, and other detrimental statements.[184] Social media varied by platform, as well. For example, content of the alternative platform *Parler*[ii] was ubiquitously anti-vaccine, offering reasons not to get vaccinated and containing false information about "side effects," links to propaganda sites, rants against government mandates, conspiracy theories, "plandemic" and other loaded language, and praise for Trump.[185]

Because of this divergence in content, what media people consumed and participated in significantly affected how they perceived COVID vaccines and their vaccination status. News consumption and COVID knowledge was positively correlation with vaccination rates.[186] The *COVID States Project* surveyed 20,669 people across the United States in June–July 2021. Results indicated that 87 percent of people who got their news from multiple sources (none of which were Facebook, Newsmax, or Fox News) were vaccinated.[187] This type of consumer was also the least likely to believe myths about COVID vaccines.[188]

People exposed to misinformation were more likely to express hesitancy about getting a vaccine.[189] In the *States Project*, when individuals listed Facebook, Newsmax, or Fox as primary sources of information, vaccinations decreased to 67 percent. Rates were lowest among

---

ii An alternative platform without gatekeeping mainly used by conservatives.

those who listed Fox News (59%), Facebook (47%), or Newsmax (42% vaccinated, with 41% stating that they would not get vaccinated).[190] Consumers of these three sources were mostly likely to believe one or more misconceptions about COVID vaccines and overwhelmingly identified as Republicans.[191] Other scholarship also identified a strong negative correlation between Fox News viewership and vaccine rates.[192] Fluctuations in the Vaccine Adverse Event Reporting System correlated with varying tones in Fox News coverage of the vaccine, suggesting that people were reporting adverse events in response to consuming media coverage.[193]

Those who identified Trump as their primary source of COVID information were among the least likely to get vaccinated.[194] This is not surprising, given that Sarah Evanega and colleagues' comprehensive study of more than thirty-eight million news articles identified Trump as the most profound spreader of COVID-related misinformation in the pandemic.[195] Confidence in the research and development process increased vaccination, which fell along partisan lines, with 87 percent of Democrats/Democrat-leaning indicated a "great deal" or "fair amount" of confidence in the COVID-19 research and development process, compared to 45 percent of Republicans/Republican-leaning.[196] Moreover, conservatives were more likely to spread misinformation and conspiracy theories on social media, including the creation of hydroxychloroquine tweets.[197] Vaccine hesitancy wasn't just a problem in the United States. In many countries, people used social media platforms to spread anti-vaccine messages and express their reluctance to get vaccinated.[198]

CONCLUSION

By 2023, at least one vaccine dose had been administered to over 72.3 percent of the world's population, with 67 percent considered fully vaccinated.[199] More than twenty-four different vaccines were used. Nine vaccines were most common:

VACCINE NAME	NUMBER OF COUNTRIES[200]
Oxford-AstraZeneca	185
Pfizer-BioNTech	165
Moderna	114
Johnson & Johnson	103
Sinopharm-Beijing	72
Sinovac	41
Gamaleya	35

Vaccination rates ranged from less than 1 percent of the population in Burundi to over 99 percent in United Arab Emirates, Qatar, Macau, and Brunei.[201] Latin America had the highest vaccination percentage (82 percent with at least one dose), whereas only 37 percent of people in Africa had received the vaccine.[202] Despite the proven effectiveness of COVID vaccines, 19.9 percent of US adults never received a single dose, some of whom chose to lose their jobs rather than get vaccinated.[203] Globally, individuals were more reluctant to get boosters than the initial vaccine series.[204] A meta-analysis of scholarly studies found that this hesitancy was due to perceived benefit/efficacy, experience with COVID-19 infections, skepticism, and other factors.[205]

Despite the emphasis of most popular and scholarly analysis on the shadows of misinformation and vaccine hesitancy, the reality is that the majority of Americans got vaccinated. Upon receiving their first doses, people expressed feeling safe, relieved, and other positive emotions.[206] The narrative of Pfizer, Moderna, and J&J is one of triumph: For the first time in history, safe, effective vaccines were developed swiftly enough to make a difference. News content informed people of vaccine progress and announced the incredibly high levels of effectiveness. Local and state health department websites updated individuals on their eligibility and guided them to nearby vaccine sites. Social media platforms enabled the sharing of vaccine information and vaccine selfies, which encouraged others to get immunized. Both traditional and digital media outlets were critical to targeted and mass vaccination campaigns. In other words, COVID vaccine development was overwhelming successful, preventing at least three million US deaths and fourteen to nineteen million worldwide.[207]

CHAPTER SEVEN

Depicting the "New Normal"

THE IMPACT OF COVID ON AND IN ENTERTAINMENT

The pandemic profoundly impacted the entertainment industry, delaying live production for more than a year and reshaping how stories would be filmed and carried out in television and movies. Production shutdowns began occurring as the virus spread. By early February, mainland China and Hong Kong had closed all theaters and stopped production and post-production.[1] Soon after, Italy became the first European country to halt entertainment, due to its early COVID surge.[2] Following the WHO pandemic declaration on March 11, many countries around the world ceased entertainment production.[3]

In the United States, although mitigation measures varied by geographic location, the entertainment industry was most impacted by restrictions in California and New York. On March 7, San Francisco temporarily banned all "non-essential activities." Two days later, Santa Clara restricted gatherings larger than 1,000 people.[4] In New York, Governor Andrew Cuomo banned gatherings over 500 people on March 12, suspending the 31 stage productions of the Broadway district.[5] On March 19, California Governor Gavin Newsom issued a statewide shelter-in-place order, enforced with penalties of $1,000 in fines or six months in jail for breaking orders.[6] New York entered its lockdown on March 20. By April 4, 2020, 42 states had issued mandatory stay-at-home orders, prohibiting all nonessential public activities.[7]

Shelter-in-place orders prohibited in-studio production. Film crews and scripted television ceased, while those working in other types of programming varied in their responses. *Queer Eye*, *The Amazing Race*, and many other reality shows stopped filming. *Keeping Up with the Kardashians* and the cooking show *Pioneer Woman* continued through new, crew-less formats, in which family members filmed the action.[8] On April 11, 2020, *Saturday Night Live* aired the first of its three at-home episodes.[9] News, daytime, and late-night shows also moved home, with reporters and late-night hosts broadcasting themselves from their kitchens, closets, bedrooms, studios, and other makeshift spaces.[10]

In April and May 2020, most scripted television production remained on hiatus. However, several COVID-themed movies and specials aired through streaming services. *Love in the Time of Corona*, *Social Distance*, and *A Parks and Recreation Special* took place during lockdown, with characters interacting over Zoom and other video chat platforms. The OWN network legal drama *All Rise* was the first regular scripted TV show to air an episode. "Dancing at Los Angeles" was filmed remotely through FaceTime and other video platforms and aired May 4, 2020. The storyline was set during the shelter-in-place orders. As such, characters (and the actors) take calls alone from their homes and wear masks if they venture outside. The episode exemplified the lockdown moment, with b-roll footage of empty streets, scenes of main characters participating in virtual and characters binge-eating Captain Crunch over video platforms. The central storyline raised questions about how to hold court proceedings virtually. Meanwhile, in Prague, Paris, Poland, Iceland, Portugal, and Spain, in-person film and television production resumed in mid-May.[11]

Around the world, TV producers, directors, actors, and crew faced a number of questions in planning for a return to in-person production. In June 2020, the Directors Guild of America, Screen Actors Guild - American Federation of Television and Radio, International Alliance of Theatrical Stage Employees, and the Teamsters' Committees for COVID-19 Safety Guidelines issued *The Safe Way Forward*, a white paper outlining necessary mitigation procedures for entertainment production to resume.[12] Even though more was known about COVID in the summer of 2020, vaccines were not yet available. Therefore, mitigation focused on regular testing of cast and crew based on a "Zone System," in which physical distancing and level of PPE that could be worn determined frequency of testing. Production sites were required to add handwashing/sanitizing stations and medical checkpoints. COVID impacted location and script decisions, such as filming more scenes outside, cutting down on group scenes, and rethinking scenes considered too risky.[13]

TO INCORPORATE THE PANDEMIC?

When crews returned from hiatus, television writers had to determine whether to incorporate pandemic elements into the upcoming season's narratives. On one hand, the integration of the current moment reinforced a realism within a fictional world. Viewers could relate to their favorite characters' donning masks and practicing precautions. Opponents, however, argued for an escape from the crisis, preferring that programs continued on as normal, as if the novel coronavirus had never emerged.[14] Given that the pandemic still raged on as episodes aired, shows with pandemic components had the potential to model or reinforce mitigation strategies, shape important COVID-related decisions, and provide catharsis as characters experienced similar struggles during the global crises. Such depictions also captured the moment, preserving the fictionalized experiences in collective memory. This chapter explores the pandemic impact on entertainment, including the extent to which fictional shows incorporated elements of the global health crisis into their storylines. Although the chapter focuses on American shows, these questions also surfaced for producers around the world.

Background: Real-life People and Events in TV

Fictional representations of real-life stories, people, and events have been a constant part of television. Biopic films have captured the lives of numerous actors, comedians, musicians, celebrities, politicians, athletes, historical figures, criminals, and ordinary people. Such depictions are far from true-life reflections, utilizing voiceovers, flashbacks of "younger selves," and other conventions specific to the genre.[15] Screenwriters determine which elements to preserve and what to change, adding a fictional love story to a historical tragedy (i.e., *Titanic*), using computer effects to incorporate actual footage of deceased figures into fictional scenes, as with John Lennon and JFK into *Forrest Gump*, or preserving the original singing of artists while actors lip sync, as in *Ray* (2004) and other biopics. In based-on-a-true-story narratives, real-life events, conversations, relationships, and other aspects are intentionally constructed to fit Hollywood storytelling but appear to hold more authenticity with audiences because they are based on actual people.[16]

Entertainment producers choose when to incorporate unexpected events into already running television realities. For example, in the mid-1980s, *Punky Brewster* was a popular sitcom about "Punky" the orphaned girl, who lives with her adoptive father and aspires to be an astronaut. After the real-life *Challenger* Space Shuttle explosion, *Punky Brewster* aired a special episode in which Punky learns about the tragedy and becomes devastated that her astronaut heroes have been killed. The fictional show included facts about the *Challenger* and a guest appearance by astronaut Edwin "Buzz" Aldrin, playing himself. According to a *Los Angeles Times* article published before the episode's airing, writer and producer David W. Duclon created the storyline "to help the young viewers who are its principal audience deal with the feelings that the disaster may have engendered, and to encourage those who are interested in the space program to continue pursuing their goals."[17]

After the September 11, 2001 (9/11) terrorist acts, producers and writers had to determine the extent to which fictional television would acknowledge that day and how shows could transition back to their realities, according to television scholar Lynn Spigel.[18] Some programs, like *The West Wing*, used 9/11-related standalone episodes, disrupting ongoing series narratives to address the contextual moment.[19] Other programs incorporated 9/11 into their initial premises. Premiering in

2004, *CSI: New York* was set in a post-9/11 New York, in which protagonist (and lead Crime Scene Investigator) Mac Taylor had lost his wife in the fall of the twin towers.[20] The show aired a special 9/11 memorial episode on the tenth anniversary, providing fictional flashbacks of the main characters' experiences on that day.[21] Fictionalizing real-world events, particularly traumatic ones, serves a purpose beyond creating quality drama. Such integration adds authenticity to a fictional storyline, helping viewers to process and cope with tragedies. They also serve to capture the moment in collective memory, as, for example, films about the Holocaust have done.[22]

THE IMPACT OF FICTIONAL STORIES

Although TV producers take varying degrees of leeway within the fictional worlds they create, such narratives can impact the audience's knowledge, perceptions, and behavior. This is especially true for certain genres—in particular, medical dramas, which have been used intentionally to educate the public and even medical students about health care-related concepts.[23] Fictional programs have also been effective in persuading viewers to modify their behavior.[24]

The theory of parasocial interaction helps to explain entertainment media's influence for its viewing audience, referring to the "seeming face-to-face relationship between spectator and performer."[25] When viewers are exposed to particular celebrities or fictional characters, they can form emotional attachments, which extend beyond viewing sessions, "much like a friendship that exists between two persons beyond their face-to-face communication sequences."[26] Overall, the relationships that viewers form with their favorite characters can magnify the potential influence of the narratives. Therefore, messages about COVID (mitigation strategies, coping with loss, etc.) shaped at least some viewers' own perceptions and behavior related to the pandemic.

Debates about incorporating real-life traumatic events are twofold. On the one hand, entertainment media serves as an escape from everyday life. We watch television to briefly forget about the problems of real life. In "Entertainment and Utopia," scholar Richard Dyer articulated TV's function as an outlet, stating, "Entertainment offers the image of 'something better' to escape into, or something we want deeply that our day-to-day lives don't provide. Alternatives, hopes, wishes—these are the stuff of utopia, the sense that things could be better, that something other than what can be imagined and maybe realized."[27] Leading up to the Fall 2020 TV season, popular writers used this rationale for writers to not construct a pandemic reality within fictional television.

On the other hand, the pandemic reality can also be theoretically justified, as television narratives already draw from real-world contexts. Scholar Stuart Hall explained in his theory of encoding and decoding:

"Though the production structures of television originate the television discourse, they do not constitute a closed system. They draw topics, treatments, agendas, events, personnel, images of the audience, 'definitions of the situation' from other sources and other discursive formations within the wider socio-cultural and political structure of which they are a differentiated part."[28]

Such connections contribute to the construction of meaningful mediated realities for viewers, helping them to make sense of their own experiences. Watching fictionalized pandemic realities then, could have helped viewers process and cope with their own experiences.

COVID AND FICTIONAL REALITIES

As crews adopted mitigation protocol, scripted shows were divided on whether to place their shows in a pre-pandemic world without masks, social distancing, and testing or in storylines set in the global health crisis. *The Rookie*, *Succession*, *American Horror Story*, *The Upshaws*, *Emily in Paris*, and other programs continued the fictional reality established before COVID, pretending the pandemic never happened. Characters mingled with each other, went to work, attended school, and traveled freely—all while showing their bare, unmasked faces. In a similar vein, *Gossip Girl*, *And Just Like That* (the *Sex and the City* revival), *Curb Your Enthusiasm* and others skipped over the pandemic, returning to a post-crisis time in which characters casually mentioned lockdowns, social distancing, supply-hoarding, and other components in past tense.

Producers that decided to incorporate the pandemic into their shows faced a slew of questions: How do you move from season finale or mid-season cliffhanger to a pandemic moment? At what point do you enter into the fictionalized pandemic timeline? What elements are carried out? And, considering the complexity and array of issues linked to this global crisis (as conveyed in the other chapters of this book), what do the programs choose to feature? For many shows, the pandemic was too big to ignore. At the same time, the program's established characters, premise, formula, and genre influenced how the pandemic would play out in its constructed world.

Most pandemic-set seasons first aired in Fall 2020 or January 2021. Fans were introduced to COVID-themed episodes through promos featuring mask-wearing characters. Season opener titles "The New Normal" (*New Amsterdam*), "The New Abnormal" (*9-1-1*), "Hero Pizza" (*Black-ish*), "Keep Truckin', Six Feet Apart" (*The Conners*), "Nothing Seems the Same" (*Station 19*), "Frontline" (*The Good Doctor*), "Remember Me in Quarantine" (*Law & Order: Special Victims Unit*), "Fever" (*The Morning Show*) and others denoted these moments as uniquely pandemic, setting them apart from the previous season.

PANDEMIC NARRATIVE: RISE OF THE CRISIS

Scripted programs vary on when the fictional storylines began in the pandemic. Season 2 of *The Morning Show* begins on the 2020 New Year's Eve celebration and progresses toward the pandemic. The newsroom characters' coverage of the real-life Democratic Party Primary debates, and rising COVID statistics mark the timeline of the fictionalized reality. In the season finale, a main character battles COVID in mid-March as the news crew prepares to broadcast from home.

The retail sitcom *Superstore* episode "Essential" starts moments before the crisis became official, in early March 2020. During a meeting, employees begin announcing the effects of the impending pandemic.

Dina declares that a waterpark is closing and says, "Seems like this coronavirus deal is spreading." Then Garrett looks at his phone and exclaims, "Whoa! The NBA just announced they're suspending the season." Mateo adds, "More cases are popping up in Oregon, Washington, New York . . ." At this point, another worker yells, "You guys, Tom Hanks has it!" Everyone gasps. The timeline jumps ahead to two weeks later, with the characters experiencing the struggles of retail work during the lockdown.

Medical dramas *The Good Doctor* and *The Resident* construct the escalation of the local crisis, moving the timeline from the first patients in their hospitals to full pandemic mode. Set in San Jose, California, *The Good Doctor* begins with the title card "February 26, 2020" and then "One week to California State of Emergency." The scene starts at a coffee shop, in which a woman coughs, dispersing zoomed-in particles into the air. She covers her mouth, touches her face, and hands money to the cashier, dropping the change in a communal jar of coins.

Later, the woman, named Mildred, is at the hospital with a temperature of nearly 101 degrees, complaining of a sore throat, body aches, and a cough. Wearing no mask or other protection, Dr. Morgan Reznick examines her, as the patient coughs throughout the hospital visit.

MILDRED: My daughter is very worried that I might have this virus from China. What's it called?"

REZNICK: Have you been to China or been around anyone who's been to China recently?

Mildred shakes her head.

REZNICK: Taken any cruises?

She shakes her head again.

REZNICK: The coronavirus doesn't cause sore throats. This is a bad case of the flu. Go home, rest, drink plenty of fluids. You'll be fine in a week or two.

The scene cuts from a close-up of the worried patient's face to the title slide "TWO WEEKS LATER." We hear intense coughing and see Mildred hooked to a high-flow oxygen machine. Outside of her isolated room, Dr. Audrey Lim tells Mildred's adult daughter, "The virus has damaged your mother's lungs. Her body is working harder and harder to breathe, but her blood oxygen levels continue to drop." The daughter responds, "She definitely has Corona?" Dr. Lim nods and says, "We're doing everything we can to help her." The shot cuts to another title slide: "This episode of *The Good Doctor* is a made-up story about a real battle still being fought. Honor the heroes: Doctors, nurses, and other frontline workers, many of whom have given their lives. Do your part. Wear a mask."

Season four of *The Resident* similarly begins with a title card: "Sometime in the future, when the COVID-19 pandemic is history . . ." and then shows Dr. Conrad Hawkins and Nurse Practitioner Nic Nevin chatting with their friends as they get dressed for their wedding. After the characters briefly discuss recent difficult times, another title card places the timeline in the moments leading up to the pandemic: "March 2, 2020." Conrad and Nic are shown chatting as they walk on crowded Atlanta streets toward the hospital. No one wears masks or mentions COVID. Inside the hospital, all have bare faces and the mood is jovial.

After the care providers greet each other, Dr. Devon Pravesh asks Dr. Hawkins for a consult: "Bay One, Carter Wiggins, 34. Headache, febrile and fatigue. Take a look at his hands over here" (as they walk toward the patient, who is near other people and not wearing a mask). The patient coughs, complains of a loss of smell, and has red lesions on his hands. Nurse Ellen Hundley determines that he has a fever.

HAWKINS: Have you traveled anywhere recently?
WIGGINS (patient): Uh, Seattle. To see my grandmother.
HAWKINS and Pravesh look at each other.
HAWKINS: Okay, we'll be right back.

Ominous music plays as the two walk back to the nurses' station. Hawkins asks the other providers, "How many cases of COVID-19 in Seattle?" They look up the information, learning that Seattle has fourteen cases and five deaths at that moment. Pravesh responds, "The symptoms fit. I think we have our first case of coronavirus."

Just then, an off-screen alarm beeps. Nurse Hundley yells, "We need a crash cart! I've lost his pulse!" She initiates CPR with her bare hands and no protective gear. Dr. Hawkins frantically tells her, "Hundley, stop! You need PPE!" Before she can put on gear, we see particles flying out of the unconscious patient's mouth as she works to resuscitate him. The scene cuts to the program's theme song and introduction.

Depicting Crisis: Spring 2020

Most medical dramas focus on Spring 2020 for their pandemic realities. *The Good Doctor* and *The Resident* both start their post-intro storyline a few weeks after the pandemic has been declared. Likewise, other medical dramas set their pandemic episodes at this entry point, when little was known about the virus and no vaccines were available. For these shows, title cards and visual cues establish the pandemic reality. *Chicago Med* begins with a close-up of a sign "Covid ICU strict infectious protocols in patient rooms. No family members," followed by shots of health professionals in full PPE.

In this new pandemic reality, COVID screenings have become a routine part of going to work at hospitals. Familiar health professional characters routinely undergo screenings and COVID tests to enter their hospitals. Dr. Hawkins and Nurse Nevin are screened upon arrival in *The Resident*—contrary to the earlier, pre-pandemic scene in which they chatted and then easily walked into the building. In *Chicago Med*, Dr. Halstead goes through screening to get into work. As he gets his temperature taken, the nurse, Doris, questions him.

DORIS (doing the screening): Any symptoms? Headache, dry cough? Nope. 98.5. Good. Let's get you tested.

HALSTEAD: I was just tested this morning.

DORIS: You went home. Nobody goes back in the E.D. without getting tested. Come on. Come up. Open up. (She swabs his nostrils).

Once at work, scenes of fictional health professionals in full PPE treating isolated patients distinguish medical dramas' representation of the early pandemic in television. As in real-life, fictional hospitals are so overrun by COVID patients that triage centers are set up in parking lots and all elective surgeries have been canceled. Regardless of physicians' usual specialties, all are tasked with COVID-related duties. Surgeons in *The Good Doctor*, *The Resident*, and *Grey's Anatomy* work on COVID floors treating patients, after the doctors' surgeries have been canceled. These characteristic moments appear in several medical dramas, as partially identified in a quantitative analysis of these shows, conducted by Cambra-Badii, Guardiola, and Baños.[29]

"Heroic Health Professionals"

Across medical dramas, health professionals are depicted as "harried medical heroes"—fatigued health professionals pushed beyond their limits to treat COVID patients in isolated wards. Their tired eyes hide beyond protective glasses, face shields or helmets, gowns, and gloves. For example, in *New Amsterdam*, the episode starts out of focus and then slowly comes into focus on a health professional in full PPE, wearing a face shield, mask, and a gown. Dramatic music plays as he walks toward the camera in one shot. Once his face fills the frame, he removes his face shield, revealing weary eyes, red marks on his cheeks, and a worn nose. All the red marks look very sore. He is wearing a surgical mask over an N95. When the nurses and doctors finally get a brief respite, the removal of their masks reveal the physical toll of pandemic care-providing. Similar scenes appear across medical dramas that construct the pandemic. Fictional health professionals are repeatedly depicted with faces marred by PPE and so fatigued that they can barely stand. In *The Good Doctor*, Surgeon Shaun Murphy tells his girlfriend that his ears hurt from wearing two masks.

Hospital staff also face the additional burdens of creating and maintaining makeshift triage areas in the parking lots, performing endless exams and COVID testing. They accomplish these tasks while short on protective equipment. As in real-life, early in the pandemic, hospitals face severe shortages of masks and other protective gear, forcing staff to reuse equipment and to get creative. In *The Resident*, Nurse Nevin has to wear the same disposable surgical mask five days in a row. And in

Grey's Anatomy, Dr. Richard Webber implements a new, more efficient way to disinfect and reuse PPE. Storylines in multiple shows address the shortage of ventilators, ECMOs, and other breathing equipment, forcing fictional doctors to prioritize patients for treatment or share ventilators.

Caring for COVID patients is emotionally taxing, as the doctors and nurses lose patient after patient, even with their excellent skill and abilities. Adding to this toll is the burden of COVID isolation. Health professionals are taxed with facilitating FaceTime and Zoom conversations with loved ones, including their final goodbyes. As viewers, we watch these fictionalized moments, including an emotional scene in *The Good Doctor* in which a patient's family says goodbye to their unconscious loved one, about to die from COVID alone.

These health professionals make sacrifices in their personal lives. Due to fears of transmitting the virus to others, the fictional characters remark on their decisions to remain separate from their families. Dr. Grey tells others that she hasn't seen her kids in two weeks because she's been working on the COVID ward. Dr. Maggie Pierce sleeps in a tent in her yard to protect her family. Dr. Atticus Lincoln sleeps in his front yard in a tent to protect his girlfriend and newborn son. In *9-1-1*, firefighters Hen and Chimney reflect on the time apart from their spouses and children. *The Good Doctor* characters also isolate themselves while working COVID shifts, as we see Sean isolate away from his girlfriend. These practices intensify the emotional toll of caring for the sick, in which fictional doctors and nurses have no one to take care of them.

Health professionals struggle emotionally with feeling powerless to help their patients. *The Resident's* Dr. Kit Voss laments, "I feel so helpless. We're surgeons. We cut. We fix. With this disease, there's so little we can do. Just hold their hands and support them. And too many are dying in these rooms alone." Similarly, in the season premiere of *Grey's Anatomy* (set in April 2020), Dr. Meredith Grey expresses her frustration at losing her fourth patient of the day. She breaks down in the supply room, knocking stuff over and sobbing heavily. A colleague asks, "Who died?" Grey replies, "EVERYONE!" Episodes later, after Meredith becomes severely ill with COVID, her colleague, Dr. Teddy Altman expresses her inability to care for her, remarking to a friend, "This virus is like a drunk uncle at a wedding. You've got no idea what it's gonna do or when it's gonna turn on you. I am reading everything on COVID because every 24 hours there's something new. And I have to keep up because there could be one drug, one procedure. It could help. It could help everyone. It could help Meredith Grey." In other words, even the best doctors and nurses are powerless against the coronavirus.

Across genres, health professionals are considered heroes, applauded by the public. *Grey's Anatomy* and *Station 19* briefly incorporate the adulation for medical personnel. Toward the end of the pandemic-focused premiere episode, uplifting music plays as the fire truck passes masked people waving and holding signs to show their support for the first responders. *The Resident* includes a similar scene. In the aptly named *Black-ish* season premiere "Hero Pizza," Dr. Rainbow Johnson and her colleagues discuss how their community provided pizza for them and other hospital employees. *All Rise* and *The Good Doctor* honor real-life medical professionals and other essential workers, with title cards thanking them for their work. This wave of gratitude reflects April 2020, in which media outlets, community outreach, and other groups understandably and repeatedly praised those in health care and other essential work, showering employees with praise, free food, and other rewards.[30]

THE RISK OF COVID, ACCORDING TO TV

TV storylines reinforce CDC guidelines on protecting oneself against COVID. Dr. Miranda Bailey sums up the advice in the *Grey's Anatomy* season premiere: "Wash your hands. Wear a mask. Stay six feet apart at all times. Work from home. Only leave the house for essential services." All programs set in a pandemic reality convey these rules in some way, addressing the importance of staying home during the shelter-in-place order, modeling mask-wearing, and reminding others to practice social distancing. To set a show during the pandemic is to model these mitigation strategies.

People shelter-at-home or mention when they had to shelter-at-home. Post-lockdown narratives incorporate many pandemic characteristics. Characters undergo temperature screenings, use sanitizer, and take COVID tests. Storylines also convey other ways that characters have modified their behavior to reduce risks, including telehealth (*This is Us* and *9-1-1*), kids participating in distance learning (*9-1-1*, *This is Us*, and *Black-ish*), exercising at home (*All Rise*), and avoiding eating at restaurants (*All Rise*, *9-1-1 Lone Star*). Characters criticize others for breaking the rules, as exemplified in *Black-ish*, when Rainbow Johnson yells at her neighbors for hosting a birthday party during lockdown.

Masks appear in every pandemic-set show, although they aren't worn consistently. Mask use and other mitigation strategies are especially inconsistent outside of medical dramas. For example, in *Law & Order: SVU's* "Remember Me in Quarantine," Detective Odafin Tutuola (played by Ice-T) dons a mask to head out into the field, but then is never shown wearing it while in public. In fact, none of the detectives wear masks while interviewing people, yet background characters are all wearing masks. Other non-medical dramas provide similar contradictory messages about mask-wearing, including characters who pull down their masks to speak or remove masks while conversing with colleagues in small spaces.

In TV's constructions, these strategies are 100 percent effective, even when set during pre-vaccination times. Children and "regular" people stay healthy, never testing positive for COVID or becoming ill. COVID cases on television are nearly always severe, leading to hospitalization or death, and almost exclusively exist in medical dramas. People with mild symptoms or who are asymptomatic are absent from fictional shows, likely because nearly all of the patients appear in medical dramas. COVID cases can be categorized into three types: Heroic health professionals, the "innocent" or vulnerable, and people who intentionally put themselves at risk.

Despite their protective gear, in this pre-vaccine era (typically set in

Spring 2020), several of the hospital staff catch COVID, facing critical or even fatal cases. Most notably, *Grey's Anatomy* spends its entire 17th season primarily following Dr. Meredith Grey's experiences, from caring for COVID patients to collapsing in the parking lot from the virus at the end of the second episode. Even while she is severely ill in the hospital, Meredith continues to be heroic. During a staffing shortage, barely conscious Meredith wearily gets out of bed and successfully resuscitates another patient, only to lose consciousness from exhaustion on her way back. She then deteriorates so much that she has to be on a ventilator for most of the season. Her colleague, Dr. Tom Koracick, also becomes ill enough to require hospitalization.

The nurse that cared for the first COVID patient in *The Resident* also becomes critically ill and nearly dies. In *The Good Doctor*, early in the pandemic, a nurse contracts COVID from a patient initially believed to have diverticulitis. The nurse later dies from the disease. In *The Resident*, Nurse Ellen Hundley contracts COVID while trying to resuscitate the index patient at her hospital (the first person to have COVID) and nearly dies from the disease. Dr. Voss becomes infected while treating patients, after her mask breaks from the PPE shortage. Hospital staff in other positions are also susceptible to COVID. At Conrad and Nic's wedding at the end of *The Resident* COVID episode, they list the various custodial workers and others from the hospital that died from COVID. The high incidence of COVID for nurses, doctors, and other care providers on television reflected real life. Especially in the early months of the pandemic, real-life health professionals were very much at risk. At least 3,607 US health professionals died from COVID between March 2020 and March 2021.[31] Nurses made up 32 percent, followed by healthcare support (20%) and physicians (17%). Sixty-four percent were health professionals of color and over half were under the age of sixty. A lack of PPE strongly contributed to infection.[32]

Heroic patients also include those who become ill because they were caring for others or held jobs requiring them to be out in public. Notably, Dr. Pravesh's father dies after catching COVID while driving his taxi in *The Resident*. Although a few characters become severely ill, television does not adequately represent the toll on the care industry or on other essential workers. Missing are depictions of deaths in under sixty nurses of color who worked in nursing homes or residential facilities—the largest group of COVID victims.[33]

Vulnerable Patients

Fictional television also features cases of COVID patients who become ill (and often die) after contracting the disease from nursing homes, prisons, or other places that put them at risk. These patients have no control over their living or working arrangements and, therefore, are not constructed as culpable when they become ill. For example, in *Grey's Anatomy*, Dr. Miranda Bailey's mother gets COVID from her assisted living facility and dies from it within the same episode. After an African American woman is arrested in *All Rise*, she expresses concern about catching COVID to her attorney, explaining that she has underlying conditions. Her worries increase as she is transferred to a crowded jail with many COVID cases. Just before her release is approved, the woman dies, leaving her children behind.

Overlapping with this group are people of color who contract COVID. Fictional health professionals struggle with racial inequity in severe COVID cases and patient deaths. Patient photographs in *The Resident* are primarily people of color. In *Chicago Med*, Nurse April Sexton (a woman of color) comments that she continues to work tirelessly because the people from her community are "dying at twice the rate." Similarly, in *Grey's Anatomy*, Dr. Maggie Pierce says that she's had fifty-three people die, "most of them Black women." In a later episode, Maggie remarks, "If COVID were killing white people at the rate that it is killing Black people, you better believe that everyone would be wearing masks because it would be the damn law." Racial disparities observed in fiction unfortunately reflected real life, with Black Americans disproportionately dying from COVID in Spring 2020 at significantly higher rates than white and other racial groups.[34] Disparities continued throughout the pandemic, with heightened deaths also among American Indian and Alaska Native and Hispanic people.[35]

Irresponsible Patients

"Irresponsible" patient characters fail to take measures to protect themselves from COVID. These patients break quarantine and sometimes refuse to follow other mitigation strategies. Therefore, they are framed as blameworthy for becoming infected. Television narratives explicitly connect the patients' actions and beliefs to them contracting COVID, and sometimes spreading the disease to their loved ones.

In *Chicago Med*, a teenage girl gets her father sick with COVID after she broke lockdown restrictions to visit her friends. After he recovers, she expresses remorse, stating, "I could have killed you! I'm so sorry." Similarly, in a *Station 19*/*Grey's Anatomy* crossover episode, teenagers get in a car accident on their way home from a party—held illegally against shelter-in-place orders. Although none of the teens get COVID, their behavior and the subsequent injuries of one teen prompt several doctors to blame them for going out in public. Privately, Dr. Avery Jackson says to his colleague, "You hear this, uh, kid was out partying with friends? I don't know what the hell these kids are thinking." She replies, "Yeah, well, people do stupid things." Later, the patient's dad blames himself, telling his son's doctor, "I had this feeling in my gut like it's not a good idea, but I figured, it's just a few kids. They'll all wear masks. No one will find out. Why didn't I say no?" The teen dies, not from COVID, but from his injuries. Still, the message is conveyed that breaking quarantine caused his untimely death since the health professionals focus on the teens attending the party more than the car accident as the reason for the boy's death.

People who deny that COVID exists and ardently oppose masking and other mitigation make up a slim number of the fictional COVID patients. *Grey's Anatomy* devotes most of one episode to such a case, which conveys the consequences of not following mitigation strategies. Paramedics bring in a white man in his forties who had collapsed while jogging. They state that his oxygen saturation is at 88 and he is having trouble breathing. As Dr. Bailey takes the man's history, he repeatedly pulls down his mask to answer her questions. The patient then claims that he has asthma and that his inhaler expired (as his mask slips under his nose).

BAILEY: Mr. Anderson, is it possible you've been exposed to COVID-19?

MAN: No. That's a no.

BAILEY (gestures) and says: Mask up. Hospital policy. (to another doctor) Move him to an isolated room and give him a full work-up. Chest x-ray, lower extremity duplex and a COVID test. Page me with the results.

MAN: Okay, hey. Doc, look. I'll take the work-up, okay, but I don't care what your little test says 'cause I know that it's not real.

BAILEY: What's not real?

MAN: COVID. Do I look like a sheep? I know it's a scam.

Later, Bailey informs him of his diagnosis.

BAILEY: Sir, I need you to listen to me. Your COVID test came back positive. Additionally, you have ground glass opacities in your lungs. That's why you're having trouble breathing. (She points to the x-ray of lungs with white splotches). And your toes aren't red because you run without socks. You have what's being referred to as 'COVID-toe.'

MAN: COVID-toe?

BAILEY: Yes.

MAN: Really? That's the best you go? COVID-toe? (Laughs). Are you guys even trying?

After Bailey tells him that he has a COVID-related blood clot in his leg, he replies, "I figured out that this little cold that y'all are so terrified of? Biggest moneymaker since crypto-currency. And speaking of, how do you get your kickbacks? I mean, is it like a flat fee from every patient that you diagnose? Or is it like a percentage deal, or . . ?"

Bailey steps out of the room to compose herself. When she returns, Bailey explains:

Your blood oxygen level is dangerously low. Your lungs are getting worse. And if untreated, the clot in your leg could travel to your lungs and kill you. We're seeing cases like yours all of the ti—. Sir, this is not just a cold. It's not asthma. This won't magically go away. Sir, please, let us admit you so that we can start you on steroids and put you on blood thinners. Look, because even if you are a little bit wrong, it could be fatal.

As the patient listens to Dr. Bailey, he looks at her skeptically with a mask around his chin.

He refuses treatment prescribed by Dr. Bailey. The episode concludes with the man signing himself out Against Medical Advice and collapsing. Despite the doctors' performing cardiopulmonary resuscitation (CPR) on him, the patient dies and they cover his body with a sheet.

BAILEY (to Dr. Teddy Altman as they stand next to the man's body): We offered him treatment. Could have saved him. Instead, he walked away. Most people never feel what it's like to be really great at something, Altman, but we do, right? *I* do. I can put broken people together with needles and string. But I can't fix this. I mean, how do I treat someone who is offered help and chooses to walk away? I want to hope, Altman. I want to believe that, you know, just a little longer, and we'll be over this brutal hill. But (Bailey throws her gloves away). I just, I just don't know.

Music plays throughout this dramatic scene, emphasizing the emotional toll of the patient's poor choices on his doctor.

Three depictions of COVID patients appear outside of medical/first-responder dramas, all of which present irresponsible people. Throughout season 11 of the Netflix drama *Shameless*, alcoholic, drug-using Frank Gallagher repeatedly shirks COVID precautions. In the season premiere, he is the only character out in public without a mask and remarks, "Everything's changing. The Prius crowd is moving in, taking advantage of the folks who lost their jobs in the Corona hoax." His attitude and beliefs contrast with other family members. For example, Frank's daughter-in-law reminds her husband, "Don't forget to wear your mask. I don't want to get that shit again."

In the same season, Frank develops alcohol-related dementia. In the final fifteen minutes of the series finale, Frank wanders the streets and becomes so confused that he picks up a dirty disposable mask from the gutter and puts it on his face. Frank collapses and is taken to the hospital. Once he is admitted, health professionals diagnose him with COVID and put him on oxygen, noting his poor state. Frank quickly declines and dies alone. We see his monitor show a flat line. The nurse turns off the monitor, takes off the electrodes. and lays him back. The episode (and series) ends with Frank floating over the city with a beer in his hand. His lifestyle, including his intentional shirking of COVID precautions, ultimately cause his sad demise.

On a similar, but lighter note, the wacky comedy *It's Always Sunny in Philadelphia* also connects behavior to illness. This show returned in December 2021, much later than other programs. In the *Always Sunny* reality, mitigation strategies have subsided. Bars have reopened, no one wears masks, and "the gang" (as they're called) freely travels to Ireland. In the episode "The Gang Goes to Ireland," the character Dennis starts coughing, runs a fever, and loses his sense of smell. When Dennis makes excuses for his coughing, his friend, Mac, says, "You definitely have COVID, man. You're the only one that didn't get vaccinated." Dennis continues to deny his symptoms and goes out in public, unmasked and coughing. "You have COVID" becomes a running joke in the Ireland-set storylines, until his condition gets progressively worse to the point of hospitalization. He also gives COVID to Charlie's estranged father, who dies from the disease.

In *The Morning Show*, news anchor Alex Levy ignores the looming pandemic, traveling to Italy in the midst of lockdown. Against restrictions, she flies back to the United States on a private plane and immediately returns to work without quarantining. Within two weeks, she tests positive for COVID. Although she does not become ill enough for hospitalization, we see Alex suffer from the virus. Over the phone, she begs her doctor to admit her to the hospital. He replies:

> But if you can breathe, don't go to the hospital. All you'd be doing is putting more people at risk. There are no treatments yet. There's not really anything they can do for you, unless you need to be intubated and put on a ventilator. But you should keep those available for people who need them.

Over two episodes, she shakes and sweats with fever, to the extent to which she curls up naked under her shower. Her misery becomes spectacle when her coworker convinces her to livestream her experiences. Alex admits on camera that she put others at risk with her trip to Italy.

Constructions of "irresponsible patients" are not new to television, but first appeared in 1990s medical dramas.[36] These representations attribute lifestyle choices to health, suggesting that one's actions shape one's health (often ignoring other contextual factors). In a pandemic era, TV storylines convey that healthy, nonessential workers who catch COVID bring it upon themselves and, therefore, suffer the consequences. Moreover, no one is shown as asymptomatic or with mild symptoms. Obviously, certain behaviors can heighten health risks. However, by only including these types of fictional patients, such narratives stigmatize people with COVID, ignoring the prevalence of the disease and overlook vaccines as mitigating factors that lessen its severity.[37]

THE PANDEMIC "REALITY" AT HOME

While medical dramas showcase the illness side of the pandemic, other genres express additional effects and experiences of the global health crisis. Most shows offer privileged perspectives—the inconvenience of Zoom calls, lockdown boredom, and annoyance with briefly donning a mask. Characters in *Black-ish*, *Last Man Standing*, and *This is Us* simply wait for the pandemic to end while the face minor challenges at home. For the most part, legal and first-responder dramas feature characters continuing their regular work, just with masks (sometimes), as exemplified in *9-1-1*, *9-1-1 Lonestar*, *All Rise*, *Station 19*, and *Law & Order: SVU*.

Few shows incorporated the economic impact of the pandemic into their storylines. In *The Conners*, a domestic sitcom about working-class suburban struggles, the family faces further challenges with the lockdown. Dan has to fire his crew. Jackie is working hard to deliver food so that she doesn't lose her restaurant. Ben and Darlene can't get advertisers for their online crime magazine. Their collective lack of income leads to the bank's threat of eviction. Ultimately, the characters take on difficult, low-paying jobs at a plastics factory so that they can buy food and pay the mortgage. Likewise, the characters in *Shameless* also suffer financially during the pandemic and are forced to find alternative means of generating income. COVID restrictions force *Always Sunny in Philadelphia* characters to close their bar, Paddy's Pub. During the temporary closure, they pair off to find alternative, humorous ways of seeking income, immediately recovering once they can reopen their bar.

These depictions are just glimpses into the economic challenges faced in real life. In April 2020, unemployment rates skyrocketed throughout the world. The US unemployment reached an all-time high of 14.8 percent.[38] More than a year later, the Census Bureau's Household Pulse Survey indicated the devastating economic impacts, with twelve million adults struggling to pay rent and almost twenty million households experiencing food scarcity, disproportionately affecting people of color.[39]

"ENDING" THE PANDEMIC

Fictional narratives regularly play with time in their pandemic realities, moving back and forth in the pandemic moment. *The Morning Show*, *Black-ish*, and *New Amsterdam* begin their seasons in or after the crisis has subsided and then revert to earlier times. Across genres, shows use "COVID scene" montages to indicate both the moment in the pandemic and time passing. The *All Rise* season premiere begins with the title slide "July 2020," followed by a montage of people wearing masks, shots of someone wiping down a keyboard and other pandemic visuals—indicating that characters have returned to work. In the news drama *The Morning Show*, the song "Return to Me" plays as a montage of drone footage shows the empty streets of a locked-down New York.

Black-ish, *9-1-1*, and other shows juxtapose "COVID" scenes to pass time, alerting audiences to the entry point into the pandemic.

Programs vary on how long shows exist within the crisis framework *New Amsterdam* condenses its pandemic reality into a four-minute montage. The song "What a Wonderful World" plays behind heartbreaking scenes of a parking lot triage center with rows of makeshift beds, a patient receiving CPR, providers scrubbing with soap, a deceased patient being covered up, a patient trying to touch a video screen of a loved one, rosary beads given to a patient, the video chat screen of a child waking up a weary doctor, a health professional slumped down as one sits next to him, and a doctor becoming ill. This montage ends with applause for a patient's recovery and the administration of the first vaccine to health professionals. The next scene is in a post-pandemic world. The Tim Allen sitcom *Last Man Standing* similarly does a time jump in the introduction, moving ahead to a "normal" setting.

Two shows introduce and conclude pandemic storylines within their season premieres. *New Amsterdam* ends the pandemic with a jump to the "near future"/post-crisis, in which friends and family gather for a wedding. Meanwhile, at the end of the two-part openers of *The Good Doctor*, actor Freddie Highmore (who plays the lead character) speaks to the camera in his native British accent, telling viewers that the storyline is moving beyond the pandemic. His speech resembles Martin Sheen's introduction to the post-9/11 episode of *The West Wing* in 2001.[40]

Most programs gradually phased out verbal and visual cues of a pandemic reality, slowly eliminating masks, references to quarantine and social distancing, and other signs that a global health crisis is going on. In a similar vein, some shows move in and out of a pandemic reality, only bringing in COVID and mitigation as it fits with the storyline. *9-1-1* and *This is Us* fade out mitigation strategies, while also incorporating vaccination as minor parts of the timeline. No programs depict fluctuating COVID rates or the tightening of restrictions (i.e., schools shifting to distance learning after reopening), likely because they wrapped up before the Delta and Omicron COVID waves began.

Three programs carry COVID throughout their seasons. As

previously discussed, *The Morning Show* COVID season begins in January and builds up to mid-March 2020. Season eleven of *Shameless* exists in a loosening pandemic reality, as mask-wearing in public gradually decreases and other changes suggest the reduction of mitigation strategies (i.e., the kids return to school and bars open). Even through the finale, though, masks are expected, as a stranger yells at Frank, "Put on a mask, asshole!," health professionals use PPE, and COVID is still a threat as Frank dies from the virus in the final moments. The entirety of *Grey's Anatomy*, season 17 takes place during COVID, directly affecting the main characters and not wavering in its mitigation strategies. From episode two through fifteen, Meredith Grey is hospitalized with COVID (most of which she is in a coma). *Grey's* pandemic reality is concluded in the season finale, spanning from August 2020 through April 2021. By devoting seventeen episodes to COVID, the show is able to adopt a more complex and in-depth look at the pandemic, incorporating discussion of racial disparities, vaccine trials and vaccination for health professionals, long COVID, and other issues.

ENTERTAINMENT AND THE PANDEMIC

Overall, fictional pandemic storylines capture at least some of the multiyear global crisis, marking this moment in time with mitigation strategies, Zoom calls, and harried, heroic health professionals. Television COVID narratives continually push forward, indicating that case rates and mitigation strategies gradually declined in the pandemic episode or season. This trajectory works well in fiction, pulling characters out of a pandemic reality so they can return to "normal" storylines. However, this steady improvement did not mirror the radical fluctuation in both rates and strategies as the coronavirus mutated into Delta, Omicron, and future waves.

Pandemic realities homogenize the crisis experience, suggesting that all communities followed the same path (lockdown, reopening with masks and social distancing, and then the removal of masks and a "return to normal"). In real life, geography and political partisanship significantly influenced shelter-in-place orders and reopening, mask mandates, schools, public gatherings, and vaccination.[41] TV assumes that nearly everyone simply accepted and adopted mitigation orders, without showing the range of resistance that was actually present. In fact, little mass resistance occurs on screen. People willingly wear masks, shift to online school, and obey shelter-in-place orders. Those who refuse exemplify lone cases and face dire consequences onscreen for their decisions. Even on the West Coast (the setting for many shows), some people protested throughout the pandemic, rallying to oppose the continued shelter-in-place requirement.[42] Television does not show the profound danger of mis/disinformation or the impact of rampant conspiracy theorists on public beliefs, perceptions, and behavior—all of which, as demonstrated earlier, profoundly shaped how the pandemic unfolded.

Also missing are fictionalized stories of disabled and Indigenous communities, as well as the unique perspectives of teachers, professors, and nearly all other occupations outside of the medical profession. Most television characters are financially stable, meaning that the socioeconomic impact of the pandemic is not portrayed. Since no children's shows incorporated pandemic storylines, COVID narratives almost exclusively center around adults, overlooking the disruptive effects on kids and teens during this time.[43]

TV's limited lens overlooks the extent of loss and mourning experienced in real life and other struggles absent from the small screen. In fact, death from COVID and mourning loss are nearly invisible from television. We do not really see how Dr. Bailey comes to terms with her mother's death or Dr. Pravesh in mourning for more than a few minutes. Outside of medical dramas, most characters don't experience permanent loss from COVID, other than Charlie losing his estranged father in *Always Sunny*. Death and grief have been left out of TV's collective memory, ignoring the magnitude of the pandemic's effects.

Long after fictional shows concluded their pandemic programming, COVID influenced production behind the scenes. On-screen and off, COVID shaped the entertainment industry. As part of the pandemic workplace safety guidelines, most major film and TV productions required vaccination plus booster shots for cast and crew to be on set.[44] Even at Fox News Corporation, known for disseminating anti-vaccination messages, over 90 percent of full-time employees were vaccinated by August 2021.[45] Actors who refused vaccination were fired or let go, and had their characters written out of their shows.[46] Furthermore, the entertainment industry (like all sectors) lost many of its people to the virus, including musicians, rappers, comedians, reality stars, stunt people, actors, crew, news anchors, journalists, magicians, songwriters, playwrights, and dialect coaches.[47] Although this chapter has primarily focused on US entertainment, the pandemic challenges were also experienced in other countries—in the shutdown, return to work, and influence on content produced during this time.[48]

COVID dramatically changed how and what entertainment people consume. In a 2021 survey conducted by the United Talent Agency, over half of participants had subscribed to additional streaming services during the pandemic and 71 percent had planned to continue these subscriptions.[49] The shelter-in-place period also prompted consumers to try out new platforms, podcasts and other types of content, genres, and perspectives, such as international programming. It increased fandom, as participants expressed more willingness to join online communities for celebrities and influencers and even pay for content.[50] In other words, while the pandemic-specific narratives in fictional television may be forgotten, COVID significantly shaped the future of the entertainment industry.

CHAPTER EIGHT

Life After Crisis

PRESERVING MEMORY AND EXPERIENCE

Today, we mark a tragic milestone: one million American lives lost to COVID-19. One million empty chairs around the dinner table. Each an irreplaceable loss. Each leaving behind a family, a community, and a Nation forever changed because of this pandemic. Jill and I pray for each of them.

On May 12, 2022, President Joe Biden made this proclamation, ordering flags at half-mast to remember the one million American deaths from COVID.[1] By the following May, 127,152 more people had died in the United States.[2] Despite not being the most populous country, the United States recorded the highest number of COVID-19 deaths of the 6,947,192 global total, followed by Brazil (703,719), and India (531,905).[3] Deaths reached the all-time pandemic high of 26,028 in the United States for the week of January 3–6, 2021.[4] Hospitalizations peaked on January 22, 2022, with the seven-day average hospitalization at 158,593 for the nation.[5] US cases varied regionally, spiking nationally in December 2020–January 2021 and December 2021–January 2022 due to the Omicron variant.[6] Studies from the CDC suggest that 77 percent of those over age 15 have been infected, some multiple times.[7] More than 15.5 million children tested positive for COVID.[8] After the acute phase passed, thousands were and continue to be diagnosed with long COVID, suffering ongoing respiratory, cardiac, or neurological symptoms.[9]

The numbers are astonishing and heartbreaking, but they do little to capture the experiences of the pandemic years. Before 2020, it was difficult to fathom what living through a pandemic might be like. Narratives of past disease experiences felt so distant. Images of mask-wearing people during SARS seemed like an impossibility. Even in February that year, the notion that schools, zoos, parks, and other public spaces would soon become vacant was nearly inconceivable, especially in the United States. Once lockdown orders almost universally kept children and nonessential workers home, we thought it would be a week or two before activities would resume. Just as unpredictable were the divisive, politically charged responses that erupted. Isolation and the dependency on social media for interaction incited partisan-aligned skepticism of each other, further driving people into their echo chambers.

Many of the themes and issues that defined the pandemic emerged in January 2020. China's delay in publicly acknowledging the rising crisis was paralleled in the United States and other countries later on. Responses to the quarantined *Diamond Princess* foreshadowed the following months. Unfounded language stigmatizing and blaming Asian culture arose across platforms, fueled by Trump. Conspiracy theories and mis/disinformation circulated almost immediately. What was said and not said about vaccine development would later impact public perceptions. For good and for bad, media channels and content played integral roles in how the global crisis unfolded, contributing to the exceptionally high number of cases and deaths in the United States and shaping public perception and behaviors. This chapter provides a macro view of media in the pandemic, first comparing similarities to past large-scale contagious scourges and then examining what made COVID unique.

Repeating History

In many ways, the COVID-19 global crisis followed patterns apparent in other epidemics and pandemics.[10] Throughout the COVID pandemic, people drew comparisons to epidemic and pandemic history, especially the "Spanish Flu" of 1918, as they tried to make sense of their current moment.[11] Paralleling past outbreaks, media consumption soared as the crisis escalated. In the spring of 2020, people turned to existing media products for information, entertainment, and community connections.[12] When school, work, leisure activities, and, essentially, most of life shut down, individuals used existing media channels to stay updated, connect with each other, and be entertained. Like the newspapers and pamphlets in eighteenth century epidemics, available media outlets (newspapers, radio, TV, and social media) served as public spaces for announcements, persuasion, blame and stigma, speculation on the disease, promotion of untested remedies, and the preservation of both mundane and tragic events (i.e., passing time in quarantine or pictures of overflowing hospitals).[13] As was evident in other recent epidemics, government leaders, public health authorities, and regular people used social media to share news stories, opinions, and experiences.[14]

Unfortunately, as was historically true, this health crisis magnified existing inequities, with marginalized groups suffering far more than those in privileged positions in terms of stigma, vulnerability and disease, health care access, and the digital divide.[15] Like the 1918 influenza pandemic, COVID cases and deaths were difficult to accurately track and record.[16] The pandemic dominated news and entertainment products, as people struggled to make sense of their new realities.[17] Writers integrated some of the pandemic experiences into popular culture, offering representations of the virus and a slice of pandemic world.

COVID AS ITS OWN ENTITY

The novel coronavirus pandemic stands alone in its magnitude and duration. Cases appeared on every inhabited continent.[18] Increased global population and travel, combined with the transmissibility of COVID, unpredictable incubation rate, sometimes asymptomatic presentation, and other variables enabled the virus to become pandemic and to remain a constant threat for multiple years.[19] A lack of stringent mitigation strategies in the United States and some other countries also contributed to high case and death rates.[20] Contemporary technology and the coordination of global public health monitoring made it easier to chart how and when the virus was spreading.[21] This pandemic was also the first to have effective treatments and vaccines developed during its course, preventing approximately 14–19 million deaths worldwide.[22]

Public reception and perception also radically differed from previous outbreaks and epidemics. As discussed in the introduction, the United States had experienced more than sixty years since its last major epidemic. People took for granted that disease was not a threat, ignoring the possibility of illness upheaving entire societies. SARS, H1N1, Ebola, and Zika had all halted before infiltrating the United States. Americans and others in the world were ill-prepared for a true health crisis. And when coronavirus first emerged, Trump and his administration downplayed its severity, delayed national responses, and undermined lockdowns, masking, vaccination, and other mitigation strategies.[23] Deeply entrenched individualism in US culture contributed to resistance against collective attempts to slow COVID's transmission.[24]

The digital climate dramatically shaped how people experienced the pandemic. Global technology enabled those outside of Wuhan, then China, then Washington state and New York City to know about the virus more than a month before cases emerged close to home. Digital communication allowed preparation for what could lie ahead. At the same time, the uncertainty also meant that the information on COVID—from WHO, the CDC, public health leaders, and news outlets—was constantly shifting. This evolution of information about the new disease in real time was often perceived as contradictory and confusing, undermining trust in science, government, and journalism.[25]

As much of the official messaging on COVID focused nationally or internationally and not locally, news content and public health guidance often seemed to conflict with real-life observations. In a print-only era, diffusion of information was limited to the speed and reach of physical newspapers and books. The "Spanish Flu" was not constructed as a pandemic until after the fact. We know that the deadly flu/pneumonia combination was evident as early as March 1918 in Kansas. However, people in 1918 were largely unaware of the epidemiological threat until it went overseas, stretched throughout Europe and Asia in the summer, and came back in August.[26] News constructed influenza as epidemic, not pandemic, meaning that the rapidly spreading disease received little attention until it was upon a town. Then local papers advised residents on rising cases, mentioning familiar names of those sick or dead from the disease. Mitigation measures (i.e., school closings, quarantines, masks) were typically easily accepted because of the visibility of the health crisis. With this local focus, newspapers provided definitive parameters of the direct crisis lasting about six to eight weeks from the first cases through the peak and subsequent decline.[27]

With COVID, the delay between learning about the potential threat and experiencing local cases varied geographically, sometimes taking months. The additional notice helped prepare for the looming crisis. And yet, it affected how people thought about the seemingly distant threat. Moreover, ongoing crisis information desensitized people, increasingly causing COVID or pandemic fatigue, even as early as April and May 2020.[28] The COVID-19 pandemic did not unfold in a linear path. Waves of outbreaks continued for more than three years, as cases ebbed and flowed in different geographic areas. Impressions of the coronavirus situation moved up and down, based on school closings, vaccination rollout, and variant outbreaks.[29] Some of its length was due to the evolving nature of the virus. The rest of the variation could be attributed to mitigation measures that delayed outbreaks of COVID and the reliance on media platforms that existed in 2020. Advanced notice was beneficial for preparation,[i] but challenging for public morale and understanding of the pandemic.

Despite the capabilities of this era, firsthand experiences and disease imagery were surprisingly scarce. COVID news coverage overwhelmingly focused on statistics and not personalized stories of the unfolding tragedy. In the past, public health decisions were difficult to question back when people read about friends and neighbors dying from a disease in the local paper, witnessed the burning of toys and clothes after a child

i Despite this notice, both the U.S. and global preparations were later found to be woefully inadequate.

was taken to the hospital, or heard the funeral bells incessantly tolling. This visible impact of COVID was much more removed from the public eye. Precautions kept journalists and media professionals from capturing stories, video, and photos in hospitals. Occasionally, doctors, nurses, and other health professionals were photographed with weary faces deeply entrenched with mask lines. Without the inclusion of regular people, though, this world seemed both separate and far away. Restrictions on patients' visitors removed additional means of experiencing and conveying the crisis as patients died alone, away from family and friends.[30] Bans on funerals and gatherings removed collective grieving and the sharing of sorrow.[31] As a result, mitigation measures may have seemed premature or unnecessary, as it was harder to imagine what a pandemic really looked like without directly encountering makeshift hospitals, coffins stacked on streets, or mass graves.

The decline and changes to local journalism also shaped this coverage.[32] In past epidemics, local papers listed names of people ill with disease and in death notices. For the COVID pandemic, this was not the case. First of all, by the twenty-first century, fewer communities had local newspapers. And, due to tension about the pandemic and stigma attached to disease, even local obituaries rarely mentioned COVID.[ii] Its victims were memorialized in the *Boston Globe*, the *New York Times*, and other large newspapers and social media groups like @FacesofCOVID. However, the absence of names in local papers meant that residents in a particular town had no idea of who had succumbed to COVID, other than well-known citizens and names shared by friends or family, making the disease seem innocuous.

Media Consumption and Effects

What people read, watched, scrolled, shared, and created in the COVID pandemic significantly affected how they perceived the crisis and what

ii Some of the omission of COVID likely also stemmed from the new ways that obituaries are disseminated. Many news outlets use *Legacy.com*, which does not usually list a person's cause of death.

they chose to do and not do. Especially in Spring 2020, consumption of local, national, and international news outlets, public health websites, social media, and entertainment skyrocketed.[33] Digital weekly and Sunday news circulation increased in 2020, as large and small news outlets removed paywalls for articles related to COVID.[34] Although local, network, and cable news audiences all experienced growth, Fox News, in particular, significantly attracted new viewers in 2020.[35] Podcasts also became more popular, as consumers turned to them for entertainment and information.[36] Over half of adults got their news from social media, listing Twitter and Facebook for the top platforms, while adults using TikTok for news also increased.[37] Science news content on social media became much more common, especially among Democrats and those with more education, and consumers talked about science news more compared to before the pandemic.[38]

Age largely determined content consumption. Older groups gravitated toward television news, while younger consumers were more likely to use social media for news and chose Snapchat and TikTok as their preferred platforms.[39] And, increasingly, people chose to solely consume media aligned with their political party, reinforcing split "media ecosystems."[40]Almost half of Democrats consumed a politically mixed news diet, tuning into CNN, then NPR, *MSNBC*, the *New York Times*, and the *Washington Post*.[41] Only 34 percent of Republications consumed mixed sources.[42] Older Republicans were more likely to consume only right-leaning media, primarily Fox News and talk radio.[43] This fragmented media consumption meant that audiences widely differed in what messaging they were receiving, and depending on one's news diet, fanned confusion and resistance to public health mitigation strategies.

Mis/disinformation

Although the spread of misleading and false COVID information (known as misinformation) was recognized as a global problem, its impact varied by region.[44] Social media's lack of monitoring facilitated the dissemination of misinformation.[45] Twitter, Facebook, and YouTube began flagging or blocking inaccurate information early on in the timeline, before the viral reach had become pandemic.[46] From April to June 2020, Meta Platforms Inc. added warnings about COVID misinformation to ninety-eight million Facebook and Instagram posts and removed seven million more for promoting fake remedies, conspiracy theories, and other harmful information.[47] Yet, social media sites had too much content spreading too fast for the gatekeepers to flag or block all potentially harmful messages.[48] Because of the use of strong emotional appeals in misinformation, it moved much more quickly than factual information.[49] In other words, people were more likely to respond to and share heavily charged material (i.e., claims about untested remedies) than fact-based scientific articles.

The intentional dissemination of false content (disinformation), conspiracy theories, and stigmatizing messages also raged due to certain politicians, anti-vaccine individuals, and companies (i.e., the "Disinformation Dozen") deliberately creating such messages.[50] Although mis/disinformation was problematic worldwide, in the United States, the Trump administration propagated much of the disinformation and xenophobia, making these issues even more prominent and problematic in the United States.[51] Trump was later quantitatively identified as the most prolific source of misinformation[iii] about the pandemic.[52] While he was president, social media platforms allowed Trump to post even false content, for example, his statements about ingesting bleach, without blocking or flagging it as misinformation.[53] Trump consistently propagated distrust in media, using the term "fake news" more than 146 times, just in 2020.[54]

Fox News and other right-wing news outlets disseminated more misinformation than mainstream or left-leaning sources, beginning early in the COVID-19 crisis.[55] Regular people also shared mis/disinformation throughout their social networks. Regardless of partisan

---

iii Twitter permanently banned Trump on February 8, 2021, in response to his tweets about the Capitol insurrection. https://blog.twitter.com/en_us/topics/company/2020/suspension. Trump was suspended for two years from Facebook and Instagram. https://about.fb.com/news/2023/01/trump-facebook-instagram-account-suspension/.

affiliation, older people shared the most misinformation, especially those over 65.[56] A study of more than 4,000 COVID misinformation tweets revealed that conservatives were more likely to spread conspiracy theories.[57] Misleading content and misinformation significantly hindered consumer trust, fueling public resistance to public health measures and COVID vaccination.[58] Mis/disinformation and politicization of COVID led to fierce divisions in public perceptions of the virus, masking, and vaccination.[59] Widely spread false claims convinced people to hoard hydroxychloroquine, ingest ivermectin, and take Borax baths to remove "nanotechnologies" from COVID vaccines, in addition to many other unproven and dangerous "remedies."[60] The effects of misinformation were highly dependent on socio-demographics, political affiliation, trust in scientists, and social media usage.[61]

Because of the type of COVID messaging distributed in conservative media outlets, those who identified as conservative were less likely to view the virus as a threat or to see themselves at risk, and more likely to believe that media exaggerated the risk or believe in conspiracy theories.[62] This identification was also correlated with difficulty in discerning between made-up and real COVID headlines and less knowledge about COVID.[63] Moreover, Republicans who used the White House and Trump as their main sources of COVID information were more likely than other Republicans to believe that the pandemic was overhyped.[64] This group was also more critical of mainstream media and showed a greater distrust in journalists.[65]

Across political affiliation and other divisive characteristics, the tail-end of the pandemic had people questioning state of news, accuracy of social media, and their own consumption habits.[66] In a 2022 Pew Research survey, only a quarter of adults believed that journalists did a good job managing or correcting information.[67] Nearly half of respondents said that they had little or no trust in the information received from news organizations.[68] It should be noted that "trust in media" -type poll results typically differ when people are asked about specific outlets and when they are given the option of "Neither trustworthy nor untrustworthy" and "don't know."[69] Moreover, social media has started to change, as TikTok has been increasingly banned, Elon Musk's purchase of Twitter (now X) has changed the site, and new social media platform alternatives have continued to emerge.[70]

Despite the many negative aspects of media channels in the pandemic, twenty-first century technology overwhelming served crucial, positive roles throughout the global crisis. WHO, the CDC, and other public health authorities were able to quickly connect and update the public. Technology allowed for many employees to work from home, attend virtual school, receive telehealth care, and engage in online shopping, and those made social distancing possible. Entertainment helped people to pass the time, cope with the stress of the pandemic, and connect with each other.[71] Digital communications allowed for quick and easy knowledge-sharing, including information that helped scientists develop multiple safe, effective vaccines. Social media guided users on why, when, and where to get vaccinated, eventually persuading most of the world to be protected against COVID-19.

REMEMBERING AND MOVING FORWARD

For three years, the COVID-19 pandemic shaped everyday life and dominated media content. Belief that the crisis was ending steadily increased from November 2021 through March 2023, in which 49 percent of Gallup survey respondents said it was over.[72] The PHEIC ended two months later, in May 2023, technically marking the end of the pandemic. Yet, it does not feel over for those who are still social distancing, learning online, or masking. Concern about catching COVID hovered around 60 percent of Gallup respondents until the vaccine rollout, dropped significantly, rose again with Omicron, and then declined to about 25 percent.[73] The majority of people stopped taking COVID precautions after they got vaccinated. However, concerns about COVID continue to wax and wane. In a February 2023 Gallup poll, 15 percent of adults were still isolating, 23 percent continued to avoid large crowds, and nearly a third of participants wore masks in public.[74] Over 60 percent of respondents believed the COVID situation was getting better. In early summer, this number increased to 71 percent and then dropped by September 2023, with only 41 percent of participants believing that COVID was improving.[75] Concerns about catching COVID had also increased by that point.[76] Demographics, health, personal experience, and other factors shaped and continue to shape perceptions of risk.

COVID changed the world. After the Spring 2020 adoption surge, more households have pets.[77] Hybrid and work-from-home jobs are much more common as employers have discovered new possibilities for remote work.[78] Video conferencing, other forms of digital communication and demand for online classes have also increased.[79] Economic hardship during the pandemic prompted numerous entrepreneurial opportunities.[80] Applications for new businesses continue to be much higher than in 2019.[81] The biggest triumph of the pandemic—effective COVID vaccines—are paving the way for effective vaccines against other diseases.[82]

It is too soon to fully gauge the multitude of negative COVID effects. School-age children are still recovering from learning loss due to school closings and interruptions.[83] People continue to struggle economically, especially those in low-income families.[84] The crisis significantly took a toll on physical and mental health. Teenagers, particularly LGBTQIA+ youth, face ongoing psychological stress and mental health issues from the pandemic, as it isolated groups from their social networks.[85] Pandemic effects were also magnified for already marginalized groups.[86] People of color still have more difficulty accessing health care.[87] Black maternal and infant mortality increased over the last three years.[88] Black Americans, Asian Americans, LGBTQIA+ communities, and other marginalized groups continue to face racism, stigma, discrimination, and legislation stripping away rights and protections.[89] The pandemic's impact on people with disabilities cannot be ignored, as they disproportionately faced challenges: disrupted regular care and services, higher risks of complications and death from the virus, and other health inequities.[90] For example, d/Deaf or hard of hearing patients and those with cognitive disabilities faced additional communication barriers, with discharge instructions not clearly communicated.[91]

Grief and mourning for the millions of lives lost to COVID continues. In 2021, artist Suzanne Brennan Firstenberg designed a temporary exhibit of more than 600,000 white flags upon the National Mall in Washington, DC, to represent the number of US COVID deaths at that time.[92] A permanent national display has not yet been created, yet various cities' murals and monuments remind residents of the pandemic victims.[93] Memorial websites and social media groups have also been created to digitally preserve memories of the deceased. TV shows and films constructed fictional narratives depicting the trauma of this moment. Are these spaces enough to cement the toll of the pandemic in collective memory? After the 1918 pandemic, people moved on, scarcely writing about their influenza experiences.[94] The "Spanish Flu" was nearly written out of history until the temporary interest in the disease sparked in 2020.

What the COVID-19 pandemic has demonstrated is that local and national government leaders must work with WHO, the CDC, and other public health authorities to issue clear, united messaging about the risk of disease and the steps toward preparation.[95] Recognizing their roles in crises, media producers, journalists, and social media gatekeepers should work together to create clear content and curb misinformation. And on the consumer side, the need for news and media literacy has never been more important.[96] Children and adults need to learn how to gather credible information and to regard social media as channels for content, not as news producers. Finally, we need to have detailed plans in place for distributing and consuming content during crises. As COVID showed the world in 2020, future pandemics are inevitable and media will play integral roles as to how the global calamity unfolds.

Notes

Preface

1 "Statement on the Fifteenth Meeting of the IHR (2005) Emergency Committee on the COVID-19 Pandemic." *News*. WHO. May 5, 2023, https://www.who.int/news/item/05-05-2023-statement-on-the-fifteenth-meeting-of-the-international-health-regulations-(2005)-emergency-committee-regarding-the-coronavirus-disease-(covid-19)-pandemic.

Chapter One: The Unexpected Crisis in the Digital Era

1 "WHO Director-General's Opening Remarks at the Media Briefing on COVID-19 - 11 March 2020." *WHO Director-General Speeches*. WHO. March 11, 2020, https://www.who.int/director-general/speeches/detail/who-director-general-s-opening-remarks-at-the-media-briefing-on-covid-19---11-march-2020.

2 Ella Koeze and Nathaniel Popper, "The Virus Changed the Way We Internet," *New York Times* (2020, April 7), https://www.nytimes.com/interactive/2020/04/07/technology/coronavirus-internet-use.html; "COVID-19: Tracking the Impact on Media Consumption," *Insights*, The Nielsen Company. (2020, June 16), https://www.nielsen.com/us/en/insights/article/2020/covid-19-tracking-the-impact-on-media-consumption/.

3 Laurie Garrett, "COVID-19: The Medium Is the Message," *The Lancet* 395, no. 10228 (2020): 942–43; Rupali Jayant Limaye, Molly Sauer, Joseph Ali, Justin Bernstein, Brian Wahl, Anne Barnhill, and Alain Labrique, "Building Trust While Influencing Online COVID-19 Content in the Social Media World," *The Lancet Digital Health* 2, no. 6 (2020): e277-e278; Saiful Islam, Tonmoy Sarkar, Sazzad Hossain Khan, Abu-Hena Mostofa Kamal, SM Murshid Hasan, Alamgir Kabir, Dalia Yeasmin et al., "COVID-19–Related Infodemic and Its Impact on Public Health: A Global Social Media Analysis," *The American Journal of Tropical Medicine and Hygiene* 103, no. 4 (2020): 1621–1629; Oberiri Destiny Apuke and Bahiyah Omar, "Fake News and COVID-19: Modelling the Predictors of Fake News Sharing

Among Social Media Users," *Telematics and Informatics* (2020): 101475; Gordon Pennycook, Jonathon McPhetres, Yunhao Zhang, Jackson G. Lu, and David G. Rand, "Fighting COVID-19 Misinformation on Social Media: Experimental Evidence for a Scalable Accuracy-Nudge Intervention," *Psychological Science* 31, no. 7 (2020): 770–80; Sheera Frenkel, Ben Decker, and Davey Alba, "How the 'Plandemic' Movie and Its Falsehoods Spread Widely Online," *New York Times*, May 5, 2020, https://www.nytimes.com/2020/05/20/technology/plandemic-movie-youtube-facebook-coronavirus.html; "Managing the COVID-19 Infodemic: Promoting Healthy Behaviours and Mitigating the Harm from Misinformation and Disinformation," WHO, September 23, 2020, https://www.who.int/news/item/23-09-2020-managing-the-covid-19-infodemic-promoting-healthy-behaviours-and-mitigating-the-harm-from-misinformation-and-disinformation; "Understanding the Infodemic and Misinformation in the Fight Against COVID-19," Pan American Health Organization, (2020), https://iris.paho.org/bitstream/handle/10665.2/52052/Factsheet-infodemic_eng.pdf?sequence=16.

4 "Statement on the Fifteenth Meeting of the IHR (2005) Emergency Committee," WHO.

5 "WHO Coronavirus (COVID-19) Dashboard," WHO, https://covid19.who.int/.

6 Lazaro Gamio, Eleanor Lutz, and Albert Sun, "As Emergency Ends, a Look at Covid's U.S. Death Toll," *New York Times*, May 11, 2023, https://www.nytimes.com/interactive/2023/05/11/us/covid-deaths-us.html.

7 Josh Holder, "Tracking Coronavirus Vaccinations Around the World," *New York Times*, March 13, 2023, https://www.nytimes.com/interactive/2021/world/covid-vaccinations-tracker.html.

8 "Naming the Coronavirus Disease (COVID-19) and the Virus that Causes It," *Technical Guidance*, WHO, 2023, https://www.who.int/emergencies/diseases/novel-coronavirus-2019/technical-guidance/naming-the-coronavirus-disease-(covid-2019)-and-the-virus-that-causes-it; "Coronavirus Press Conference," WHO, February 11, 2020. Transcript, https://www.who.int/docs/default-source/coronaviruse/transcripts/who-audio-emergencies-coronavirus-full-press-conference-11feb2020-final.pdf?sfvrsn=e2019136_2.

9 Manas Pustake, Isha Tambolkar, Purushottam Giri, and Charmi Gandhi, "SARS, MERS and COVID-19: An Overview and Comparison of Clinical, Laboratory and Radiological Features," *Journal of Family Medicine and Primary Care* 11, no. 1 (2022): 10.

10 "Symptoms," *Coronavirus Disease 2019 (COVID-19)*, CDC, April 17, 2020, https://web.archive.org/web/20200417213406/https://www.cdc.gov/coronavirus/2019-ncov/symptoms-testing/symptoms.html.

11 Hualei Xin, Jessica Y. Wong, Caitriona Murphy, Amy Yeung, Sheikh Taslim Ali, Peng Wu, and Benjamin J. Cowling, "The Incubation Period Distribution of Coronavirus Disease 2019: A Systematic Review and Meta-Analysis," *Clinical Infectious Diseases* 73, no. 12 (2021): 2344–352.

12 Yu Wu, Liangyu Kang, Zirui Guo, Jue Liu, Min Liu, and Wannian Liang, "Incubation Period of COVID-19 Caused by Unique SARS-CoV-2 Strains: A Systematic Review and Meta-Analysis," JAMA network open 5, no. 8 (2022): e2228008-e2228008; Diana Duong, "Alpha, Beta, Delta, Gamma: What's Important to Know about SARS-CoV-2 Variants of Concern?" (2021): E1059-E1060.

13 Yu Wu, Liangyu Kang, Zirui Guo, Jue Liu, Min Liu, and Wannian Liang, "Incubation period of COVID-19.

14 "Symptoms," CDC.

15 "Symptoms," CDC.

16 "Symptoms," CDC.

17 Jingjing He, Yifei Guo, Richeng Mao, and Jiming Zhang, "Proportion of Asymptomatic Coronavirus Disease 2019: A Systematic Eeview and Meta-analysis," *Journal of Medical Virology* 93, no. 2 (2021): 820–30; Weijing Shang, Liangyu Kang, Guiying Cao, Yaping Wang, Peng Gao, Jue Liu, and Min Liu, "Percentage of Asymptomatic Infections among SARS-CoV-2 Omicron Variant-Positive Individuals: A Systematic Review and Meta-Analysis." *Vaccines* 10, no. 7 (2022): 1049.

18 "Similarities and Differences between Flu and COVID-19," *Influenza*, CDC, September 28, 2022, https://www.cdc.gov/flu/symptoms/flu-vs-covid19.htm.

19 "Similarities and Differences between Flu and COVID-19," *Influenza*, CDC, "Multisystem Inflammatory Syndrome (MIS)," CDC, January 3, 2023, https://www.cdc.gov/mis/; V. Rajesh, Jolsana Augustine, R. Divya, and Melcy Cleetus, "COVID-19 Presenting as Acute Transient Flaccid Limb Paralysis," *Journal of Family Medicine and Primary Care* 10, no. 4 (2021): 1789; Sameer K. Mehta and Ashok Sunder, "Getting Paralysed after COVID: Guillain–Barre Syndrome," *Journal of Family Medicine and Primary Care* 10, no. 7 (2021): 2706; Hanganu, Andreea-Raluca, Alexandru Constantin, Elena-Sonia Moise, Cristian-Mihail Niculae, Ioana Diana Olaru, Cristian Băicuș, and Adriana Hristea, "Peripheral Nervous System Involvement Associated with COVID-19. A Systematic Review of Literature." *PLoS ONE* 18, no. 4 (2023): e0283827.

20 "People with Certain Medical Conditions," *COVID-19*, CDC, May 11, 2023, https://www.cdc.gov/coronavirus/2019-ncov/need-extra-precautions/people-with-medical-conditions.html.

21 "Long COVID or Post-COVID Conditions," *COVID-19*, CDC, December 16, 2022, https://www.cdc.gov/coronavirus/2019-ncov/long-term-effects/index.html.

22 "Risk for COVID-19 Infection, Hospitalization, and Death by Age Group," CDC, May 30, 2023, https://www.cdc.gov/coronavirus/2019-ncov/covid-data/investigations-discovery/hospitalization-death-by-age.html.

23 "Provisional COVID-19 Deaths: Focus on Ages 0–18 Years," *Data*. CDC. June 21, 2023, https://data.cdc.gov/NCHS/Provisional-COVID-19-Deaths-Focus-on-Ages-0-18-Yea/nr4s-juj3.

24 "FDA Takes Key Action in Fight Against COVID-19 by Issuing Emergency Use Authorization for First COVID-19 Vaccine." *FDA News Release*. December

11, 2020, https://www.fda.gov/news-events/press-announcements/fda-takes-key-action-fight-against-covid-19-issuing-emergency-use-authorization-first-covid-19; “Moderna Announces FDA Authorization of Moderna COVID-19 Vaccine in U.S.” *Moderna Press Release*. December 18, 2020, https://investors.modernatx.com/news/news-details/2020/Moderna-Announces-FDA-Authorization-of-Moderna-COVID-19-Vaccine-in-U.S/default.aspx.

25 Nick Andrews, Elise Tessier, Julia Stowe, Charlotte Gower, Freja Kirsebom, Ruth Simmons, Eileen Gallagher et al. “Duration of Protection Against Mild and Severe Disease by COVID-19 Vaccines,” *New England Journal of Medicine* 386, no. 4 (2022): 340–50.

26 “What Are the Possible Treatment Options for COVID-19?” *Administration for Strategic Preparedness & Response*, U.S. Department of Health & Human Services, https://aspr.hhs.gov/COVID-19/Treatments/Pages/Possible-Treatment-Options-for-COVID19.aspx.

27 Nobuyuki Horita, and Takeshi Fukumoto, “Global Case Fatality Rate from COVID-19 Has Decreased by 96.8 Percent during 2.5 Years of the Pandemic,” *Journal of Medical Virology* (2022).

28 Jared Diamond, *Guns, Germs, and Steel: The Fates of Human Societies* (New York: W. W. Norton & Company, 1999); Hays, *The Burdens of Disease*; McNeill, *Plagues and Peoples*; Rosenberg, *Explaining Epidemics*; Sheldon J. Watts, *Epidemics and History: Disease, Power and Imperialism* (New Haven, Connecticut: Yale University Press, 1997); Foss, Katherine A, *Constructing the Outbreak: Epidemics in Media and Collective Memory* (Amherst: University of Massachusetts Press, 2020).

29 Foss, *Constructing the Outbreak.*

30 Carol R. Byerly, “The US Military and the Influenza Pandemic of 1918–1919,” *Public Health Reports* 125, no. 3_suppl (2010): 81–91.

31 Abdul Rahim Shaik, and Arakkal Maniyat Shemjaz, “The Rise of Physical Therapy: A History in Footsteps.” *Archives of Medicine and Health Sciences* 2, no. 2 (2014): 257–60; Verville, Richard Emery, and John F. Ditunno Jr. “Franklin Delano Roosevelt, Polio, and the Warm Springs Experiment: Its Impact on Physical Medicine and Rehabilitation,” *PM&R* 5, no. 1 (2013): 3–8.

32 Donald R. Hopkins, *The Greatest Killer: Smallpox in History* (Chicago: University of Chicago Press, 2002).

33 Howard Markel and Alexandra Minna Stern, “The Foreignness of Germs: The Persistent Association of Immigrants and Disease in American Society,” *The Milbank Quarterly* 80, no. 4 (2002): 757–88; Moore, Harriet, “Contagion from Abroad: US Newspaper Framings of Immigrants and Epidemics, 1891 to 1893,” *Atlanta Review of Journalism History* 8 (2009).

34 Samuel K. Cohn Jr, “The Black Death and the Burning of Jews,” *Past and Present* 196, no. 1 (2007): 3–36.

35 Alan M. Kraut, *Silent Travelers: Germs, Genes, and the Immigrant Menace* (JHU Press, 1995), 3.

36 Alan M. Kraut, *Silent Travelers.*

37 Judith Walzer Leavitt, *Typhoid Mary: Captive to the Public's Health* (Beacon Press, 1997).

38 Gregory M. Herek and Eric K. Glunt, "An Epidemic of Stigma: Public Reactions to AIDS," *American Psychologist* 43, no. 11 (1988).

39 Kraut, *Silent Travelers.*

40 Laura Eichelberger, "SARS and New York's Chinatown: the Politics of Risk and blame during an epidemic of fear." *Social science & medicine* 65, no. 6 (2007): 1284–1295.

41 Sarah Monson, "Ebola as African: American Media Discourses of Panic and Otherization," *Africa Today* 63, no. 3 (2017): 3–27; Crystal Chang, Anthony Salerno, and Edbert B. Hsu, "Perspectives on Xenophobia during Epidemics and Implications for Emergency Management," *Journal of Emergency Management* 18, no. 7 (2020): 23–29; Trevor Hoppe, "'Spanish flu': When Infectious Disease Names Blur Origins and Stigmatize those Infected," *American Journal of Public Health* 108, no. 11 (2018): 1462–1464.

42 Foss, *Constructing the Outbreak.*

43 "Section 11: Epidemic Disease Occurrence," CDC, 2012, https://www.cdc.gov/csels/dsepd/ss1978/lesson1/section11.html.

44 "Disease Outbreaks," *Health Topics*, WHO, 2023, https://www.emro.who.int/health-topics/disease-outbreaks/index.html.

45 "Section 11: Epidemic Disease Occurrence"; David Morens, Gregory K. Folkers, and Anthony S. Fauci, "What Is a Pandemic?" *Journal of Infectious Diseases* 200, no. 7 (2009): 1018–21.

46 WHO. International Health Regulations (2005). WHO, 2008. See especially p. 43.

47 Annelies Wilder-Smith and Sarah Osman, "Public Health Emergencies of International Concern: A Historic Overview," *Journal of Travel Medicine* 27, no. 8 (2020): taaa227; "Statement on the Fifteenth Meeting of the IHR (2005) Emergency Committee," WHO; "Statement of the Thirty-Fifth Polio IHR Emergency Committee," *News* (WHO. May 12, 2023, https://www.who.int/news/item/12-05-2023-statement-of-the-thirty-fifth-polio-ihr-emergency-committee; "Fifth Meeting of the International Health Regulations (2005) (IHR) Emergency Committee on the Multi-Country Outbreak of mpox (monkeypox)," *News* (WHO. May 11, 2023), https://www.who.int/news/item/11-05-2023-fifth-meeting-of-the-international-health-regulations-(2005)-(ihr)-emergency-committee-on-the-multi-country-outbreak-of-monkeypox-(mpox).

48 W. K. Lam, N. S. Zhong, and W. C. Tan, "Overview on SARS in Asia and the World," *Respirology* 8 (2003): S2-S5.

49 "2014–2016 Ebola Outbreak in West Africa," *Outbreaks* (CDC, March 8, 2019), https://www.cdc.gov/vhf/ebola/history/2014-2016-outbreak/index.html.

50 Celine Klemm, Enny Das, and Tilo Hartmann, "Swine Flu and Hype: A

Systematic Review of Media Dramatization of The H1N1 Influenza Pandemic." *Journal of Risk Research* 19, no. 1 (2016): 1–20; Monson, Sarah. "Ebola as African: American Media Discourses of Panic and Otherization." *Africa Today* 63, no. 3 (2017): 3–27.

51 Abigail Johnson Hess, "A Sobering Stat During Coronavirus Fears—90 Percent of Employees Admit They Have Gone to Work When Sick," *CNBC*. First published November 3, 2019. Updated February 28, 2020, https://www.cnbc.com/2019/11/03/90percent-of-employees-say-they-come-to-work-sickheres-how-to-fix-that.html.

52 Daniel J. Wilson, "A Crippling Fear: Experiencing Polio in the Era Of FDR," *Bulletin of the History of Medicine* 72, no. 3 (1998): 464–95.

53 Foss, *Constructing the Outbreak*.

54 Bo Bian, Jingjing Li, Ting Xu, and Natasha Z. Foutz, "Individualism During Crises," *The Review of Economics and Statistics* 104, no. 2 (2022): 368–85.

55 Sylvia Noble Tesh, *Hidden Arguments: Political Ideology and Disease Prevention Policy* (Rutgers University Press, 1988).

56 "Summary of the Affordable Care Act." *Health Reform*. Kaiser Family Foundation. April 25, 2013, https://www.kff.org/health-reform/fact-sheet/summary-of-the-affordable-care-act/; Jennifer Tolbert, Patrick Drake, and Anthony Damico, "Key Facts About the Uninsured Population," *Uninsured*, Kaiser Family Foundation. December 19, 2022, http://tinyurl.com/ytub9ra5; Amy E. Cha and Cohen, Robin A. Cohen "Reasons for Being Uninsured Among Adults Aged 18–64 in the United States, 2019," *Data Briefs*, National Center for Health Statistics. September 2020, https://www.cdc.gov/nchs/products/databriefs/db382.htm#:~:text=In percent202019 percent2C percent20the percent20percentage percent20of,in percent20fair percent20or percent20poor percent20health.

57 Rachel Garfield, Kendal Orgera, and Anthony Damico, "The Uninsured and the ACA: A Primer—Key Facts about Health Insurance and the Uninsured amidst Changes to the Affordable Care Act," *Uninsured*, Kaiser Family Foundation. January 25, 2019, https://www.kff.org/report-section/the-uninsured-and-the-aca-a-primer-key-facts-about-health-insurance-and-the-uninsured-amidst-changes-to-the-affordable-care-act-how-does-lack-of-insurance-affect-access-to-care/.

58 James B. Kirby and Toshiko Kaneda, "Unhealthy and Uninsured: Exploring Racial Differences in Health and Health Insurance Coverage Using a Life Table Approach," Demography 47, no. 4 (2010): 1035–51.

59 "American Views: Trust, Media and Democracy: A Gallup/Knight Foundation Survey," *Gallup* (2018). Standard_Template_WithCover_040617 (knightfoundation.org).

60 Lisa Shearer, "Social Media Outpaces Print Newspapers in the U.S. As A News Source," *Social Media & the News*, Pew Research Center (December 10, 2018), https://www.pewresearch.org/short-reads/2018/12/10/social-media-outpaces-print-newspapers-in-the-u-s-as-a-news-source/.

61 Shearer, "Social Media Outpaces Print Newspapers in the U.S. As A News Source."

62 Penelope Muse Abernathy, *The Expanding News Desert*. A Report of the Center for Innovation and Sustainability in Local Media (University of North Carolina at Chapel Hill: 2018), https://www.usnewsdeserts.com/reports/expanding-news-desert/.

63 Abernathy, *The Expanding News Desert.*

64 Abernathy, *The Expanding News Desert.*

65 Abernathy, *The Expanding News Desert.*

66 Andrew Perrin and Monica Andersen, "Share of U.S. Adults Using Social Media, Including Facebook, Is Mostly Unchanged Since 2018." *Social Media*. Pew Research Center. April 10, 2019, https://www.pewresearch.org/short-reads/2019/04/10/share-of-u-s-adults-using-social-media-including-facebook-is-mostly-unchanged-since-2018/.

67 Perrin and Andersen, "Share of U.S. Adults Using Social Media."

68 Perrin and Andersen, "Share of U.S. Adults Using Social Media."

69 Perrin and Andersen, "Share of U.S. Adults Using Social Media."

70 John Herman, "How TikTok is Rewriting the World," *New York Times*, March 10, 2009; "TikTok: How Fast Is It Growing in the US, And Who's Using It?" *Marketing Charts*, May 6, 2019. TikTok: How Fast Is It Growing in the US, And Who's Using It? - Marketing Charts.

71 Foss, *Constructing the Outbreak.*

72 Tanya R. Berry, Joan Wharf-Higgins, and P. J. Naylor, "SARS Wars: An Examination of the Quantity and Construction of Health Information in The News Media," *Health Communication* 21, no. 1 (2007): 35–44.

73 Seth Motel, "Ebola Ranks Among Highest in News Interest Since 2010," *News Coverage*. Pew Research Center. October 21, 2014, https://www.pewresearch.org/short-reads/2014/10/21/ebola-ranks-among-highest-in-news-interest-since-2010/; "Ebola Worries Rise, But Most Are 'Fairly' Confident in Government, Hospitals to Deal With Disease," *Report* (Pew Research Center: October 21, 2014), https://www.pewresearch.org/politics/2014/10/21/ebola-worries-rise-but-most-are-fairly-confident-in-government-hospitals-to-deal-with-disease/.

74 Rumi Chunara, Jason R. Andrews, and John S. Brownstein, "Social and News Media Enable Estimation of Epidemiological Patterns Early in the 2010 Haitian Cholera Outbreak," *The American Journal of Tropical Medicine and Hygiene* 86, no. 1 (2012): 39; Aron Culotta, "Detecting Influenza Outbreaks by Analyzing Twitter Messages," *arXiv preprint arXiv:1007.4748* (2010); Eiji Aramaki, Sachiko Maskawa, and Mizuki Morita, "Twitter Catches the Flu: Detecting Influenza Epidemics Using Twitter," In *Proceedings of the 2011 Conference on Empirical Methods in Natural Language Processing* (2011): 1568–1576.

75 Stuart E. Middleton, Lee Middleton, and Stefano Modafferi, "Real-time Crisis Mapping of Natural Disasters Using Social Media," *IEEE Intelligent Systems* 29, no. 2 (2013): 9–17.

76 Andrew McNeill, Peter R. Harris, and Pam Briggs, "Twitter Influence on UK Vaccination and Antiviral Uptake During The 2009 H1N1 Pandemic," *Frontiers In Public Health* 4 (2016): 26; Michael S. Deiner, Cherie Fathy, Jessica Kim, Katherine Niemeyer, David Ramirez, Sarah F. Ackley, Fengchen Liu, Thomas M. Lietman, and Travis C. Porco. "Facebook And Twitter Vaccine Sentiment in Response to Measles Outbreaks," *Health Informatics Journal* 25, No. 3 (2019): 1116–132.

77 Foss, *Constructing the Outbreak.*

78 "American Views: Trust, Media and Democracy," *Gallup*.

79 Philipp Müller, Pascal Schneiders, and Svenja Schäfer. "Appetizer or Main Dish? Explaining the Use of Facebook News Posts as a Substitute for Other News Sources," *Computers In Human Behavior* 65 (2016): 431–41.

80 Maksym Gabielkov, Arthi Ramachandran, Augustin Chaintreau, and Arnaud Legout, "Social Clicks: What and Who Gets Read on Twitter?," In *Proceedings of the 2016 ACM SIGMETRICS International Conference On measurement and modeling of computer science*, 179–92. 2016.

81 "Journalism, 'Fake News' and Disinformation." UNESCO Handbook for Journalism Education and Training. 2018, https://en.unesco.org/sites/default/files/journalism_fake_news_disinformation_print_friendly_0.pdf.

82 Anita Desikan, Taryn MacKinney, Casey Kalman, Jacob M. Carter, Genna Reed, and Gretchen T. Goldman, "An Equity and Environmental Justice Assessment of Anti-Science Actions During the Trump Administration," *Journal of Public Health Policy* 44, No. 1 (2023): 147–62; Peter J. Hotez, "Anti-Science Extremism in America: Escalating and Globalizing," *Microbes And Infection* 22, No. 10 (2020): 505–7; Michael D. Shear, Maggie Haberman, Nicholas Confessore, Karen Yourish, Larry Buchanan, and Keith Collins. "How Trump Reshaped the Presidency in Over 11,000 Tweets," *New York Times*, November 2, 2019, https://www.nytimes.com/interactive/2019/11/02/us/politics/trump-twitter-presidency.html.

83 Shear, Haberman, Confessore, Yourish, and Collins, "How Trump Reshaped the Presidency in Over 11,000 Tweets."

84 Search of "Donald J. Trump" and "Fake News." *The American Presidency Project*, https://www.presidency.ucsb.edu/advanced-search?field-keywords= percent22fake+news percent22&field-keywords2=&field-keywords3=&from percent5Bdate percent 5D=01-11-2017&to percent5Bdate percent5D=12-31-2019&person2=200301&items_per_page=100; "American Views: Trust, Media and Democracy," *Gallup*.

85 Edson C. Tandoc Jr., Wei Lim Zheng, and Richard Ling, "Defining "Fake News" A Typology of Scholarly Definitions," *Digital Journalism* 6, no. 2 (2018): 137–53.

86 Angie Drobnic Holan, "The Media's Definition of Fake News vs. Donald's Trump's, *Politifact*, The Poynter Institute. October 18, 2017, https://www.politifact.com/article/2017/oct/18/deciding-whats-fake-medias-definition-fake-news-vs/.

87 Emily Van Duyn and Jessica Collier, "Priming and Fake News: The Effects of Elite Discourse on Evaluations of News Media," *Mass Communication and Society* 22, no. 1 (2019): 29–48.

88 The conservative *Fox News* cable channel established itself as a channel for Trump's ideologies. Jane Mayer, "The Making of the Fox News White House." *The New Yorker* 11 (2019), https://newsliteracymatters.commons.gc.cuny.edu/wp-content/blogs.dir/8164/files/2019/08/The-Making-of-the-Fox-News-White-House-The-New-Yorker.pdf.

89 "American Views: Trust, Media and Democracy," *Gallup*.

90 Lauren Weber, Sudden Departure of White House Global Health Security Head Has Experts Worried," *The Atlantic*, May 10, 2018, https://www.huffpost.com/entry/tim-ziemer-global-health-security-leaves_n_5af37dfbe4b0859d11d02290.

91 Klaus Bruhn Jensen, "Humanistic Scholarship as Qualitative Science: Contributions to Mass Communication Research," In *A Handbook of Qualitative Methodologies for Mass Communication Research*, 17–43. Routledge, 2002.

92 Peter L. Berger, and Thomas Luckmann, *The Social Construction of Reality: A Treatise in the Sociology of Knowledge*, Anchor, 1967.

Chapter Two: Diffusion from Wuhan

1 "WHO-convened Global Study of Origins of SARS-CoV-2: China Part," *Joint WHO-China Study*, 14 January-10 February 2021, file:///C:/Users/ktabe/Downloads/Final-joint-report_origins-studies-6-April-201.pdf.

2 "WHO-convened Global Study of Origins of SARS-CoV-2: China Part," *Joint WHO-China Study*.

3 "WHO-convened Global Study of Origins of SARS-CoV-2: China Part," *Joint WHO-China Study*.

4 Everett M. Rogers, *Diffusion of Innovations*, Simon and Schuster, 2010, p. 5.

5 Rogers, *Diffusion of Innovations*.

6 Delbert C. Miller, "A Research Note on Mass Communication," *American Sociological Review* 10, no. 5 (1945): 691–94.

7 Miller, "A Research Note on Mass Communication."

8 Delbert C. Miller, "A Research Note on Mass Communication," *American Sociological Review* 10, no. 5 (1945): 691–94; Paul B. Sheatsley and Jacob J. Feldman, "The Assassination of President Kennedy: A Preliminary Report on Public Reactions and Behavior," *Public Opinion Quarterly* 28, no. 2 (1964): 189–215; M. L. DeFleur, The Growth and Decline of Research on the Diffusion of the News, 1945–1985. *Communication Research, 14*(1), 109–30; Michael E. Mayer, William B. Gudykunst, Norman K. Perrill, and Bruce D. Merrill, "A Comparison of Competing Models of the News Diffusion Process." *Western Journal of Communication (includes Communication Reports)* 54, no. 1 (1990): 113–23; Michael D. Basil and William J. Brown, "Interpersonal Communication in News Diffusion: A Study of "Magic" Johnson's Announcement," *Journalism Quarterly* 71, no. 2 (1994): 305–20.

9 Jooho Kim, Juhee Bae, and Makarand Hastak, "Emergency Information Diffusion

on Online Social Media During Storm Cindy in US," *International Journal of Information Management* 40 (2018): 153–65.

10 Foss, *Constructing the Outbreak.*

11 G. Eysenbach, "Infodemiology: Tracking Flu-Related Searches on the Web for Syndromic Surveillance," In: *AMIA Annual Symposium Proceedings.* American Medical Informatics Association, 2006, p. 244; Emily H. Chan, Vikram Sahai, Corrie Conrad, and John S. Brownstein, "Using Web Search Query Data to Monitor Dengue Epidemics: A New Model for Neglected Tropical Disease Surveillance," *Plos Neglected Tropical Diseases* 5, no. 5 (2011): e1206; Samantha Cook, Corrie Conrad, Ashley L. Fowlkes, and Matthew H. Mohebbi, "Assessing Google Flu Trends Performance in the United States During the 2009 Influenza Virus A (H1N1) Pandemic," *Plos One* 6, no. 8 (2011): e23610; Donald R. Olson, Kevin J. Konty, Marc Paladini, Cecile Viboud, and Lone Simonsen, "Reassessing Google Flu Trends Data for Detection of Seasonal and Pandemic Influenza: A Comparative Epidemiological Study at Three Geographic Scales," *Plos Computational Biology* 9, no. 10 (2013): e1003256.

12 Alessio Signorini, Alberto Maria Segre, and Philip M. Polgreen, "The Use of Twitter to Track Levels of Disease Activity and Public Concern in the US During the Influenza A H1N1 Pandemic," *Plos One* 6, no. 5 (2011): e19467; Andrews Chunara and Brownstein, "Social and News Media Enable Estimation of Epidemiological Patterns"; Sherry Towers, Shehzad Afzal, Gilbert Bernal, Nadya Bliss, Shala Brown, Baltazar Espinoza, Jasmine Jackson et al., "Mass Media and the Contagion of Fear: The Case of Ebola in America," *PloS One* 10, no. 6 (2015): e0129179.

13 Towers, Afzal, Bernal, Bliss, Brown, Espinoza, Jackson et al., "Mass Media and the Contagion of Fear."

14 Towers, Afzal, Bernal, Bliss, Brown, Espinoza, Jackson et al., "Mass Media and the Contagion of Fear"; Michelle Odlum, and Sunmoo Yoon, "Health Information Needs and Health Seeking Behavior During the 2014–2016 Ebola Outbreak: A Twitter Content Analysis," *PLoS currents* 10 (2018).

15 "Update 95—SARS: Chronology of a Serial Killer," WHO, July 4, 2003, https://www.who.int/csr/don/2003_07_04/en/.

16 "CDC SARS Response Timeline," *CDC*, April 26, 2013. CDC SARS Response Timeline | About | CDC; WHO, *Consensus document on the epidemiology of severe acute respiratory syndrome (SARS).* No. WHO/CDS/CSR/GAR/2003.11. WHO, 2003.

17 Peter Washer, "Representations of SARS in the British Newspapers," *Social Science & Medicine* 59, no. 12 (2004): 2561–571.

18 Eichelberger, "SARS and New York's Chinatown"; Patrick Wallis and Brigitte Nerlich, "Disease Metaphors in New Epidemics: The UK Media Framing of the 2003 SARS epidemic," *Social Science & Medicine* 60, no. 11 (2005): 2629–639.

19 "WHO-convened Global Study of Origins of SARS-CoV-2: China Part," *Joint WHO-China Study*, 14 January-10 February 2021, file:///C:/Users/ktabe/Downloads/Final-joint-report_origins-studies-6-April-201.pdf.

20 Wenjun Wang, Yikai Wang, Xin Zhang, Xiaoli Jia, Yaping Li, and Shuangsuo Dang, "Using WeChat, a Chinese Social Media App, for Early Detection of the COVID-19 Outbreak in December 2019: Retrospective Study," *JMIR mHealth and uHealth* 8, no. 10 (2020): e19589.

21 As quoted in "Xinhua Headlines: Chinese Doctor Recalls First Encounter with Mysterious Virus," *XinhuaNet*, April 16, 2020, http://www.xinhuanet.com/english/2020-04/16/c_138982435.htm.

22 Xixing Li, Weina Cui, and Fuzhen Zhang, "Who Was the First Doctor to Report the COVID-19 Outbreak in Wuhan, China?" *Journal of Nuclear Medicine* 61, no. 6 (2020): 782–83; Sudhvir Singh, Christine McNab, Rose McKeon Olson, Nellie Bristol, Cody Nolan, Elin Bergstrøm, Michael Bartos et al., "How An Outbreak Became a Pandemic: A Chronological Analysis of Crucial Junctures and International Obligations in the Early Months of the COVID-19 Pandemic," *The Lancet* 398, no. 10316 (2021): 2109–124.

23 Li, Cui, and Zhang, "Who Was the First Doctor to Report the COVID-19 Outbreak?"

24 "Chinese Doctor Recalls First Encounter with Mysterious Virus," *New China TV*, April 16, 2020, https://www.youtube.com/watch?v=tqXvmWk-1W8.

25 Chinese Doctor Recalls First Encounter with Mysterious Virus," *New China TV*.

26 Li, Cui, and Zhang, "Who Was the irst doctor to report the COVID-19 outbreak?"

27 "Circular on the Investigation of Dr. Li Wenliang's Situation Reported by the Masses," *CCTV News*, March 19, 2020, http://m.news.cctv.com/2020/03/19/ARTIrEO6nz5wKzeVnNlyBgTM200319.shtml.

28 "Circular on the Investigation of Dr. Li Wenliang's Situation," *CCTV News*.

29 Li, Cui, and Zhang. "Who was the First Doctor to Report the COVID-19 Outbreak?"

30 "Circular on the Investigation of Dr. Li Wenliang's Situation," *CCTV News*.

31 Andrew Green. "Li Wenliang," *The Lancet* 395, no. 10225 (2020): 682.

32 Green, "Li Wenliang"; "Circular on the Investigation of Dr. Li Wenliang's Situation," *CCTV News*.

33 https://news.ltn.com.tw/news/world/breakingnews/3025267.

34 Panda@DCheng36387164, (Translated from Chinese), "SARS/Suspected SARS outbreak in Wuhan, China," *Twitter*, December 30, 2019, http://tinyurl.com/mpnhndb2.

35 自由亚洲电台@RFA_Chinese【紧急通知】(Translated from Chinese), "emergency [*sic.*] notice] [Pneumonia of unknown cause appears in Wuhan] . . ." *Twitter*, December 30, 2019, https://twitter.com/RFA_Chinese/status/1211830443063922689.

36 Maryn McKenna, "How ProMed Crowdsourced the Arrival of COVID-19 and SARS," *Wired*, March 23, 2020, https://www.wired.com/story/how-promed-crowdsourced-the-arrival-of-covid-19-and-sars/.

37 McKenna, "How ProMed Crowdsourced the Arrival of COVID-19 and SARS."

38 "Undiagnosed Pneumonia," *ProMED*, December 30, 2019, https://promedmail.org/promed-post/?id=20191230.6864153.

39 "Undiagnosed Pneumonia," *ProMED*.

40 Singh, McNab, Olson, Bristol, Nolan, Bergstrøm, Bartos et al., "How An Outbreak Became a Pandemic."

41 "Wuhan Municipal Health Commission's Briefing on the Current Situation of Pneumonia in Our City," Wuhan Municipal Health Commission, December 31, 2019, https://web.archive.org/web/20200106064908/http://wjw.wuhan.gov.cn/front/web/showDetail/2019123108989.

42 Weng Ziquian, "Always Know | Sudden Unexplained Pneumonia? Don't Panic! All You Need to Know is Here," *RedNet.cn*, December 31, 2019, https://hn.rednet.cn/content/2019/12/31/6495266.html.

43 Viral Pneumonia Cases Reported in Central China." *The People's Daily*. December 31, 2019.

44 "Wuhan Patients with Unexplained Pneumonia and Their Onset Sites have been Isolated and Many Hospitals Hold a Special Meeting on Prevention and Treatment," *21st Century Business Herald 21*, December 31, 2019; Yuanzhou, Cheng, "27 Cases of Viral Pneumonia Found in Wuhan, 7 in Critical Condition," *The Beijing News*. December 31, 2019.

45 "Patients with Unknown Cause of Pneumonia," *ProMed*, December 31, 2019, https://promedmail.org/promed-post/?id=6864153.

46 https://www.info.gov.hk/gia/general/201912/31/P2019123100667.htm.

47 Mandy Zuo, Lilian Cheng, Alice Yan, and Cannix Yau, "Hong Kong Takes Emergency Measures as Mystery 'Pneumonia' Infects Dozens in China's Wuhan City," *South China Morning Post*, December 31, 2019, http://web.archive.org/web/20200201154848/https://www.scmp.com/news/china/politics/article/3044050/mystery-illness-hits-chinas-wuhan-city-nearly-30-hospitalised.

48 "WHO-convened Global Study of Origins of SARS-CoV-2: China Part," *Joint WHO-China Study*, 14 January-10 February 2021, file:///C:/Users/ktabe/Downloads/Final-joint-report_origins-studies-6-April-201.pdf.

49 "WHO-convened Global Study of Origins of SARS-CoV-2: China Part," *Joint WHO-China Study*.

50 "WHO-convened Global Study of Origins of SARS-CoV-2: China Part," *Joint WHO-China Study*.

51 "WHO-convened Global Study of Origins of SARS-CoV-2: China Part," *Joint WHO-China Study*.

52 "COVID-19 and China: A Chronology of Events (December 2019-January 2020)," *Congressional Research Service*, May 13, 2020, https://sgp.fas.org/crs/row/R46354.pdf.

53 Jane Dalton, "Mystery Illness in Chinese City Affects Nearly 30 People," *The Independent* (London, England), Jan. 1, 2020.

54 Dalton, "Mystery Illness in Chinese City Affects Nearly 30 People."

55 Associated Press, "Hong Kong Steps Up Response to Mystery Disease from China," *South China Morning Post*. January 3, 2020.

56 Associated Press, "Cases of Mystery Respiratory Illness in China Rise to 44," *Corpus Christi Caller Times* (Corpus Christi, TX), Jan. 4, 2020.

57 "Hong Kong Steps Up Response to Mystery Disease from China," *The Garden Island* (Lihue, Hawaii), Jan. 4, 2020.

58 "Disease Outbreak News" (DONs), WHO, https://www.who.int/emergencies/disease-outbreak-news.

59 WHO, "Pneumonia of Unknown Cause—China," *Disease Outbreak News*, (Jan. 5, 2020), https://www.who.int/emergencies/disease-outbreak-news/item/2020-DON229.

60 "Wuhan Municipal Health Commission's Briefing on Unexplained Viral Pneumonia," Wuhan Municipal Health Commission. January 5, 2020, http://wjw.wuhan.gov.cn/front/web/showDetail/2020010509020.

61 "Wuhan Municipal Health Commission's Briefing on Unexplained Viral Pneumonia." Wuhan Municipal Health Commission. January 5, 2020.

62 "Hong Kong Activates Serious Response Level for Infectious Disease," *People's Daily*, January 5, 2020.

63 "Mystery Illness Cases in China Numbers 44," *Fort Collins Coloradan*, January 4, 2020; "Mysterious lung infection stirs alert," *Atlanta Constitution* (Atlanta, GA), Jan. 5, 2020; "China Officials: Mysterious Illness isn't SARS," *Bellingham Herald*, Jan. 6, 2020.

64 Sui-Lee Wee and Vivian Wang, "China Grapples with Mystery Pneumonia-like Illness," *New York Times*. January 6, 2020, https://www.nytimes.com/2020/01/06/world/asia/china-SARS-pneumonialike.html?searchResultPosition=1.

65 Photo by Andy Wong.

66 "China Publishes Timeline on COVID-19 Information Sharing, Int'l Cooperation," Xinhua, April 6, 2020, http://www.xinhuanet.com/english/2020-04/06/c_138951662.htm; Fan Wu, Su Zhao, Bin Yu et al., "A New Coronavirus Associated with Human Respiratory Disease in China," *Nature*, February 3, 2020, https://www.nature.com/articles/s41586-020-2008-3.pdf.

67 Natasha Khan, "New Virus Discovered by Chinese Scientists Investigating Pneumonia Outbreak." *Wall Street Journal*. January 8, 2020.

68 "Undiagnosed Pneumonia—China (HU) (05): Novel Coronavirus Identified." *ProMed*, January 8, 2020, https://promedmail.org/promed-post/?id=6877694.

69 Xinhua News Agency, "Preliminary Progress in the Etiological Identification of the Unexplained Viral Pneumonia Epidemic in Wuhan," *CCTV*, January 9, 2020, http://news.cctv.com/2020/01/09/ARTIMxiGSClHAjC4B1Gy2VcP200109.shtml?spm=C94212.P4YnMod9m2uD.ENPMkWvfnaiV.102.

70 Zhuang Pinghui and Elizabeth Cheung, "China 'Must Find Source' After Identifying Wuhan Pneumonia as New Virus From SARS Family, *South China Morning Post*, January 9, 2020, https://www.scmp.com/news/china/society/article/3045288/china-confirms-new-coronavirus-it-investigates-mystery-wuhan?utm_content=article&utm_medium=Social&utm_source=Twitter#Echobox=1578538388.

71 Associated Press, "Chinese Report Says Illnesses May Be from New Coronavirus, *The Monitor*, January 9, 2020.
72 Gerry Shih and Lena H. Sun, "China Identifies New Strain of Coronavirus as Source of Pneumonia Outbreaks" *Washington Post*, January 9, 2020.
73 Gerry Shih, and Lena H. Sun, "Pneumonia Outbreak Tied to New Coronavirus Strain," *The Star Tribune* (Minneapolis, MN), Jan. 10, 2020.
74 Sakun Boon-Itt and Yukolpat Skunkan, "Public Perception of the COVID-19 Pandemic on Twitter: Sentiment Analysis and Topic Modeling Study," *JMIR Public Health and Surveillance* 6, no. 4 (2020): e21978.
75 CDC, "Outbreak of Pneumonia of Unknown Etiology (PUE) in Wuhan, China," *Health Alert Network*, Jan. 8, 2020, https://emergency.cdc.gov/han/HAN00424.asp.
76 CDC, "Outbreak of Pneumonia of Unknown Etiology (PUE) in Wuhan, China,"
77 CDC. "Outbreak of Pneumonia of Unknown Etiology (PUE) in Wuhan, China."
78 Yanan Wang, "China Working to Contain Outbreak of New Virus," *The Fresno Bee* (Fresno, CA), Jan. 10, 2020.
79 WHO, "WHO Advice for International Travel and Trade in Relation to the Outbreak of Pneumonia Caused by a New Coronavirus in China," *Newsroom*, Jan. 10, 2020, https://www.who.int/news-room/articles-detail/who-advice-for-international-travel-and-trade-in-relation-to-the-outbreak-of-pneumonia-caused-by-a-new-coronavirus-in-china/.
80 Zaheer Allam, "The First 50 Days of COVID-19: A Detailed Chronological Timeline and Extensive Review of Literature Documenting the Pandemic," *Surveying The COVID-19 Pandemic and Its Implications* (2020): 1.
81 "WHO Says No Clear Evidence of Human-to-Human Transmission of Novel Coronavirus," *The People's Daily*, January 15, 2020, https://web.archive.org/web/20200115230738/http://en.people.cn/n3/2020/0115/c90000-9648971.html.
82 "WHO Says No Clear Evidence," *The People's Daily*.
83 "Japan Confirms 1st Case of Pneumonia Linked to Coronavirus," *The People's Daily*, January 16, 2020.
84 https://cdc.gov/coronavirus/novel-coronavirus-2019.html.
85 https://twitter.com/MixedTheKid/status/1217612618447380485.
86 Dhivya Karmegam and Bagavandas Mapillairaju, "What People Share about the COVID-19 Outbreak on Twitter? An Exploratory Analysis," *BMJ Health & Care Informatics* 27, no. 3 (2020).
87 Lily Kuo, "China Confirms Human-to-Human Transmission of Coronavirus, *The Guardian*, January 19, 2020, https://www.theguardian.com/world/2020/jan/20/coronavirus-spreads-to-beijing-as-china-confirms-new-cases. "COVID-19 and China: A Chronology of Events (December 2019-January 2020), *Congressional Research Service*. May 13, 2020, https://sgp.fas.org/crs/row/R46354.pdf.
88 https://twitter.com/WHO/status/1219317208205209600.
89 Susan V Lawrence, "COVID-19 and China: A Chronology of Events (December

2019-January 2020)," *Congressional Research Service*, May 13, 2020; "All-out Efforts Ordered to Curb Spread of Virus," *The People's Daily*, January 21, 2020, https://web.archive.org/web/20200121173830/http://en.people.cn/n3/2020/0121/c90000-9650576.html

90 "First Travel-related Case of 2019 Novel Coronavirus Detected in the United States," *CDC Newsroom Releases*, January 21, 2020, https://www.cdc.gov/media/releases/2020/p0121-novel-coronavirus-travel-case.html.

91 See https://twitter.com/CDCgov/status/1219725632906694663.

92 https://twitter.com/CDCgov/status/1219725632906694663.

93 Matthew J. Belvedere, "Trump Says He Trusts China's Xi on Coronavirus and the US Has It 'Totally Under Control,'" *CNBC*, January 22, 2020, https://www.cnbc.com/2020/01/22/trump-on-coronavirus-from-china-we-have-it-totally-under-control.html.

94 Charles F. Parker and Eric K. Stern, "The Trump Administration and the COVID-19 Crisis: Exploring the Warning-Response Problems and Missed Opportunities of a Public Health Emergency," *Public Administration* (2022).

95 Associated Press, "Virus Hits Travel and Lodging Industries Hard," *The Olympian*, January 22, 2020.

96 WHO, "WHO Director-General's Statement on the Advice of the IHR Emergency Committee on Novel Coronavirus," *Detail*, Jan. 23, 2020, https://www.who.int/director-general/speeches/detail/who-director-general-s-statement-on-the-advice-of-the-ihr-emergency-committee-on-novel-coronavirus.

97 WHO, "WHO Director-General's Statement."

98 CDC, "Second Travel-related Case of 2019 Novel Coronavirus Detected in the United States," *CDC Newsroom Releases*, Jan. 24, 2020, https://www.cdc.gov/media/releases/2020/p0124-second-travel-coronavirus.html; Reuters Staff, "In his own words: Trump and the coronavirus," *Reuters*, October 2, 2020, https://www.reuters.com/article/health-coronavirus-usa-trump-comments-ti/in-his-own-words-trump-and-the-coronavirus-idUSKBN26N0U7.

99 Jacopo Cerri, Emiliano Mori, Leonardo Ancillotto, Danilo Russo, and Sandro Bertolino, "COVID-19, Media Coverage of Bats and Related Web Searches: A Turning Point for Bat Conservation?," *Mammal Review* 52, no. 1 (2022): 16–25.

100 Cerri, Mori, Ancillotto, Russo, and Bertolino, "COVID-19, Media Coverage of Bats and Related Web Searches."

101 Fatemeh Tahmasbi, Leonard Schild, Chen Ling, Jeremy Blackburn, Gianluca Stringhini, Yang Zhang, and Savvas Zannettou, "'Go eat a bat, Chang!': On the Emergence of Sinophobic Behavior on Web Communities in the Face of COVID-19," In *Proceedings of the Web Conference 2021*, 1122–133.

102 WHO, "Novel Coronavirus (2019-nCOV) Situation Report-5," Jan. 25, https://www.who.int/docs/default-source/coronaviruse/situation-reports/20200125-sitrep-5-2019-ncov.pdf.

103 WHO, "Novel Coronavirus (2019-nCOV) Situation Report-6," Jan. 26, https://www.who.int/docs/default-source/coronaviruse/situation-reports/20200126-sitrep-6-2019--ncov.pdf.

104 WHO, "Novel Coronavirus (2019-nCOV) Situation Report-8," Jan. 28, https://www.who.int/docs/default-source/coronaviruse/situation-reports/20200128-sitrep-8-ncov-cleared.pdf.

105 CDC, "HHS and CDC Supporting Safe, Expedient Departure of US Citizens," *CDC Newsroom Releases*, Jan. 28, 2020, https://www.cdc.gov/media/releases/2020/s0128-wuhan-departure.html.

106 CDC, "CDC Confirms Person-to-Person Spread of New Coronavirus in the United States." *CDC Newsroom Releases*, Jan. 30, 2020, https://www.cdc.gov/media/releases/2020/p0130-coronavirus-spread.html.

107 "Novel Coronavirus (2019-nCOV) Situation Report—10," WHO, January 30, 2020, https://www.who.int/docs/default-source/coronaviruse/situation-reports/20200130-sitrep-10-ncov.pdf?sfvrsn=d0b2e480_2.

108 "Novel Coronavirus (2019-nCOV) Situation Report—10," WHO, January 30, 2020, https://www.who.int/docs/default-source/coronaviruse/situation-reports/20200130-sitrep-10-ncov.pdf?sfvrsn=d0b2e480_2.

109 Helen Regen, Jessie Yeung, Steve George, and Fernando Alfonso, "January 31 Coronavirus News," *CNN*, February 4, 2020, https://www.cnn.com/asia/live-news/coronavirus-outbreak-01-31-20-intl-hnk/index.html.

110 James Griffiths and Amy Woodyatt, "China Goes into Emergency Mode as Number of Confirmed Wuhan Coronavirus Cases Reaches 2,700," *CNN*, January 27, 2020, https://www.cnn.com/2020/01/26/asia/wuhan-coronavirus-update-intl-hnk/index.html.

111 "Public Facilities to Close in Virus Fight," *News.gov.hk*, January 28, 2020, https://www.news.gov.hk/eng/2020/01/20200128/20200128_130523_425.html; "Gov't Staff to Work From Home," *News.gov.hk*, January 28, 2020, https://www.news.gov.hk/eng/2020/01/20200128/20200128_114401_545.html.

112 Caroline Kantis, Samantha Kiernan, Jason Socrates Bardi, and Lillian Posner, "Updated: Timeline of the Coronavirus," *Think Global Health*, https://www.thinkglobalhealth.org/article/updated-timeline-coronavirus.

113 Laura Stanthanam, "Most Americans Think Novel Coronavirus is a Real Threat, Poll Says," *PBS*, February 4, 2020, https://www.pbs.org/newshour/health/most-americans-think-novel-coronavirus-is-a-real-threat-poll-says.

114 Stanthanam, "Most Americans Think Novel Coronavirus is a Real Threat."

115 "Virus," *Google Trends*, https://trends.google.com/trends/explore?date=2020-01-01percent202020-02-02&geo=US&q=virus.

116 Lawrence, "COVID-19 and China: A Chronology of Events."

117 Lawrence, "COVID-19 and China: A Chronology of Events."

118 Keir Simmons, Jennifer Jett, Amy Perrette, and Elizabeth Kuhr, "A Reporter Risked Her Life to Show the World Covid in Wuhan. Now She May Not Survive Jail, *NBC*

News, December 18, 2021, https://www.nbcnews.com/news/china/reporter-zhang-zhan-risked-life-show-world-covid-wuhan-now-may-not-sur-rcna9212.

119 Aravind Sesagiri Raamkumar, Soon Guan Tan, and Hwee Lin Wee. "Measuring the Outreach Efforts of Public Health Authorities and The Public Response on Facebook During the COVID-19 Pandemic in Early 2020: Cross-Country Comparison," *Journal of Medical Internet Research* 22, no. 5 (2020): e19334.

120 Priyanka Khatri, Shweta R. Singh, Neeta Kesu Belani, Yin Leng Yeong, Rahul Lohan, Yee Wei Lim, and Winnie ZY Teo, "YouTube as Source of Information on 2019 Novel Coronavirus Outbreak: A Cross-Sectional Study of English and Mandarin Content," *Travel Medicine and Infectious Disease* 35 (2020): 101636; Qiang Chen, Chen Min, Wei Zhang, Xiaoyue Ma, and Richard Evans, "Factors Driving Citizen Engagement with Government Tiktok Accounts During the COVID-19 Pandemic: Model Development and Analysis," *Journal of Medical Internet Research* 23, no. 2 (2021): e21463.

121 Daniel A. González-Padilla, and Leonardo Tortolero-Blanco, "Social Media Influence in the COVID-19 Pandemic," *International Brazilian Journal of Urology* 46 (2020): 120–24; Jessica Guynn, "Coronavirus Outbreak: Social Media Platforms Scramble to Contain Misinformation," *TechXplore*, January 31, 2020, https://techxplore.com/news/2020-01-coronavirus-outbreak-social-media-platforms.html.

122 Dhivya Karmegam and Bagavandas Mapillairaju, "What People Share About the COVID-19 Outbreak on Twitter? An Exploratory Analysis," *BMJ Health & Care Informatics* 27, no. 3 (2020); Philip D. Waggoner, "Community Detection in Google Searches Related to 'Coronavirus,'" *Journal of Data Science* 19, no. 2 (2021): 334–47.

123 Jacopo Cerri, Emiliano Mori, Leonardo Ancillotto, Danilo Russo, and Sandro Bertolino. "COVID-19, Media Coverage of Bats and Related Web Searches: A Turning Point for Bat Conservation?," *Mammal Review* 52, no. 1 (2022): 16–25.

124 "WHO-convened Global Study of Origins of SARS-CoV-2: China Part," *Joint WHO-China Study*, 14 January-10 February 2021, file:///C:/Users/ktabe/Downloads/Final-joint-report_origins-studies-6-April-201.pdf.

125 "WHO Coronavirus (COVID-19) Dashboard." WHO.

Chapter Three: "Like Sitting Ducks"

1 David Abel, "Diamond Dave and Princess Sally. Diamond Princess cruise. Quarantine. Yokohama. Video 3." *YouTube*. February 14, 2020. First appeared on *Facebook Live*, https://www.youtube.com/watch?v=Var8Pmlsk_s&t=13s.

2 Leah F. Moriarty, Mateusz M. Plucinski, Barbara J. Marston, Ekaterina V. Kurbatova, Barbara Knust, Erin L. Murray, Nicki Pesik et al., "Public Health Responses to COVID-19 Outbreaks on Cruise Ships—Worldwide, February–March 2020," *Morbidity and Mortality Weekly Report* 69, no. 12 (2020): 347.

3 Kevin Brown, *Poxed and Scurvied: The Story of Sickness & Health at Sea*. Seaforth Publishing, 2011.

4 Brown, *Poxed and Scurvied.*

5 Brown, *Poxed and Scurvied*; Vivian Nutton, "Medicine in Medieval Western Europe, 1000–1500," in *The Western Medical Tradition: 800 BC to AD 1800*, edited by Lawrence I. Conrad, Michael Neve, Vivian Nutton, Roy Porter and Andrew Wear, Cambridge University Press, 139–98, 1995.

6 Mark Harrison, *Disease and the Modern World: 1500 to the Present Day* (John Wiley & Sons, 2013).

7 Brown, *Poxed and Scurvied.*

8 Brown, *Poxed and Scurvied.*

9 Brown, *Poxed and Scurvied*; Kraut, *Silent Travelers.*

10 "Transport News and Notes. Atlantic Ship Passenger Drop Shown as Airline Use Increased in 1959," *New York Times*, January 9, 1960; Patsy Morgan and Lisa Power. "Cruise Tourism and the Cruise Industry," In *Research Themes for Tourism*, edited by Peter Robinson, Sine Heitmann, and Peter U. C. Dieke, 276–300, CABI.

11 Travis W. Heggie and Tracey Burton-Heggie, "Death at Sea: Passenger and Crew Mortality on Cruise Ships," *International Journal of Travel Medicine and Global Health* 8, no. 4 (2020): 146–51.

12 Heggie and Burton-Heggie, "Death at Sea: Passenger and Crew Mortality on Cruise Ships."

13 Heggie and Burton-Heggie, "Death at Sea: Passenger and Crew Mortality on Cruise Ships."

14 Heggie and Burton-Heggie, "Death at Sea: Passenger and Crew Mortality on Cruise Ships"; "2020 State of the Cruise Industry Outlook," Cruise Lines International Association (CLIA), https://cruising.org/-/media/research-updates/research/state-of-the-cruise-industry.ashx.

15 Arézou Minooee and Leland S. Rickman, "Infectious Diseases on Cruise Ships," *Clinical Infectious Diseases* 29, no. 4 (1999): 737–43.

16 Minooee and Rickman, "Infectious Diseases on Cruise Ships."

17 "Operational Safety," *Cruise Industry Policies*, Cruise Lines International Association, 2022, https://cruising.org/en/about-the-industry/policy-priorities/cruise-industry-regulation.

18 "Cruise Industry Regulation," *Policy Priorities.*

19 "About the Vessel Sanitation Program," CDC. August 29, 2019, https://www.cdc.gov/nceh/vsp/desc/aboutvsp.htm.

20 Nan Zhang, Ruosong Miao, Hong Huang, and Emily YY Chan, "Contact Infection of Infectious Disease Onboard a Cruise Ship," *Scientific Reports* 6, no. 1 (2016): 1–13.

21 Helen Regen, Jessie Yeung, Steve George, and Fernando Alfonso, "January 31 Coronavirus News," *CNN*, February 4, 2020, https://www.cnn.com/asia/live-news/coronavirus-outbreak-01-31-20-intl-hnk/index.html.

22 "Novel Coronavirus (2019-nCOV) Situation Report—10," WHO, January 30, 2020, https://www.who.int/docs/default-source/coronaviruse/situation-reports/20200130-sitrep-10-ncov.pdf?sfvrsn=d0b2e480_2.

23 Associated Press, "Virus Hits Travel and Lodging Industries Hard," *The Olympian*, 22 January 2020 (and other newspapers); Patti Domm, "New China Virus Spooks Global Markets but Analysts Say It May Not Be As Bad as SARS," *CNBC*, January 21, 2020, https://www.cnbc.com/2020/01/21/new-china-virus-spooks-global-markets-but-analysts-say-it-may-not-be-as-bad-as-sars.html.

24 Anne Kalosh, "China's Coronavirus Outbreak Will Be Something to Closely Monitor as It Relates to the Cruise Industry But at Present is Not Likely to be a Material Headwind, Wells Fargo Securities Said in a Note," *Seatrade Cruise News*, January 21, 2020, https://www.seatrade-cruise.com/news/coronavirus-not-currently-seen-significant-cruise-threat.

25 Michael Juliano, "Coronavirus 'Not Likely a Material Headwind' for Cruise," *TradeWinds*, January 21, 2020, https://www.tradewindsnews.com/cruise-and-ferry/coronavirus-not-likely-a-material-headwind-for-cruise/2-1-741797.

26 Olivia Sharpe, "China Virus Latest: Is It Safe to Travel to China?" *World of Cruising*, January 22, 2020, https://www.worldofcruising.co.uk/cruise-news/coronavirus-china-travel-safe-advice-cruise.

27 Teresa Ooi, "Coronavirus—How to Avoid the Disease That Has 4,500," *Cruise Passenger*, January 25, 2020, https://cruisepassenger.com.au/news/cortonavirus-cruise-lines-are-best-equipped-to-tackle-risk/.

28 "Cruise Lines Race to React to Coronavirus," *Cruise Industry News*, January 22, 2020, https://www.cruiseindustrynews.com/cruise-news/22301-cruise-lines-race-to-react-to-coronavirus.html.

29 "Cruise Lines Increase Passenger Screening After Coronavirus Outbreak," *Ship Technology*, January 23, 2020, https://www.ship-technology.com/news/cruise-lines-passenger-screening-coronavirus-outbreak/.

30 Rob Gill, "Coronavirus: Operators and Cruise Lines Take Action Over Outbreak," *Travel Trade Gazette*, January 23, 2020, https://www.ttgmedia.com/news/coronavirus-operators-and-cruise-lines-take-action-over-outbreak-20981.

31 Mikhail Voytenko, "Major Cruise Lines Banning Tourists from Wuhan and Hebei, to Prevent Coronavirus," *Maritime Bulletin*, January 24, 2020, http://www.maritimebulletin.net/2020/01/24/major-cruise-lines-banning-tourists-from-wuhan-and-hebei-to-prevent-coronavirus/.

32 "Cruise Lines Act on Coronavirus Risk," *The Maritime Executive*, January 26, 2020, https://maritime-executive.com/article/cruise-lines-act-on-coronavirus-risk.

33 R. Ali, Royal Caribbean, MSC, others cancel China Cruises Due to Coronavirus Outbreak." *USA Today*, January 26, 2020, https://www.usatoday.com/story/travel/cruises/2020/01/26/coronavirus-outbreak-royal-caribbean-msc-cruises-canceled-china/4581361002/.

34 Harriet Mallinson, "Coronavirus: Major Cruise Lines Cancel Multiple Cruises as

Virus Spreads—41 Dead. *Daily Express*, January 27, 2020, https://www.express.co.uk/travel/cruise/1233695/coronavirus-cruise-cancelled-cruises-china-royal-caribbean-msc-news-latest.

35 Cortney Moore, "Cruise Lines Suspend China Operations Amid Coronavirus Outbreak," *Fox Business*, January 26, 2020, https://www.foxbusiness.com/lifestyle/cruise-lines-china-coronavirus.

36 "Coronavirus Fallout: Luxury Cruise with More Than 5,000 Onboard Quarantined in Shenzhen," *Hindustan Times*, January 27, 2020, https://www.hindustantimes.com/world-news/coronavirus-fallout-luxury-cruise-with-more-than-5000-onboard-quarantined-in-shenzhen/story-ZJYx3dCA6VjsyP9zngvR8O.html.

37 Mikhail Voytenko, "Some 5,000 Cruise Passengers and 1,200 Crew Screened for Coronavirus, 148 Isolated. *Maritime Bulletin*, January 26, 2020, http://www.maritimebulletin.net/2020/01/26/some-5000-cruise-passengers-and-1200-crew-screened-for-coronavirus-148-isolated/.

38 "We Received the Following Message . . ." *Crew Center Facebook* group, Shared on *Twitter*, February 6, 2020, https://m.facebook.com/story.php?story_fbid=2684951171583066&id=221802457897962.

39 "We Received the Following Message . . ." *Crew Center Facebook* group.

40 Frédérick Auvray, "Coronavirus Crisis Freezes Cruises in China," *Le Marin*, January 28, 2020, https://lemarin.ouest-france.fr/secteurs-activites/shipping/35861-la-crise-du-coronavirus-gele-la-croisiere-en-chine?sfns=mo.

41 "Multiple Cruise Lines Suspend Chinese Sailings. *Cruise Industry News*. January 25, 2020, https://www.cruiseindustrynews.com/cruise-news/22321-multiple-cruise-lines-suspend-chinese-sailings.html.

42 Joanna Rose Aglibot, "No Stopping of Cruise Ships' Arrival in Subic Amid Coronavirus Alert," *The Philippines Daily Inquirer*, January 24, 2020, https://newsinfo.inquirer.net/1219127/no-stopping-of-cruise-ships-arrival-in-subic-amid-coronavirus-alert?utm_source=dlvr.it&utm_medium=twitter.

43 "In a Good Position: CLIA," *Cruise Weekly*, January 24, 2020, https://www.cruiseweekly.com.au/trade-issue-thursday/cw-for-fri-24-jan-2020/61466.

44 "In a Good Position: CLIA," *Cruise Weekly*.

45 Orlando Martinez, "Timeline: 2020–2021 Cruise Industry Shutdown," *CruiseRadio.Net*, September 2, 2021, https://cruiseradio.net/timeline-2020-cruise-ship-industry-shutdown/.

46 Helen Regen, Jessie Yeung, Steve George, and Fernando Alfonso, "January 31 Coronavirus News," *CNN*, February 4, 2020, https://www.cnn.com/asia/live-news/coronavirus-outbreak-01-31-20-intl-hnk/index.html.

47 Takuya Yamagishi, Hajime Kamiya, Kensaku Kakimoto, Motoi Suzuki, and Takaji Wakita, "Descriptive Study of COVID-19 Outbreak Among Passengers and Crew on Diamond Princess Cruise Ship, Yokohama Port, Japan, 20 January to 9 February 2020." *Eurosurveillance* 25, no. 23 (2020): 2000272.

48 Yamagishi, Kamiya, Kakimoto, and Wakita, "Descriptive Study of COVID-19

Outbreak Among Passengers and Crew"; "Early Spring Southeast Asia Voyage 16 Days," *Princess Cruises*, Retrieved on July 11, 2022, https://web.archive.org/web/20180725003613/https://www.princesscruises.jp/voyage/M003/.

49 Yamagishi, Kamiya, Kakimoto, Suzuki, and Wakita, "Descriptive Study of COVID-19 Outbreak Among Passengers and Crew."

50 Yamagishi, Kamiya, Kakimoto, Suzuki, and Wakita, "Descriptive Study of COVID-19 Outbreak Among Passengers and Crew."

51 Anne Kalosh, "Diamond Princess Held in Yokohama on Coronavirus Precaution." *Seatrade Cruise News*. February 3, 2020, https://www.seatrade-cruise.com/news/diamond-princess-held-yokohama-coronavirus-precaution.

52 Yamagishi, Kamiya, Kakimoto, Suzuki, and Wakita, Descriptive Study of COVID-19 Outbreak Among Passengers and Crew."

53 "Captain's Announcement—New Cases Confirmed," *Diamond Princess—M002A & M003*, February 6, 2020.

54 "Diamond Princess Cruise Ship," *Princess*, 2022, https://www.princess.com/ships-and-experience/ships/di-diamond-princess/.

55 "Diamond Princess Oceanview Stateroom," *Princess Cruises*, https://www.princess.com/html/global/popups/metas/di/di_oceanview.html.

56 "Diamond Princess Balcony Stateroom," *Princess Cruises*, https://www.princess.com/html/global/popups/metas/di/di_balcony.html.

57 "Diamond Princess: Grand Suite with Balcony," *Princess Cruises*, https://www.princess.com/html/global/book/ships/di/submeta/S1/.

58 "Early Spring Southeast Asia Voyage 16 Days," *Princess Cruises*, Retrieved on July 11, 2022, https://web.archive.org/web/20180725003613/https://www.princesscruises.jp/voyage/M003/.

59 Yamagishi, Kamiya, Kakimoto, Suzuki, and Wakita, Descriptive Study of COVID-19 Outbreak Among Passengers and Crew."

60 Yamagishi, Kamiya, Kakimoto, Suzuki, and Wakita, Descriptive Study of COVID-19 Outbreak Among Passengers and Crew."

61 Hillary Leung, "Inside Life on the Crew Decks on Coronavirus-stricken Diamond Princess Cruise Ship," *Time*, February 17, 2020, https://time.com/5784190/diamond-princess-cruise-crew-coronavirus/.

62 Mateusz M. Plucinski, Megan Wallace, Anna Uehara, Ekaterina V. Kurbatova, Farrell A. Tobolowsky, Zachary D. Schneider, Atsuyoshi Ishizumi et al., "Coronavirus disease 2019 (COVID-19) in Americans aboard the Diamond Princess Cruise Ship," *Clinical Infectious Diseases* 72, no. 10 (2021): e448-e457.

63 Kenji Mizumoto and Gerardo Chowell, "Transmission Potential of the Novel Coronavirus (COVID-19) Onboard the Diamond Princess Cruises Ship, 2020," *Infectious Disease Modelling* 5 (2020): 264–70. Hillary Leung, "Inside Life on the Crew Decks on Coronavirus-stricken Diamond Princess Cruise Ship," *Time*, February 17, 2020, https://time.com/5784190/diamond-princess-cruise-crew-coronavirus/.

64 "Japan Quarantines 3,500 on Cruise Ship Diamond Princess Over Coronavirus," *Kyodo News*, February 4, 2020, https://english.kyodonews.net/news/2020/02/084cd1b786d8-abe-says-japan-developing-rapid-test-kit-for-new-coronavirus.html; Hannah Yasharoff, "Coronavirus: Princess Cruise to Stay Under Quarantine After 10 More Passengers Test Positive," *USA Today*, February 4, 2020, https://www.usatoday.com/story/travel/news/2020/02/04/coronavirus-diamond-princess-cruise-quarantined-passenger-diagnosed/4625907002/; "As China Clamps Down on Negative News, Quarantines on Land and Sea." *New York Times*, February 5, 2020.

65 "Captain's Announcement." *Diamond Princess—Voyages M002A & M003. Princess Cruises*, February 9, 2020.

66 "Update from President Jan Swarz." *Princess Cruises, YouTube*, February 8, 2020, https://www.youtube.com/watch?v=PbFpEuTaZRE.

67 "Message to U.S. Citizen Diamond Princess Passengers," Message from U.S. Embassy Tokyo—February 6, email, February, 6, 2020.

68 Excerpt from a letter from the CDC to passengers and crew aboard the Diamond Princess, February 8, 2020, https://www.princess.com/news/pdfs/alert-cdc-letter-for-diamond-princess.pdf.

69 Associated Press, "Japan Quarantines Cruise Ship as Toll of New Virus Grows," *The Whitehorse Daily Star*, February 5, 2020.

70 Associated Press, "China Opens Virus Hospital, Market Plunges as Toll Grows," *The Whitehorse Daily Star*, February 3, 2020; Ryan Tumilty and Sharon Kirkey, "Canada to Expats: Leave China," *The Leader-Post*. February 6, 2020; Dee-Ann Durbin, "Global Tourism Takes Hit Amid Virus Outbreak," *The News-Press*, February 9, 2020; Nicholas Cecil and Ross Lydall, "Emergency Powers to Stop Fatal Virus Spreading," *Evening Standard*, February 10, 2020.

71 Doug Stanglin and Charles Ventura, "Death of US Citizen First to be Linked with Virus," *USA Today*, February 9, 2020.

72 Stephen Prescott, "Wuhan Coronavirus and the History of Quarantines," *The Daily Oklahoman Sun*, February 9, 2020.

73 Eric Cheung, "This is Where Coronavirus Cases Have Been Confirmed Worldwide," *CNN*, February 10, 2020, https://www.cnn.com/asia/live-news/coronavirus-outbreak-02-10-20-intl-hnk/h_4c3787a6b61756d91d1be00c321d2d9a.

74 Ken Moritsugu and Mari Yamaguchi, "Chinese Leaders Face Public Anger Over Virus," *USA Today*, February 8, 2020; Joe McDonald, "Virus Cases Surge in China," Associated Press, *Philadelphia Inquirer*, February 10, 2020; Associated Press, "China Mostly Closed Down as Virus Deaths Pass 1,000," *The Marshall News Messenger*, February 12, 2020.

75 Ryan W. Miller, and Grace Hauck, "Pangolins May Have Spread Coronavirus to Humans: What to Know," *USA Today*, February 7, 2020, https://www.usatoday.com/story/news/health/2020/02/07/coronavirus-pangolin-virus-host-who-virus-update-friday/4688785002/.

76 Mychel Matthews, "Buhl Man on Coronavirus Quarantined Cruise Ship in Tokyo," *The Idaho Statesmen*, February 10, 2020.

77 Mark Ladao, "6 Hawaii Residents on Ship Quarantined," *Honolulu Star Advertiser*, February 5, 2020; Joanne Lee-Young, "Concern Grows for Canadians on Cruise Ship," *Vancouver Sun*. February 6, 2020; Lora Grindlay, "B.C. Couple Under 'Cabin Arrest,'" *Calgary Herald*, February 8, 2020; Annette Cary, "Richland Couple Quarantined on Cruise Ship in Japan," *Tri-City Herald*, February 14, 2020; Rolf Boone, "Olympia Woman Now Stuck on Quarantined Cruise Ship in Japan," *The News Tribune*, February 12, 2020; Langston Taylor, "Citrus County Residents Quarantined in Japan," *Tampa Bay Times*, February 9, 2020; Lindsey Holden, "Coronavirus Quarantine Traps Paso Robles Woman," *The Tribune*, February 12, 2020; Lora Grindlay. "B.C. Couple Under 'Cabin Arrest,'" *Calgary Herald*, February 8, 2020.

78 Grindlay, Lora. "Coronavirus Threat Strands B.C. Couple." *The Province Sun*. February 9, 2020.

79 Rich, Motoko and Yamamitsu, Eimi. "Jump in Coronavirus Cases on Ship Poses a Critical Test for Japan." *New York Times*. February 7, 2020.

80 Dubé, Jacob. "Quarantined Passengers Under 'Cabin Arrest." *National Post*. February 7, 2020.

81 Associated Press. "Fear, Boredom, Adventure Fill Days of Passengers, Crew." Printed in *Marshall News Messenger* and other outlets. February 14, 2020.

82 Gay Coulter, "Our Cruise Ship was Quarantined for Coronavirus. It's Been 9 Days of Surrealism," *Washington Post*, February 14, 2020, https://www.washingtonpost.com/opinions/2020/02/14/coronavirus-dispatch-life-quarantined-cruise-ship-is-like-groundhog-day/.

83 Spencer Fehrenbacher, "American Quarantined on the Diamond Princess: The Worst is Over, Let's Choose Optimism," *USA Today*, February 15, 2020, https://www.usatoday.com/story/opinion/2020/02/15/americans-quarantined-diamond-princess-coronavirus-column/4763240002/.

84 Ben Dooley and Motoko Rich, "Cruise Ship's Coronavirus Outbreak Leaves Crew Nowhere to Hide," *New York Times*, February 10, 2020.

85 Dooley and Motoko, "Cruise Ship's Coronavirus Outbreak Leaves Crew Nowhere to Hide."

86 "Captain's Announcement," *Diamond Princess—Voyages M002A & M003*. *Princess Cruises*, February 13, 2020.

87 "Captain's Announcement," *Diamond Princess—Voyages*.

88 Helena Oliviero, "Virus Derails Cruise for Local Couple," *The Atlanta Constitution*, February 13, 2020.

89 Ken Moritsugu and Mari Yamaguchi, "Japan Finds 41 More Cases on Ship," Associated Press, Printed in *Daily Hampshire Gazette*, February 7, 2020.

90 Associated Press, "Virus Cases Increase As More Preventive Measures Taken," *Sun-Journal*, February 9, 2020; Motoko Rich and Eimi Yamamitsu, "Trapped on Ship, Anxiety Runs High," *New York Times*, February 10, 2020.

91 Yamagishi, Kamiya, Kakimoto, Suzuki, and Wakita, "Descriptive Study of COVID-19 Outbreak Among Passengers and Crew."

92 Jamey Keaten and Maria Cheng, "Experts Meet to Fight Coronavirus," Associated Press, *The Montana Standard.* February 12, 2020; Mari Yamaguchi, "44 More Cases of Virus on Ship," Associated Press, *The Daily Sentinel.* February 13, 2020.

93 "Message to U.S. Citizen Diamond Princess Passengers," Message from U.S. Embassy Tokyo—February 12, email, February, 12, 2020.

94 Taylor Dolven, "How Quarantined Cruise Passengers Got Medications," *The Miami Herald*, February 16, 2020.

95 Motoko Rich, and Eimi Yamamitsu, "As Virus Cases Rise on Quarantined Cruise Ship, Passengers are on Edge," *New York Times*, February 9, 2020.

96 Motoko Rich, "As Passenger Angst Grows, Japan to Let Some Off Ship, but Fewer Than Hoped," *New York Times*, February 13, 2020.

97 Aaron Derfel, "'Get Us Out of Here,' Scared Montreal Couple Pleads," *The Gazette* (Montreal), February 13, 2020.

98 Derfel, "'Get Us Out of Here.'"

99 Editorial Board. "Coronavirus Cruise Ship: Evacuate the More Than 400 American Passengers Home," *USA Today*, February 11, 2020.

100 Editorial Board, "Coronavirus Cruise Ship: Evacuate the More Than 400 American Passengers Home."

101 State Department's Bureau of Consular Affairs, "State Department: We Do Not Anticipate Staging New Coronavirus Evacuations at This Time," *USA Today*, February 12, 2020.

102 Jamey Keaten and Maria Cheng, "Experts Meet to Fight Coronavirus"; Associated Press, *The Montana Standard.* February 12, 2020.

103 Excerpt from a letter from the CDC to passengers and crew aboard the Diamond Princess. February 12, 2020, https://www.princess.com/news/pdfs/cdc-letter-diamond-princess-021220.pdf.

104 "Diamond Princess Repatriation," *CDC Newsroom*, CDC, February 15, 2020, https://www.cdc.gov/media/releases/2020/s0215-Diamond-Princess-Repatriation.html.

105 Benjy Egel, "Americans on Coronavirus Cruise Will Ship to Travis AFB," *Sacramento Bee*, February 16, 2020.

106 Motoko Rich and Edward Wong, "They Escaped an Infected Ship, But the Flight Home Was No Haven," *New York Times*, February 17, 2020. Lena H. Sun, Lenny Bernstein, Shibani Mahtani, and Joel Achenbach, "Coronavirus-infected Americans Flown Home Against CDC's Advice," *Washington Post*, February 20, 2020, https://www.washingtonpost.com/health/coronavirus-diamond-princess-cruise-americans/2020/02/20/b6f54cae-5279-11ea-b119-4faabac6674f_story.html.

107 David Oliver, "Fauci: Cruise Ship Quarantine Failed," *USA Today*, February 18, 2020.

108 Hanako Jimi and Gaku Hashimoto, "Challenges of COVID-19 Outbreak on

the Cruise Ship Diamond Princess Docked at Yokohama, Japan: a Real-World Story," *Global Health & Medicine* (2020).

109 Yu-Ching Chou, Yu-Ju Lin, Shian-Sen Shie, Hung-Bin Tsai, and Wang-Huei Sheng, "A Major Outbreak of COVID-19 in the Diamond Princess Cruise Ship," *Research Square* (2020).

110 "Princess Cruises Announces a Voluntary and Temporary Pause of Global Operations (60 Days)," *Princess*, March 12, 2020, https://www.princess.com/news/news_releases/2020/03/princess-cruises-announces-a-voluntary-and-temporary-pause.html.

111 Hannah Sampson, "HBO Documentary Highlights Agony of Diamond Princess Crew," *Washington Post*. April 1, 2021, https://www.washingtonpost.com/travel/2021/04/01/diamond-princess-hbo-documentary-covid/.

112 Tudor A. Codreanu, Sera Ngeh, Abigail Trewin, and Paul K. Armstrong, "Successful Control of an Onboard COVID-19 Outbreak Using the Cruise Ship as a Quarantine Facility, Western Australia, Australia," *Emerging Infectious Diseases* 27, no. 5 (2021): 1279.

113 Codreanu, Ngeh, Trewin, and Armstrong. "Successful Control of an Onboard COVID-19 Outbreak."

Chapter Four: "Essential" or Sheltered in Place?

1 Uber's slogan for its Spring 2020 campaign. Ann-Christine Diaz, "Uber Thanks People For Not Riding with Uber," *AdAge*, April 10, 2020, https://adage.com/creativity/work/uber-thank-you-not-riding/2249401.

2 Nicole Winfield, "Many Failures Combined to Unleash Death on Italy's Lombardy," *AP News*, April 26, 2020, https://apnews.com/article/health-ap-top-news-rome-international-news-virus-outbreak-de2794327607a3a67ed551f0b6b71404.

3 "Trends in Number of COVID-19 Cases and Deaths in the US Reported to CDC, by State/Territory," *COVID Data Tracker*, CDC, https://covid.cdc.gov/covid-data-tracker/#trends_totalcases_select_00.

4 Mike Snider, "Coronavirus Concerns Lead to Hoarding, Panic Buying to Stock 'Panic Pantries,' Nielsen Says." *USA Today*, Updated March 5, 2020, https://www.usatoday.com/story/money/2020/03/04/coronavirus-us-spurs-panic-buying-stock-pandemic-pantries/4950835002/.

5 Russell Redman, "Coronavirus Fears Trigger Grocery Shopper Scramble," *Supermarket News*, March 2, 2020, https://www.supermarketnews.com/retail-financial/coronavirus-fears-trigger-grocery-shopper-scramble.

6 Kelly Tyko, Jessica Guynn, and Mike Snider, "Coronavirus Fears Empty Store Shelves of Toilet Paper, Bottled Water, Masks as Shoppers Stock Up." *USA Today*. February 28, 2020, https://www.usatoday.com/story/money/2020/02/28/coronavirus-2020-preparation-more-supply-shortages-expected/4903322002/.

7 Rolf Boone, "Coronavirus Prompts Local Sanitizer, Toilet Paper Shortages," *The*

Olympian, March 4, 2020, https://www.newspapers.com/image/643841034/?terms = percent22toilet percent20paper percent20shortage percent22&match=1.

8 "Toilet Paper," *Google Trends*, https://trends.google.com/trends/explore ?date=2020-02-01 percent202020-03-31&geo=US&q=toilet percent20paper.

9 "WHO Director-General's Opening Remarks at the Media Briefing on COVID-19," *WHO Director-General Speeches*.

10 "WHO Director-General's Opening Remarks at the Media Briefing on COVID-19," *WHO Director-General Speeches*.

11 Tomhanks, *Instagram* post, March 11, 2020, https://www.instagram.com /p/B9nVasnBNF5/?hl=en.

12 Jessica Gall Myrick and Jessica Fitts Willoughby, "A Mixed Methods Inquiry into the Role of Tom Hanks' COVID-19 Social Media Disclosure in Shaping Willingness to Engage in Prevention Behaviors," *Health Communication* 37, no. 7 (2022): 824–32.

13 Steve Aschburner, "Coronavirus Pandemic Causes NBA to Suspend Season After Player Tests Positive," *NBA.com*, March 12, 2020, https://www.nba.com /news/coronavirus-pandemic-causes-nba-suspend-season; Tom Brew, "Breaking: NCAA Cancels All College Sports Through End of School Year," *FanNation*, March 12, 2020, https://www.si.com/college/indiana/basketball/ncaa-cancels-bas ketball-tournaments-spring-sports.

14 "Trends in Number of COVID-19 Cases and Deaths in the US Reported to CDC, by State/Territory." *COVID Data Tracker*. CDC, https://covid.cdc.gov/covid-da ta-tracker/#trends_totalcases_select_00; Cory Turner and Anya Kamenetz, "When Should Schools Close for Coronavirus?" *NPR*, March 11, 2020, https://www.npr. org/2020/03/11/814438424/when-should-schools-close-for-coronavirus.

15 Ally J. Levine, "State By State, COVID-19 Grinds U.S. to a Halt, *Reuters*, March 24, 2020, https://graphics.reuters.com/HEALTH-CORONAVIRUS-USA /0100B5LQ46H/index.html.

16 "Trending Words on 15th March, 2020," *Trend Calendar*, 2022, https://us.trend-cal endar.com/trend/2020-03-15.html.

17 "Trends in Number of COVID-19 Cases and Deaths in the US Reported to CDC, by State/Territory," *COVID Data Tracker*, CDC, https://covid.cdc.gov/covid -data-tracker/#trends_totalcases_select_00.

18 "Coronavirus: The World in Lockdown in Maps and Charts," *BBC News*, April 7, 2020, https://www.bbc.com/news/world-52103747.

19 "Coronavirus: The World in Lockdown," *BBC News*.

20 Hannah Miller, "Reopening America: A State-by-state Breakdown of the Status of Coronavirus Restrictions," *CNBC*, April 30, 2020, https://www.cnbc.com /2020/04/30/coronavirus-states-lifting-stay-at-home-orders-reopening-busi nesses.html.

21 Sarah Mervosh, Denise Lu, and Vanessa Swales, "See Which States and Cities Have Told Residents to Stay at Home," *New York Times*, April 20, 2020, https:// www.nytimes.com/interactive/2020/us/coronavirus-stay-at-home-order.html.

22 Scott Harris, "Order of the State Health Officer Suspending Certain Public Gatherings Due to Risk of Infection by COVID-19," Alabama, April 3, 2020, https://governor.alabama.gov/assets/2020/04/Final-Statewide-Order-4.3.2020.pdf.

23 "Executive Order N-33–20," *Executive Department State of California*, https://covid19.ca.gov/img/Executive-Order-N-33-20.pdf.

24 "Emergency Order #12 Safer At Home Order," State of Wisconsin Department of Health Services, March 24, 2020, https://evers.wi.gov/Documents/COVID19/EMO12-SaferAtHome.pdf.

25 Miller, "Reopening America: A State-by-state Breakdown."

26 Sarah Mervosh, Denise Lu, and Vanessa Swales, "See Which States and Cities Have Told Residents to Stay at Home," *New York Times*, April 20, 2020, https://www.nytimes.com/interactive/2020/us/coronavirus-stay-at-home-order.html.

27 "The US Now has 1,267 Cases of the Coronavirus," *CNN*, March 11, 2020, https://www.cnn.com/world/live-news/coronavirus-outbreak-03-11-20-intl-hnk/index.html?tab=United percent20States; "Nearly 80,000 People have Died in the US From Coronavirus," *CNN*, May 11, 2020, https://www.cnn.com/world/live-news/coronavirus-pandemic-05-11-20-intl/index.html?tab=Cases; Joanna Gaitens, Marian Condon, Eseosa Fernandes, and Melissa McDiarmid, "COVID-19 and Essential Workers: A Narrative Review of Health Outcomes and Moral Injury," *International Journal of Environmental Research and Public Health* 18, no. 4 (2021): 1446.

28 Foss, *Constructing the Outbreak.*

29 Foss, *Constructing the Outbreak.*

30 Foss, *Constructing the Outbreak.*

31 "U.S. Department of Homeland Security, Cybersecurity & Infrastructure Security Agency Advisory Memorandum on Identification of Essential Critical Infrastructure Workers during COVID-19 Response." Cybersecurity & Infrastructure Security Agency, October 21, 2020, https://www.cisa.gov/critical-infrastructure-sectors.

32 "U.S. Department of Homeland Security," Cybersecurity & Infrastructure Security Agency.

33 "Coronavirus Pandemic," Gallup Poll, 2022, https://news.gallup.com/poll/308222/coronavirus-pandemic.aspx.

34 Rogers, Tiana N., Charles R. Rogers, Elizabeth VanSant-Webb, Lily Y. Gu, Bin Yan, and Fares Qeadan. "Racial Disparities in COVID-19 Mortality Among Essential Workers in the United States." *World Medical & Health Policy* 12, no. 3 (2020): 311–27.

35 Rogers, Rogers, VanSant-Webb, Gu, Yan, and Qeadan. "Racial Disparities in COVID-19 Mortality Among Essential Workers."

36 Felix Richter, "COVID-19 has Caused a Huge Amount of Lost Working Hours," *COVID-19*, World Economic Forum, February 4, 2021, https://www.weforum.org/agenda/2021/02/covid-employment-global-job-loss/.

37 "Unemployment Rates During the COVID-19 Pandemic," *Congressional Research Service*, August 20, 2021, https://sgp.fas.org/crs/misc/R46554.pdf.

38 "Unemployment Rates During the COVID-19 Pandemic," *Congressional Research Service.*

39 Kate Power, "The COVID-19 Pandemic Has Increased the Care Burden of Women and Families," *Sustainability: Science, Practice and Policy* 16, no. 1 (2020): 67–73.

40 Amy Houtrow, Debbi Harris, Ashli Molinero, Tal Levin-Decanini, and Christopher Robichaud, "Children with Disabilities In the United States and the COVID-19 Pandemic," *Journal of Pediatric Rehabilitation Medicine* 13, no. 3 (2020): 415–24.

41 Abigail Johnson Hess, "How Coronavirus Dramatically Changed College for Over 14 Million Students," *CNBC*, March 26, 2020, https://www.cnbc.com/2020/03/26/how-coronavirus-changed-college-for-over-14-million-students.html.

42 Peter Whoriskey, Maria Sacchetti, and Richard A. Webster, "Coronavirus Cases Surge at Nursing Homes as Workers Battle 'Almost Perfect Killing Machine,'" *Washington Post*, March 21, 2020, https://www.washingtonpost.com/business/2020/03/21/nursing-home-coronavirus-deaths/.

43 "The Nielsen Total Audience Report: April 2020," *Insights*. Nielsen. April 2020, https://www.nielsen.com/insights/2020/the-nielsen-total-audience-report-april-2020/; Koeze and Popper, "The Virus Changed the Way We Internet"; Isabel Cabrera, "World Reading Habits in 2020," *Global English Editing*, November 6, 2020, https://geediting.com/world-reading-habits-2020/.

44 "The Nielsen Total Audience Report: April 2020," *Insights*, Nielsen, April 2020, https://www.nielsen.com/insights/2020/the-nielsen-total-audience-report-april-2020/; Koeze and Popper, "The Virus Changed the Way We Internet."

45 "The Nielsen Total Audience Report: April 2020," *Insights*, Nielsen, April 2020, https://www.nielsen.com/insights/2020/the-nielsen-total-audience-report-april-2020/.

46 "COVID-19: Tracking the Impact," Nielsen.

47 A. J. Katz, "April 2020 Study: 2 in 3 Americans Say Watching the News Causes Anxiety, and 67 percent Experience 'Burnout,'" *TVNewser*, June 8, 2020, https://www.adweek.com/tvnewser/april-2020-study-2-in-3-americans-say-watching-the-news-causes-anxiety-and-67-experience-burn-out/443945/.

48 Katz, "April 2020 Study: 2 in 3 Americans Say Watching the News Causes Anxiety."

49 Katz, "April 2020 Study: 2 in 3 Americans Say Watching the News Causes Anxiety."

50 Koeze and Popper, "The Virus Changed the Way We Internet."

51 Koeze and Popper, "The Virus Changed the Way We Internet."

52 "COVID-19 Dashboard," Center for Systems Science and Engineering (CSSE) at Johns Hopkins University (JHU), https://www.arcgis.com/apps/dashboards/bda7594740fd40299423467b48e9ecf6.

53 "Coronavirus," *Google Trends*, https://trends.google.com/trends/explore?date=2020-01-31 percent202020-05-01&q=coronavirus; "COVID-19," *Google Trends*, https://trends.google.com/trends/explore?date=2020-01-31 percent202020-05-01&q=covid-19.

54 Koeze and Popper, "The Virus Changed the Way We Internet."

55 "This New York Hospital has Become 'The Epicenter of the Epicenter' of the Coronavirus Outbreak," *Washington Post*, March 26, 2020, https://www.youtube.com/watch?v=IW6gccYMplw.

56 "First TV Ad for Coronavirus Public Information Campaign," *The Telegraph*, March 19, 2020, https://www.youtube.com/watch?v=PBpjOIXlnUE; "Government of Spain Launches Campaign #Estevirusloparamosunidos [#We Will Stop This Virus Together] So That Whole Country Unites to Fight Coronavirus and Incentivise Measures to Keep Social Distance," *News*, March 15, 2020, https://www.lamoncloa.gob.es/lang/en/gobierno/news/Paginas/2020/20200315covid19-campaign.aspx.

57 Governor Newsom Launches Campaign to Protect Health and Well-Being of Older Californians During COVID-19 Pandemic," Office of Governor Gavin Newsom, March 31, 2020, https://www.gov.ca.gov/2020/03/31/governor-newsom-launches-campaign-to-protect-health-and-well-being-of-older-californians-during-covid-19-pandemic/; "Hawai'i Department of Health Launches COVID-19 Public Awareness Campaign Featuring Frank De Lima," *Newsroom*, State of Hawaii, Department of Health, March 30, 2020, https://health.hawaii.gov/news/newsroom/hawaii-department-of-health-launches-covid-19-public-awareness-campaign-featuring-frank-de-lima/; Wm. Steven Humphrey, "Gov. Brown and Wieden+Kennedy Release "Stay Home, Save Lives" Ad Campaign," *Portland Mercury*, March 28, 2020, https://www.portlandmercury.com/news/2020/03/28/28210661/gov-brown-and-wiedenkennedy-release-stay-home-save-lives-ad-campaign; "State of Tennessee Launches 'Do Your Part, Stay Apart' Campaign," *Newsroom*, TN Office of the Governor, March 26, 2020, https://www.tn.gov/governor/news/2020/3/26/state-of-tennessee-launches--do-your-part--stay-apart--campaign.html; "Washington State Launches Spread the Facts Public Awareness Campaign," *Newsroom*, Washington State Department of Health. April 3, 2020, https://doh.wa.gov/newsroom/washington-state-launches-spread-facts-public-awareness-campaign.

58 "16 National Health Care Leaders"; "The Best Thing Everyday Americans Can Do to Fight Coronavirus? #StayHome, Save Lives, *USA Today*. March 15, 2020, https://www.usatoday.com/story/opinion/2020/03/15/coronavirus-stay-home-hel-america-save-lives-column/5054241002/; Liberty Vittert, "Liberty Vittert: Social Distancing for Coronavirus Will Save Lives—Look at These Numbers," *Fox News*, March 17, 2020, https://www.foxnews.com/opinion/liberty-vittert-social-distancing-for-coronavirus-will-save-lives-look-at-these-numbers; Maria Goody, " Flattening A Pandemic's Curve: Why Staying Home Now Can Save Lives," *NPR*, March 13, 2020, https://www.npr.org/sections/health-shots/2020/03/13/815502262/flattening-a-pandemics-curve-why-staying-home-now-can-save-lives; Sigal Samuel, " How You Can Keep Thousands of People from Getting Coronavirus, In One GIF," *Vox*, March 26, 2020, https://www.vox.com/future-perfect/2020/3/26/21193851/coronavirus-covid-19-staying-home-social-distancing.

59 Andrew Hutchinson, "Instagram Launches 'Stay Home' Sticker and Story to

Encourage Social Distancing Amid COVID-19 Outbreak," *Social Media Today*, March 21, 2020, https://www.socialmediatoday.com/news/instagram-launches-stay-home-sticker-and-story-to-encourage-social-distan/574628/.

60 Andrew Hutchinson, "Instagram Launches New Co-Watching Feature."

61 Andrew Hutchinson, "TikTok Launches Celebrity-hosted Daily Live-streams to Entertain Users Amid COVID-19 Lockdowns," *Social Media Today*, March 27, 2020, https://www.socialmediatoday.com/news/tiktok-launches-celebrity-hosted-daily-live-streams-to-entertain-users-ami/574970/.

62 "U.S. Soccer Launches 'Bend the Curve. Stay at Home.' Campaign," *Federation News*, April 1, 2020, https://www.ussoccer.com/stories/2020/04/us-soccer-launches-bend-the-curve-stay-at-home-campaign.

63 Rick Stroud, "Tom Brady, NFL Help Raise Coronavirus Awareness with StayHomeStayStrong Campaign," *Tampa Bay Times*, March 26, 2020, https://www.tampabay.com/sports/bucs/2020/03/26/tom-brady-nfl-help-raise-coronavirus-awareness-with-stayhomestaystrong-campaign/.

64 Lisa Respers France, "Kevin Bacon and Others Want You Six Degrees for #IStayHomeFor Challenge," *CNN*, March 20, 2020, https://www.cnn.com/2020/03/20/entertainment/i-stay-home-for-celebs-trnd/index.html.

65 "Best Viral PR Campaign Advertising, Media & PR," *The Webby Awards*, https://winners.webbyawards.com/winners/advertising-media-pr/pr/best-viral-pr-campaign?years=1.

66 Bilir Gozde, "Memorable Stay Home Ad Campaigns by Brands for COVID-19," *Digital Ad Campaigns*, Digital Agency Network, June 6, 2020, https://digitalagencynetwork.com/memorable-stay-home-ad-campaigns-by-brands-for-covid-19/.

67 Mari Salazar, "'We Stay Here for You, Please Stay Home for Us' | Medical Professionals Start Social Media Campaign," *KVUE ABC News*, March 31, 2020, https://www.kvue.com/article/news/health/coronavirus/we-stay-here-for-you-please-say-home-for-us-medical-professionals-start-social-media-campaign/269-c145e15f-2723-42b2-ab52-a3b6510048bd.

68 "Governor Ivey Announces Ribbons of Hope Campaign," *Newsroom*, The Offices of Governor Kay Ivey, April 7, 2020, https://governor.alabama.gov/newsroom/2020/04/governor-ivey-announces-ribbons-of-hope-campaign/.

69 "#ThanksHealthHeroes,"#SafeHands Challenge, WHO, https://www.who.int/campaigns/connecting-the-world-to-combat-coronavirus/safehands-challenge/thankshealthheroes.

70 Hayden Brooks, "Elton John-Hosted iHeart Living Room Concert for America Raises $10 Million," *iHeart*, April 1, 2020, https://news.iheart.com/featured/living-room-concert/content/2020-04-01-elton-john-hosted-iheart-living-room-concert-for-america-raises-8-million/.

71 Brooks, "Elton John-Hosted iHeart Living Room Concert."

72 Jelisa Castrodale, Coronavirus Has Led to a Surge in Popularity for the 2011 Movie 'Contagion'." *Vice*, January 31, 2020, https://www.vice.com/en_us/article/qjdv7m/coronavirus-has-led-to-a-surge-in-popularity-for-the-2011-movie-contagion;

"Outbreak movie," *Google Trends*, https://trends.google.com/trends/explore?date=2020-01-05 percent202020-05-31&geo=US&q=outbreak percent20movie; "Contagion movie," *Google Trends*, https://trends.google.com/trends/explore?date=2020-01-05 percent202020-05-31&geo=US&q=contagion percent20movie.

73 Chris Lindahl, "Beyond 'Contagion': Interest in Outbreak Movies, Podcasts, and More Surges Across the Internet," *IndieWire*, March 17, 2020, https://www.indiewire.com/2020/03/contagion-pandemic-outbreak-movies-coronavirus-1202218477/.

74 For example, see Liang, Shu Ting, Lin Ting Liang, and Joseph M. Rosen, "COVID-19: A Comparison to the 1918 Influenza and How We Can Defeat It," *Postgraduate Medical Journal* 97, no. 1147 (2021): 273–74. Yan, Holly, "The 1918 Flu Pandemic Killed 50 Million People. These Lessons Could Help Avoid a Repeat with COVID-19," *CNN*, April 16, 2020, https://www.cnn.com/2020/04/16/health/spanish-flu-coronavirus-lessons-learned/index.html; Becky Little, "When Mask-Wearing Rules in the 1918 Pandemic Faced Resistance," *History.com*, May 6, 2020, https://www.history.com/news/1918-spanish-flu-mask-wearing-resistance.

75 Lucio Reis Filho, "No Safe Space: Zombie Film Tropes during the COVID-19 Pandemic," *Space and Culture* 23, no. 3 (2020): 253–58; Jessecae K. Marsh, Nick D. Ungson, and Dominic J. Packer, "Of Pandemics and Zombies: The Influence of Prior Concepts on COVID-19 Pandemic-related Behaviors," *International Journal of Environmental Research and Public Health* 18, no. 10 (2021): 5207.

76 "Most Americans Say Coronavirus Outbreak Has Impacted Their Lives," *Coronavirus Disease (COVID-19)*. Pew Research Center, March 30, 2020, https://www.pewresearch.org/social-trends/2020/03/30/most-americans-say-coronavirus-outbreak-has-impacted-their-lives/.

77 "Most Americans Say Coronavirus Outbreak Has Impacted Their Lives," Pew Research Center.

78 "Most Americans Say Coronavirus Outbreak Has Impacted Their Lives," Pew Research Center.

79 "3, 2, 1 Go! Video Gaming is at an All-Time High During COVID-19," *Media*. Nielsen. June 2020, https://www.nielsen.com/insights/2020/3-2-1-go-video-gaming-is-at-an-all-time-high-during-covid-19/.

80 Todd Spangler, "'Tiger King' Ranks as TV's Most Popular Show Right Now, According to Rotten Tomatoes," *Variety*, March 29, 2020, https://variety.com/2020/digital/news/tiger-king-most-popular-tv-show-netflix-1203548202/.

81 Naomi Gleit, "2020 Year in Review and Top Pop Culture Moments," *Meta*, December 7, 2020, https://about.fb.com/news/2020/12/2020-year-in-review/.

82 Koeze and Popper, "The Virus Changed the Way We Internet."

83 Andrew Hutchinson, "Snapchat Launches New 'Here for You' Mental Health Resource Ahead of Time in Response to COVID-19," *Social Media Today*, March 20, 2020, https://www.socialmediatoday.com/news/snapchat-launches-new-here-for-you-mental-health-resource-ahead-of-time-i/574507/.

84 Jenny Crawford, "Social Media on Lockdown: What were the Most Viewed

Videos in March?" *Data Insights*, https://pex.com/blog/social-media-on-lock down-most-viewed-videos-march/.

85 Tracy McGraw, "Spending 2020 Together on Twitter," *Insights*, December 7, 2020, https://blog.twitter.com/en_us/topics/insights/2020/spending-2020-together -on-twitter.

86 "Jimmy Fallon Talks About Producing 'Tonight Show' From Home," *Today*, March 19, 2020, https://www.today.com/video/jimmy-fallon-talks-about-producing-tonight -show-from-home-80964677538.

87 Jon Caramanica, "This 'Imagine' Cover Is No Heaven," *New York Times*, Updated March 23, 2020, https://www.nytimes.com/2020/03/20/arts/music/coronavirus -gal-gadot-imagine.html.

88 Travis M. Andrews, "Gal Gadot, Mark Ruffalo and Other Celebrities Asked us to 'Imagine' in a Viral Video. It Did Not Go Well," *Washington Post*, March 19, 2020, https://www.washingtonpost.com/arts-entertainment/2020/03/19/gal-gadot -imagine-viral-video/.

89 Heather Schwedel," A Video of Celebrities Singing "Imagine" So Bad It Can Bring Us All Together in Hatred," *Slate*, March 19, 2020, https://slate.com/culture /2020/03/celebrities-singing-imagine-video-explained.html.

90 Hannah Brown, "Gal Gadot's Imagine Video Draws Snarky Social-Media Backlash," *The Jerusalem Post*, March 21, 2020, https://www.jpost.com/israel-news /culture/gal-gadots-imagine-video-draws-snarky-social-media-backlash-621715.

91 Brian Moylan, "Gal Gadot's 'Imagine' Instagram video Was Peak Cringe. A Year Later, Here's What's Changed," *Think*, *NBC News*, March 21, 2021, https://www .nbcnews.com/think/opinion/gal-gadot-s-imagine-instagram-video-was-peak -cringe-year-ncna1261685.

92 Laura Brown, "Going There with Gal Gadot," *InStyle*, January 4, 2022, https:// www.instyle.com/celebrity/gal-gadot/february-2022-cover.

93 Daron James, "Learn How *Some Good News* Sends Positive Vibes While Social Distancing," *No Film School*, April 28, 2020, https://nofilmschool.com/sgn-news-show.

94 Nicole Lyn Pesce, "John Krasinski Tries Explaining to Furious Fans Why He Sold 'Some Good News' to CBS," *MarketWatch*, May 28, 2020, https://www .marketwatch.com/story/john-krasinski-tries-explaining-to-furious-fans-why -he-sold-some-good-news-to-cbs-2020-05-28.

95 Nicole Lyn Pesce, "John Krasinski Tries Explaining to Furious Fans Why He Sold 'Some Good News' to CBS," *MarketWatch*, May 28, 2020, https://www .marketwatch.com/story/john-krasinski-tries-explaining-to-furious-fans-why -he-sold-some-good-news-to-cbs-2020-05-28.

96 Mariah Carey, "Mariah Carey—Hero (Live at Home Tribute)," *YouTube*, April 10, 2020, https://www.youtube.com/watch?v=LXAIAl3ZcWg.

97 Carey. "Mariah Carey—Hero (Live at Home Tribute)."

98 Jenny Crawford, "Social Media on Lockdown: What were the Most Viewed Videos in March?" *Data Insights*, https://pex.com/blog/social-media-on-lockdown -most-viewed-videos-march/.

99 Crawford, "Social Media on Lockdown: What were the Most Viewed Videos in March?"

100 "YouTube During COVID-19." *YouTube Culture & Trends.* June 25, 2020, https://www.youtube.com/trends/articles/what-it-means-to-stayhome-on-youtube/.

101 "YouTube During COVID-19." *YouTube Culture & Trends.*

102 "YouTube During COVID-19." *YouTube Culture & Trends.*

103 "YouTube During COVID-19." *YouTube Culture & Trends*; "Watching the Pandemic: What YouTube Trends Reveal About Human Needs During COVID-19." *YouTube Culture & Trends.* May 1, 2020, https://www.youtube.com/trends/articles/covid-impact/.

104 "YouTube During COVID-19." *YouTube Culture & Trends.*

105 Melissa Locker, "Families Travel Back in Time with Childhood Photos for the 'I'm Just a Kid' Challenge," *Time*, April 15, 2020, https://time.com/5821238/im-just-a-kid-challenge-explained/.

106 Koeze and Popper, "The Virus Changed the Way We Internet."

107 "YouTube During COVID-19." *YouTube Culture & Trends.*

108 Crawford, "Social Media on Lockdown: What were the Most Viewed Videos in March?"

109 "YouTube During COVID-19." *YouTube Culture & Trends.*

110 HotandFlashy. How To Look Good on Video Calls. Zoom FaceTime Skype. Blogger Secrets." *YouTube*, March 31, 2020, https://www.youtube.com/watch?v=ACNGhPKnmok.

111 Itscaitlinhello. May 5, 2020, https://www.tiktok.com/@itscaitlinhello/video/6824228103624183046?is_from_webapp=v1&item_id=6824228103624183046.

112 Claire Glecewicz, "Few Americans Say Their House of Worship is Open, But a Quarter Say Their Faith Has Grown Amid Pandemic," *Pew Research Center*, April 30, 2020, https://www.pewresearch.org/fact-tank/2020/04/30/few-americans-say-their-house-of-worship-is-open-but-a-quarter-say-their-religious-faith-has-grown-amid-pandemic/.

113 Glecewicz, "Few Americans Say Their House of Worship is Open."

114 McLanahan, Paige, and Debra Kamin, "52 Places, Virtually," *New York Times*, Updated July 27, 2020, https://www.nytimes.com/2020/04/14/travel/52-places-to-go-virtual-travel.html.

115 McLanahan and Kamin, "52 Places, Virtually."

116 Andrew Cohen, "The NBA Launches Social Media Campaign "NBA Together" in Response to COVID-19," *Sport Techie*, March 23, 2020, https://www.sporttechie.com/nba-social-media-campaign-nba-together-coronavirus-covid-19/.

117 "Coronavirus Pandemic," Gallup Poll, 2022, https://news.gallup.com/poll/308222/coronavirus-pandemic.aspx.

118 "Coronavirus Pandemic," Gallup Poll.

119 Washington Post Staff, "Where States Reopened and Cases Spiked After the U.S. Shutdown," *Washington Post*, Updated September 11, 2020, https://www.washingtonpost.com/graphics/2020/national/states-reopening-coronavirus-map/.

120 "Coronavirus Pandemic," Gallup Poll, 2022, https://news.gallup.com/poll/308222/coronavirus-pandemic.aspx.

121 Farrow, Hannah. "Reporters Navigate Remote-Work Challenges During Pandemic." *Local News Initiative*. Northwestern. May 19, 2020, https://localnewsinitiative.northwestern.edu/posts/2020/05/19/remote-reporting/.

122 Naomi Forman-Katz and Katerina Eva Matsa, "News Platform Fact Sheet." *Fact Sheet*. September 20, 2022, https://www.pewresearch.org/journalism/fact-sheet/news-platform-fact-sheet/.

123 "Social Media Fact Sheet," *Research Topics*, Pew Research Center, April 7, 2021, https://www.pewresearch.org/internet/fact-sheet/social-media/#panel-b14b718d-7ab6-46f4-b447-0abd510f4180.

124 Rogers, Rogers, VanSant-Webb, Gu, Yan, and Qeadan, "Racial Disparities in COVID-19 Mortality Among Essential Workers"; Sarah R. Jordan, Andrea E. Daddato, Hemali P. Patel, and Christine D. Jones. "Forgotten Frontline Workers: Environmental Health Service Employees' Perspectives on Working During the COVID-19 Pandemic," *Journal of Hospital Medicine* 17, no. 3 (2022): 158–68; Lisa de Saxe Zerden, Erica L. Richman, Brianna Lombardi, and Alexandria B. Forte, "Frontline, Essential, and Invisible: The Needs of Low-Wage Workers in Hospital Settings During COVID-19," *Workplace Health & Safety* (2022): 21650799221108490; Julie A. Cederbaum, Abigail M. Ross, Lisa de Saxe Zerden, Lilly Estenson, Jennifer Zelnick, and Betty J. Ruth. "'We are on the Frontlines Too": A Qualitative Content Analysis of US Social Workers' Experiences During the COVID-19 Pandemic." *Health & Social Care in the Community* (2022); "The Plight of Essential Workers During the COVID-19 Pandemic," *Lancet (London, England)* 395, no. 10237 (2020): 1587.

125 Robin Stein and Caroline Kim, "'People Are Dying': 72 Hours Inside a N.Y.C. Hospital Battling Coronavirus," *New York Times*, March 25, 2020, https://www.nytimes.com/video/nyregion/100000007052136/coronavirus-elmhurst-hospital-queens.html; Al Tompkins, "Why It's So Difficult for Journalists to Get Inside Hospitals to Document COVID-19 Cases," *Poynter*, January 6, 2021, https://www.poynter.org/reporting-editing/2021/why-its-so-difficult-for-journalists-to-get-inside-hospitals-to-document-covid-19-cases/.

126 Alejandra Victoria Capozzo, "Dying Alone Due to COVID-19: Do the Needs of the Many Outweigh the Rights of the Few—Or the One?" *Frontiers in Public Health* 8 (2020): 593464, https://www.frontiersin.org/articles/10.3389/fpubh.2020.593464/full.

127 Katz, "April 2020 Study: 2 in 3 Americans Say Watching the News Causes Anxiety."

128 Anne C. Krendl and Brea L. Perry, "The Impact of Sheltering in Place During The COVID-19 Pandemic on Older Adults' Social and Mental Well-Being," *The Journals of Gerontology: Series B* 76, no. 2 (2021): e53-e58; Emily Leslie and Riley Wilson, "Sheltering in Place and Domestic Violence: Evidence from Calls for Service During COVID-19." *Journal of public economics* 189 (2020): 104241;

Killgore, William DS, Sara A. Cloonan, Emily C. Taylor, Matthew C. Allbright, and Natalie S. Dailey, "Trends in Suicidal Ideation Over the First Three Months of COVID-19 Lockdowns." *Psychiatry Research* 293 (2020): 113390.

Chapter Five: Not In It Together

1 "Two Years and Thousands of Voices: What Community-Generated Data Tells Us About Anti-AAPI Hate," *Stop AAPI Hate*, 2022, https://stopaapihate.org/wp-content/uploads/2022/07/Stop-AAPI-Hate-Year-2-Report.pdf.

2 "Two Years and Thousands of Voices," *Stop AAPI Hate*.

3 Antonio Gramsci, *Prison Notebooks Volume 2*. Vol. 2. Columbia University Press, 2011; Stuart Hall, "The Spectacle of the Other," *Representation: Cultural representations and signifying practices* 7 (1997);

4 Douglas M. Kellner and Meenakshi Gigi Durham, "Adventures in Media and Cultural Studies: Introducing the Keyworks," *Media and Cultural studies: Keyworks* (2001): 1–29.

5 Kraut, *Silent Travelers*.

6 John Harvey Powell and Karl Tiedemann, *Bring Out Your Dead*, Philadelphia: University of Pennsylvania Press, 1949.

7 Lucy Jarosz, "Constructing the Dark Continent: Metaphor as Geographic Representation of Africa," *Geografiska Annaler: Series B, Human Geography* 74, no. 2 (1992): 105–15.

8 Kraut, *Silent Travelers*.

9 Markel, Howard. *Quarantine!: East European Jewish immigrants and the New York City Epidemics of 1892*. JHU Press, 2022.

10 Sang Hea Kil, "Fearing Yellow, Imagining White: Media Analysis of The Chinese Exclusion Act of 1882," *Social Identities* 18, no. 6 (2012): 663–77; Charles McClain, "Of Medicine, Race, and American Law: The Bubonic Plague Outbreak of 1900," *Law & Social Inquiry* 13, no. 3 (1988): 447–513; Joan B. Trauner, "Chinese as Medical Scapegoats, 1870–1905," Joan B. Trauner, "Chinese as Medical Scapegoats, 1870–1905," *California History Magazine*, 57, no. 8. (1978): 70–87.

11 Moore, "Contagion from Abroad: US Newspaper Framings of Immigrants and Epidemics."

12 Eichelberger, "SARS and New York's Chinatown."

13 Mary J. Dobson, "Mortality Gradients and Disease Exchanges: Comparisons from Old England and Colonial America," *Social History of Medicine* 2, no. 3 (1989): 259–97.

14 Isaac Cathrall, *A Medical Sketch of the Synochus Maligna or Malignant Contagious Fever*, Philadelphia: Richard Folwell. 1796; Absalom Jones and Richard Allen, "A Narrative of the Proceedings of the Black People during the Late Awful Calamity in Philadelphia in the Year 1793," *American Journal of Public Health* 109, no. 10 (2019): 1336–337.

15 J. A. Faison, "Tuberculosis in the Colored Race." *Medical Record (1866–1922)* 55, no. 10 (1899): 375; Coleman, Thomas D. "The Susceptibility of the Negro to Tuberculosis." *Transactions of the American Climatological Association* 19 (1903): 122. Coleman, Thomas D. "The Susceptibility of the Negro to Tuberculosis." *Transactions of the American Climatological Association* 19 (1903): 122.

16 Naomi Rogers, "Race and the Politics of Polio: Warm Springs, Tuskegee, and the March of Dimes," *American Journal of Public Health* 97, no. 5 (2007): 784–95.

17 Trevor Hoppe, "'Spanish Flu': When Infectious Disease Names Blur Origins and Stigmatize Those Infected," *American Journal of Public Health* 108, no. 11 (2018): 1462–1464; "WHO issues best practices for naming new human infections," *Health Topics*, WHO, May 8, 2015, https://www.who.int/news/item/08-05-2015-who-issues-best-practices-for-naming-new-human-infectious-diseases; Lawrence Altman, "New Homosexual Disorder Worries Health Officials," *New York Times*, May 11, 1982, https://www.nytimes.com/1982/05/11/science/new-homosexual-disorder-worries-health-officials.html.

18 Wenshan Jia and Fangzhu Lu, "US Media's Coverage of China's Handling of COVID-19: Playing the Role of the Fourth Branch of Government or the Fourth Estate?" *Global Media and China* 6, no. 1 (2021): 8–23.

19 David Moser, "A Fearful Asymmetry: COVID-19 and America's Information Deficit with China," *Asia-Pacific Journal-Japan Focus* (2020).

20 Jia and Lu, "US Media's Coverage of China's Handling of COVID-19."

21 Casey Ryan Kelly, "Donald J. Trump and the Rhetoric of White Ambivalence," *Rhetoric and Public Affairs* 23, no. 2 (2020): 195–223; Rose Cuison Villazor and Kevin R. Johnson, "The Trump Administration and the War on Immigration Diversity," *Wake Forest L. Rev.* 54 (2019): 575; .

22 "Wuhan Municipal Health Commission's Briefing on the Current Situation of Pneumonia in Our City," Wuhan Municipal Health Commission, December 31, 2019.

23 Weng Ziquian, "Always Know | Sudden Unexplained Pneumonia? Don't Panic! All You Need To Know Is Here," *RedNet.cn*, December 31, 2019, https://hn.rednet.cn/content/2019/12/31/6495266.html; Viral Pneumonia Cases Reported in Central China," *The People's Daily*, December 31, 2019; "Wuhan Patients with Unexplained Pneumonia and Their Onset Sites Have Been Isolated and Many Hospitals Hold a Special Meeting on Prevention and Treatment," *21st Century Business Herald 21*, December 31, 2019; Cheng Yuanzhou, "27 Cases of Viral Pneumonia Found in Wuhan, 7 in Critical Condition," *The Beijing News*. December 31, 2019.

24 WHO, Tweet, January 15, 2020, https://twitter.com/WHO/status/1217480368829489154/photo/1.

25 Stephen Chen, "Coronavirus Weaker Than SARS But May Share Link to Bats, Chinese Scientists Say," *South China Morning Post*, January 22, 2020, https://www.scmp.com/news/china/science/article/3047114/coronavirus-weaker-sars-may-share-link-bats-chinese-scientists.

26 Chen, "Coronavirus Weaker Than SARS."
27 Chen, "Coronavirus Weaker Than SARS."
28 Cho Xie, Jane Cai, and Guo Rui. "Why Wild Animals are a Key Ingredient in China's Coronavirus Outbreak," *South China Morning Post*, January 22, 2020, https://www.scmp.com/news/china/society/article/3047238/why-wild-animals-are-key-ingredient-chinas-coronavirus-outbreak?utm_term=Autofeed&utm_medium=Social&utm_content=article&utm_source=Twitter#Echobox=1579703660.
29 Xie, Cai, and Rui, "Why Wild Animals are a Key Ingredient in China's Coronavirus Outbreak
30 陈秋实 Chen Qiushi@chenqiushi404. Tweet. January 22, 2020, https://twitter.com/chenqiushi404/status/1219885244670607361.
31 Jing Wang and Li Li, "Bats, Virus, and Racism: The Myth and the Science," *Asian Voices Matter*, March 18, 2020, https://medium.com/asian-voices-matter/bats-virus-and-racism-the-myth-and-the-science-7b9ece21fa4c.
32 Ben Cost, "Revolting Video Shows Woman Devouring Bat Amid Coronavirus Outbreak," *New York Post*. January 23, 2020, https://nypost.com/2020/01/23/revolting-video-shows-woman-devouring-bat-amid-coronavirus-outbreak/.
33 Billie Thomson, "Revolting Footage Shows Chinese Woman Eating a Whole Bat at a Fancy Restaurant as Scientists Link the Deadly Coronavirus to the Flying Mammals," *Daily Mail.com*. January 24, 2020, https://www.dailymail.co.uk/news/article-7920573/Revolting-footage-shows-Chinese-woman-eating-bat-scientists-link-coronavirus-animal.html.
34 Bhavya Sukheja, "'Coronavirus Could be Linked to Fruit Bats': Scientists as Bat Soup Videos Emerge Online," *Republic World*, January 23, 2020, https://www.republicworld.com/world-news/rest-of-the-world-news/scientists-believe-bats-could-be-linked-to-sars-like-virus.html; Shelby Talcott, "Is This Objectively Disgusting Soup What's Causing China's Disease Outbreak?" *Daily Caller*, January 23, 2020, https://dailycaller.com/2020/01/23/bat-soup-china-coronavirus-cause/; Niamh Cavanagh, "Stomach-churning Recipe for Bat Soup as Animals Named as Possible Coronavirus Host," *Daily Star*, January 23, 2020, https://www.dailystar.co.uk/news/world-news/stomach-churning-recipe-bat-soup-21345300.
35 "Bat Soup," *Google Trends*, https://trends.google.com/trends/explore?date=2020-01-15 percent202020-01-30&geo=US&q= percent22bat percent20soup percent22.
36 "Bat Soup," *Google Trends*.
37 Shiv Kumar, "Chinese Food Outlets Hit by WhatsApp Rumours on Coronavirus," *The Tribune* (India), February 9, 2020, https://www.tribuneindia.com/news/nation/chinese-food-outlets-hit-by-whatsapp-rumours-on-coronavirus-38310.
38 Laura Zhou, "'Sorry About the Tasty Bat': Chinese Online Host Apologises for Travel Show Dining Advice as Wuhan Virus Spread," *South China Morning Post*, January 26, 2020, https://www.scmp.com/news/china/society/article/3047683/sorry-about-tasty-bat-chinese-online-host-apologises-travel-show.
39 James Palmer, "Don't Blame Bat Soup for the Coronavirus," *Foreign Policy*, January 27,

2020, https://foreignpolicy.com/2020/01/27/coronavirus-covid19-dont-blame-bat-soup-for-the-virus/; Gaynor, Gerren Keith, "Coronavirus: Outrage Over Chinese Blogger Eating 'Bat Soup' Sparks Apology," *Fox News*, January 28, 2020, https://www.foxnews.com/food-drink/coronavirus-chinese-blogger-eats-bat-soup; Jane Stevenson, "Infamous Bat Soup-Eating Video Got Us Thinking About Other 'Delicacies,'" *Toronto Sun*, February 1, 2020, https://torontosun.com/news/world/infamous-bat-soup-eating-video-got-us-thinking-about-other-delicacies.

40 Liselotte Mas, "Is Bat Soup a Delicacy in China? We Debunk a Rumour on the Origin of the Coronavirus," *France 24*. March, 2, 2020, https://observers.france24.com/en/20200203-china-coronavirus-bat-soup-debunk-videos-viral-palau-indonesia.

41 BBC Monitoring, "China Coronavirus: Misinformation Spreads Online About Origin and Scale." *BBC*. January 30, 2020, https://www.bbc.com/news/blogs-trending-51271037.

42 "Bat Soup," *Google Trends*.

43 Duncan Hooper, "'I'm Delighted,' Says Teacher Who Began #jenesuispasunvirus Anti-racism Trend," *CGTN*, January 30, 2020, https://newseu.cgtn.com/news/2020-01-30/Twitter-users-in-France-complain-of-racist-abuse-over-coronavirus-NELcFWI5Y4/index.html.

44 Steve Jones, "Chinese Student Attacked in Sheffield Over Coronavirus," *The Star*, January 31, 2020, https://www.thestar.co.uk/news/crime/chinese-student-attacked-sheffield-over-coronavirus-1381837; Victoria Lindrea and Francesca Gillet, "Coronavirus: British Chinese People Reveal Prejudice Amid Outbreak," *BBC*. February 3, 2020, https://www.bbc.com/news/uk-51348593.

45 "Two Women Attack 23-year-old at Beusselstrasse S-Bahn Station," *Der Tagesspiegel* (*The Daily Mirror*), February 1, 2020, https://www.tagesspiegel.de/berlin/polizei-justiz/chinesin-in-berlin-rassistisch-beleidigt-zwei-frauen-gehen-auf-23-jaehrige-an-s-bahnhof-beusselstrasse-los/25498396.html.

46 Sarah Al-Arshani, "A Costco Sample-Stand Worker Turned Away a Kid Wearing a Face Mask Because She Thought He was From China and Could Give Her the Coronvirus," *Insider*, January 29, 2020, https://www.insider.com/wuhan-coronavirus-kid-turned-away-food-samples-at-costco-2020-1.

47 Rachel Clayton, Racist Coronavirus Event at Melbourne Nightclub Pawn & Co Cancelled After Backlash," *ABC News*, February 5, 2020, https://www.abc.net.au/news/2020-02-06/racist-coronavirus-event-mr-chans-pawn-and-co-melbourne/11934426.

48 Victoria Lindrea and Francesca Gillet, "Coronavirus: British Chinese People Reveal Prejudice Amid Outbreak," *BBC*, February 3, 2020, https://www.bbc.com/news/uk-51348593; Adrian Ma, "Coronavirus Fears Take Toll on Chinatown Businesses," *WBUR*. February 7, 2020, https://www.wbur.org/news/2020/02/07/new-coronavirus-slows-chinatown-business; Natasha Frost, "Coronavirus Rumors are Hurting Chinatowns Around the World," *Quartz*, February 6, 2020,

https://qz.com/1798597/coronavirus-rumors-are-hurting-popular-chinese-restaurants/; Desmond Brown, "As Fear of Coronavirus Spreads, Business Drops More Than 30 percent at Toronto Chinese Restaurant." *CBC*, February 6, 2020, https://www.cbc.ca/news/canada/toronto/yueh-tung-restaurant-coronavirus-fears-decrease-in-customers-1.5455224; Reeba Zachariah, "Coronavirus Scare: Chinese Restaurants in Mumbai Face Heat Over Imported Ingredients," *Times of India*, February 9, 2020, https://timesofindia.indiatimes.com/city/mumbai/ncov-scare-chinese-restaurants-face-heat-over-imported-ingredients/articleshow/74034322.cms; Vanessa Misciagna, "Coronavirus Fears Impacting Businesses in Seattle's Chinatown-International District," *King 5*, February 5, 2020, https://www.king5.com/article/news/local/coronavirus-fears-impact-business-seattle-international-district/281-d0250731-41d5-4641-bf50-1be4a0f7ed95; Samuel Yang and Christina Zhou, "Why You're Not Likely to Catch Coronavirus from Your Favorite Dumpling Restaurant," *ABC News*, February 6, 2020, https://www.abc.net.au/news/2020-02-06/coronavirus-catch-chinese-restaurant-australia-box-hill/11933186; Olson, Alexandra and Tang, Terry. "Misguided Virus Fears Hitting Asian American Businesses." Associated Press. Hawaii Tribune-Herald. February 19, 2020.

49 Amir Vera, "2 Cruise Lines Bar People with Chinese, Hong Kong or Macau Passports from Boarding Their Ships as Coronavirus Spreads," *CNN*, February 7, 2020, https://www.cnn.com/2020/02/07/us/coronavirus-cruise-ships-protocol/index.html.

50 "Coronavirus Disease 2019 (COVID-19) Situation Report-35," WHO, February 24, 2020, https://www.who.int/docs/default-source/coronaviruse/situation-reports/20200224-sitrep-35-covid-19.pdf?sfvrsn=1ac4218d_2.

51 Social Stigma Associated with COVID-19: A Guide to Preventing and Addressing Social Stigma," WHO, February 24, 2020, https://cdn.who.int/media/docs/default-source/epi-win/stigma/covid19-stigma-guide.pdf?sfvrsn=48f6ac1_2&download=true.

52 Russell Jeung, Sara Growing, and Kara Takasaki, "News Accounts of COVID-19 Discrimination 2/9–3/7/20," *A Report for A3PCON and CAA*, March 7, 2020, https://drive.google.com/file/d/1mzNEU2ebTF_5OZUon-ovrt36x22nXcuE/view.

53 Jeung, Growing, and Takasaki, "News Accounts of COVID-19 Discrimination 2/9–3/7/20,"

54 Jeung, Growing, and Takasaki, "News Accounts of COVID-19 Discrimination 2/9–3/7/20."

55 Mattha Busby, "Vietnamese Curator Dropped Because of 'Coronavirus Prejudice,'" *The Guardian*, March 5, 2020, https://www.theguardian.com/world/2020/mar/05/vietnamese-curator-dropped-because-of-coronavirus-prejudice.

56 Jeung, Growing, and Takasaki, "News Accounts of COVID-19 Discrimination 2/9–3/7/20."

57 Jeung, Growing, and Takasaki, "News Accounts of COVID-19 Discrimination 2/9–3/7/20."

58 Walter Russell Mead, "China is the Real Sick Man of Asia," *Wall-Street Journal*, February 3, 2020, https://www.wsj.com/articles/china-is-the-real-sick-man-of-asia-11580773677.

59 Walter Russell Mead, "China is the Real Sick Man of Asia," *Wall-Street Journal*, February 3, 2020, https://www.wsj.com/articles/china-is-the-real-sick-man-of-asia-11580773677.

60 Jia and Lu, "US Media's Coverage of China's Handling of COVID-19."

61 David Choi, "'They are a Very Hungry People': Fox News Host Fuels Racist Tropes About Chinese Over Coronavirus Outbreak," *Insider*, March 2, 2020, https://www.businessinsider.com/fox-news-jesse-watters-chinese-demands-apology-racism-2020-3.

62 Jennifer Hansler and Veronica Stracqualursi, "Pompeo is 'Confident' the US Will Handle Coronavirus 'Better Than Any Nation in the World,'" *CNN*, March 6, 2020, https://www.cnn.com/2020/03/06/politics/mike-pompeo-us-coronavirus-outbreak/index.html.

63 Paul Gosar@DrPaulGosar, Tweet, March 8, 2020, https://twitter.com/DrPaulGosar/status/1236821135964004352?s=20.

64 Max Rizzuto, "U.S. Politicians Exploit Coronavirus Fears with Anti-Chinese Dog Whistles, *Medium*, DFR Lab, March 17, 2020, https://medium.com/dfrlab/u-s-politicians-exploit-coronavirus-fears-with-anti-chinese-dog-whistles-ff61c9d7e458.

65 Rizzuto, "U.S. Politicians Exploit Coronavirus Fears with Anti-Chinese Dog Whistles."

66 Kevin McCarthy@GOPLeader, Tweet, March 9, 2020, https://twitter.com/GOPLeader/status/1237165063565447168?s=20.

67 Charlie Kirk@charliekirk11, Tweet on March 10, 2020, https://twitter.com/charliekirk11/status/1237306970429775872.

68 James Fallows, "2020 Time Capsule #5: The 'Chinese Virus,'" *The Atlantic*, March 18, 2020, https://www.theatlantic.com/ideas/archive/2020/03/2020-time-capsule-5-the-chinese-virus/622116/.

69 Kimmy Yam, "Trump Tweets About Coronavirus Using Term 'Chinese Virus," *NBC News*, March 16, 2020, https://www.nbcnews.com/news/asian-america/trump-tweets-about-coronavirus-using-term-chinese-virus-n1161161?cid=sm_npd_nn_tw_ma.

70 HuffPost@HuffPost, Tweet, March 18, 2020, https://twitter.com/HuffPost/status/1240340944714526721.

71 Rizzuto, "U.S. Politicians Exploit Coronavirus Fears with Anti-Chinese Dog Whistles."

72 "Twitter Trends on 17th March, 2020," *Trend Calendar*, 2022, https://us.trend-calendar.com/trend/2020-03-17.html.

73 "Chinese Virus," *Factbase*, Search for 1/14/2020 to 3/31/2020, https://factba.se/trump/search# percent22chinese percent2Bvirus percent22; Allan Smith, "Photo of Trump Remarks Shows 'Corona' Crossed Out and Replaced with 'Chinese' Virus,"

NBC News, March 19, 2020, https://www.nbcnews.com/politics/donald-trump/photo-trump-remarks-shows-corona-crossed-out-replaced-chinese-virus-n1164111; Jérôme Viala-Gaudefroy, and Dana Lindaman, "Donald Trump's 'Chinese virus': The Politics of Naming," *The Conversation*, April 21, 2020, https://theconversation.com/donald-trumps-chinese-virus-the-politics-of-naming-136796.

74 Tahmasbi, Schild, Ling, Blackburn, Stringhini, Zhang, and Zannettou,""Go Eat a Bat, Chang!'"

75 Sean Darling-Hammond, Eli K. Michaels, Amani M. Allen, David H. Chae, Marilyn D. Thomas, Thu T. Nguyen, Mahasin M. Mujahid, and Rucker C. Johnson, "After "The China Virus" Went Viral: Racially Charged Coronavirus Coverage and Trends in Bias Against Asian Americans," *Health Education & Behavior* 47, no. 6 (2020): 870–79.

76 Sabrina Tavernise and Richard A. Oppel Jr., "Spit On, Yelled, Attacked: Chinese-Americans Fear for Their Safety," *New York Times*, March 23, 2020, https://www.nytimes.com/2020/03/23/us/chinese-coronavirus-racist-attacks.html.

77 Sophia Chang, "NYPD Investigating Hate Crime After Asian Woman Allegedly Punched for Not Wearing Face Mask," *Gothamist*, March 11, 2020, https://gothamist.com/news/nypd-investigating-hate-crime-after-asian-woman-allegedly-punched-not-wearing-face-mask.

78 Caitlin Yoshiko Kandil, "Asian Americans Report Over 650 Racist Acts Over Last Week, New Data Says," *NBC News*, March 26, 2020, https://www.nbcnews.com/news/asian-america/asian-americans-report-nearly-500-racist-acts-over-last-week-n1169821.

79 Kandil, "Asian Americans Report Over 650 Racist Acts Over Last Week."

80 Jérôme Viala-Gaudefroy and Dana Lindaman, "Donald Trump's 'Chinese virus': The Politics of Naming," *The Conversation*, April 21, 2020, https://theconversation.com/donald-trumps-chinese-virus-the-politics-of-naming-136796.

81 "China Virus," *Factbase*, https://factba.se/trump/search# percent22china percent2Bvirus percent22.

82 "Trump Calls the Coronavirus the 'Kung Flu," Video of a Trump Rally in Tulsa, Oklahoma, posted to *YouTube* by the *Los Angeles Times*, June 20, 2020, https://www.youtube.com/watch?v=fN2tgtcKGck.

83 Barry Sautman, "Big Thunder, Little Rain: The Yellow Peril Framing of the Pandemic Campaign Against China," *Chinese Journal of International Law* 20, no. 2 (2021): 395–424.

84 Sarah Midkiff, "Marsha Blackburn's Stop COVID Act is Rooted in Xenophobia," *Refinery29*, May 6, 2020, https://www.refinery29.com/en-us/2020/05/9784868/marsha-blackburn-stop-covid-act-china-twitter.

85 "Blackburn Reintroduces the Stop COVID Act to Hold China Accountable for Spreading COVID-19," *News*, Marsha Blackburn U.S. Senator for Tennessee website, June 10, 2021, https://www.blackburn.senate.gov/2021/6/blackburn

-reintroduces-the-stop-covid-act-to-hold-china-accountable-for-spreading-covid-19/6e4ef395-f8f3-4c4e-93cf-4693c2a7741e.

86 Iliana Magra and Christine Hasuser, "Lululemon Fires Employee Over 'Bat Fried Rice' Shirt," *New York Times*, April 22, 2020, https://www.nytimes.com/2020/04/22/business/lululemon-bat-fried-rice-shirt-coronavirus.html.

87 Ariadna Matamoros-Fernández and Aleesha Rodriguez, "Not Just a Joke: We Scoured Tiktok for Anti-Asian Humour During the Pandemic, and Found Too Many Disappointing Memes," *The Conversation*, September 29, 2022, https://theconversation.com/not-just-a-joke-we-scoured-tiktok-for-anti-asian-humour-during-the-pandemic-and-found-too-many-disappointing-memes-184166.

88 Matamoros-Fernández and Rodriguez, "Not Just a Joke."

89 Posted by FireRed, "Kung Flu Fighting by Steven Crowder," March 23, 2020, https://www.youtube.com/watch?v=xKh-pJlxkDs.

90 Su Zhaohui, Dean McDonnell, Junaid Ahmad, Ali Cheshmehzangi, Xiaoshan Li, Kylie Meyer, Yuyang Cai, Ling Yang, and Yu-Tao Xiang, "Time to Stop the Use of 'Wuhan Virus','China Virus' or 'Chinese Virus' Across the Scientific Community," *BMJ Global Health* 5, no. 9 (2020): e003746.

91 Guangting Zeng, Linlin Wang, and Zanling Zhang, "Prejudice and xenophobia in COVID-19 research manuscripts," *Nature Human Behaviour* 4, no. 9 (2020): 879–79.

92 Jia and Lu, "US Media's Coverage of China's Handling of COVID-19."

93 Michelle King, "Say No to Bat Fried Rice: Changing the Narrative of Coronavirus and Chinese Food," *Food and Foodways* 28, no. 3 (2020): 237–49; Moser, David. "A Fearful Asymmetry: COVID-19 and America's Information Deficit with China." *Asia-Pacific Journal-Japan Focus* (2020).

94 Laura Silver, Kat Devlin, and Christine Huang, "Americans Fault China for Its Role in the Spread of COVID-19," *Health Policy*, Pew Research Center, July 30, 2020, https://www.pewresearch.org/global/2020/07/30/americans-fault-china-for-its-role-in-the-spread-of-covid-19/.

95 Silver, Devlin, and Huang, "Americans Fault China for Its Role in the Spread of COVID-19."

96 Silver, Devlin, and Huang, "Americans Fault China for Its Role in the Spread of COVID-19."

97 Neil G. Ruiz, Juliana Horowitz, and Christine Tamir, "Many Black and Asian Americans Say They Have Experienced Discrimination Amid the COVID-19 Outbreak," *Pew Research Center*, July 2020,

98 Ruiz, Horowitz, and Tamir, "Many Black and Asian Americans Say They Have Experienced Discrimination."

99 Ruiz, Horowitz, and Tamir, "Many Black and Asian Americans Say They Have Experienced Discrimination."

100 Stephanie L. Haft and Qing Zhou, "An Outbreak of Xenophobia: Perceived Discrimination and Anxiety in Chinese American College Students Before and During the COVID-19 Pandemic," *International Journal of Psychology* 56, no. 4 (2021): 522–31.

101 "Report to the Nation: Anti-Asian Prejudice & Hate Crime," Center for the Study of Hate & Extremism, April 28, 2021.

102 "Two Years and Thousands of Voices: What Community-Generated Data Tells Us About Anti-AAPI Hate," *Stop AAPI Hate*. 2022, https://stopaapihate.org/wp-content/uploads/2022/07/Stop-AAPI-Hate-Year-2-Report.pdf.

103 "Two Years and Thousands of Voices: What Community-Generated Data Tells Us About Anti-AAPI Hate," *Stop AAPI Hate*.

104 Joel Rose, "Some Republicans Claimed Migrants Fueled a COVID-19 Surge. Doctors Say It's Not True," *NPR*, August 9, 2021, https://www.npr.org/2021/08/09/1026207555/some-republicans-claimed-migrants-fueled-a-covid-19-surge-doctors-say-its-not-tr; "Sen. Cruz: South Texas COVID Rates are Rising Because of the Biden-Harris Border Crisis," *Ted Cruz U.S. Senator for Texas Press Release*, July 14, 2021, https://www.cruz.senate.gov/newsroom/press-releases/sen-cruz-south-texas-covid-rates-are-rising-because-of-the-biden-harris-border-crisis.

105 Hamel, Liz, Lopes, Lunna, Sparks, Grace, Kirzinger, Ashley, Kearney, Audrey, Stokes, Mellisha, and Brodie, Mollyann, "KFF COVID-19 Vaccine Monitor: September 2021," *Kaiser Family Foundation*, September 28, 2021, https://www.kff.org/coronavirus-covid-19/poll-finding/kff-covid-19-vaccine-monitor-september-2021/.

106 Hans Henri P. Kluge, Zsuzsanna Jakab, Jozef Bartovic, Veronika d'Anna, and Santino Severoni, "Refugee and Migrant Health in the COVID-19 Response," *The Lancet* 395, no. 10232 (2020): 1237–239.

107 Cato T. Laurencin and Aneesah McClinton, "The COVID-19 Pandemic: A Call to Action to Identify and Address Racial and Ethnic Disparities," *Journal of Racial and Ethnic Health Disparities* 7, No. 3 (2020): 398–402; Reyes, Maritza Vasquez, "The Disproportional Impact Of COVID-19 on African Americans," *Health and Human Rights* 22, no. 2 (2020): 299.

108 "Investigate Rates of COVID-19 in the United States," *Health Equity Tracker*, August 2022, https://healthequitytracker.org/exploredata?gclid=CjoKCQjwpeaYBhDXARIsAEzItbEfV6pt5DgQ1otyadSDtoHsiAZ72p3pd6pEWG95M233GAZJfOpbYTAaAmpYEALw_wcB.

109 Laurencin and McClinton, "The COVID-19 Pandemic: A Call to Action to Identify and Address Racial and Ethnic Disparities"; Reyes, "The Disproportional Impact Of COVID-19 on African Americans."

110 Adam J. Milam, Debra Furr-Holden, Jennifer Edwards-Johnson, Birgete Webb, John W. Patton III, Nnayereugo C. Ezekwemba, Lekiesha Porter et al., "Are Clinicians Contributing to Excess African American COVID-19 Deaths? Unbeknownst to Them, They May Be," *Health Equity* 4, no. 1 (2020): 139–41; Tegan K. Boehmer, Emily H. Koumans, Elizabeth L. Skillen, Michael D. Kappelman, Thomas W. Carton, Aditiben Patel, Euna M. August et al., "Racial and Ethnic Disparities in Outpatient Treatment of COVID-19 — United States, January–July 2022," *Morbidity and Mortality Weekly Report* 71, no. 43 (2022): 1359.

111 Danbi Lee, Paula M. Kett, Selina A. Mohammed, Bianca K. Frogner, and Janice

Sabin. "Inequitable Care Delivery Toward COVID-19 Positive People of Color and People with Disabilities," *PLOS Global Public Health* 3, no. 4 (2023): e0001499.

112 Lee, Kett, Mohammed, Frogner, and Sabin," "Inequitable Care Delivery."

113 Lee, Kett, Mohammed, Frogner, and Sabin," "Inequitable Care Delivery."

114 Frederiksen, Brittni, Ranji, Usha, and Salganicoff, Alina, and Long, Michelle. "Women's Experiences with Health Care During the COVID-19 Pandemic: Findings from the KFF Women's Health Survey. 2021," *Kaiser Family Foundation*, https://www.kff.org/womens-health-policy/issue-brief/womens-experiences-with-health-care-during-the-covid-19-pandemic-findings-from-the-kff-womens-health-survey/.

115 Hill, Evan, Tiefenthäler, Ainara, Triebert, Christiaan, Jordan, Drew, Willis, Haley and Stein, Robin. "How George Floyd Was Killed in Police Custody," *New York Times*, Updated January 24, 2022; Leonard E. Egede and Rebekah J. Walker, "Structural Racism, Social Risk Factors, And COVID-19—a Dangerous Convergence for Black Americans," *New England Journal of Medicine* 383, no. 12 (2020): e77, https://www.nytimes.com/2020/05/31/us/george-floyd-investigation.html.

116 Audra D. S. Burch, Amy Harmon, Sabrina Tavernise, and Emily Badger, "The Death of George Floyd Reignited a Movement. What Happens Now?" *New York Times*, Updated June 23, 2023, https://www.nytimes.com/2021/04/20/us/george-floyd-protests-police-reform.html.

117 Larry Buchanan, Quoctrung Bui, and , Jugel K. Patel, "Black Lives Matter May Be the Largest Movement in U.S. History," *New York Times*, July 3, 2020, https://www.nytimes.com/interactive/2020/07/03/us/george-floyd-protests-crowd-size.html.

118 Yiwei Xu, Elizabeth K. Farkouh, Caroline A. Dunetz, Sravya L. Varanasi, Sophia Mathews, Sarah E. Gollust, Erika Franklin Fowler, Steven Moore, Neil A. Lewis Jr, and Jeff Niederdeppe, "Local TV News Coverage of Racial Disparities in COVID-19 During the First Wave of the Pandemic, March–June 2020," *Race and Social Problems* 15, No. 2 (2023): 201–13; Mia Moody-Ramirez, Gabriel Tait, and Dorothy Bland, "An Analysis of George Floyd-Themed Memes: A Critical Race Theory Approach to Analyzing Memes Surrounding the 2020 George Floyd Protests," *Journal of Social Media in Society* 10, No. 2 (2021): 373–401.

119 Lindsey Dawson, Ashley Kirzinger, and Jennifer Kates. "The Impact of the COVID-19 Pandemic on LGBT People," *San Francisco, CA: The Kaiser Family Foundation* (2021), https://www.kff.org/coronavirus-covid-19/poll-finding/the-impact-of-the-covid-19-pandemic-on-lgbt-people/.

120 The Trevor Project, 2021 National Survey on LGBTQ Youth Mental Health. West Hollywood, California: The Trevor Project (2021), https://www.thetrevorproject.org/survey-2021/?section=ResearchMethodology.

121 The Trevor Project, "2021 National Survey on LGBTQ Youth Mental Health."

122 Federica Previtali, Laura D. Allen, and Maria Varlamova, "Not Only Virus Spread: The Diffusion of Ageism During the Outbreak of COVID-19," *Journal of Aging & Social Policy* 32, no. 4–5 (2020): 506–14.

123 "Impact Report: COVID-19 and Domestic Violence," *Council on Criminal Justice*, February 23, 2021, https://counciloncj.org/impact-report-covid-19-and-domestic-violence-trends/; Office of Inspector General, "National Snapshot of Trends in the National Domestic Violence Hotline's Contact Data Before and During the COVID-19 Pandemic," U.S. Department of Health & Human Services, April 2022, https://oig.hhs.gov/oas/reports/region9/92106000RIB.pdf.

124 Tiago S. Jesus, Sutanuka Bhattacharjya, Christina Papadimitriou, Yelena Bogdanova, Jacob Bentley, Juan Carlos Arango-Lasprilla, Sureshkumar Kamalakannan, and Refugee Empowerment Task Force, International Networking Group of the American Congress of Rehabilitation Medicine, "Lockdown-related Disparities Experienced by People with Disabilities During the First Wave of the COVID-19 Pandemic: Scoping Review With Thematic Analysis," *International Journal of Environmental Research and Public Health* 18, no. 12 (2021): 6178.

125 John Lai and Nicole O. Widmar, "Revisiting the Digital Divide in the COVID-19 Era," *Applied Economic Perspectives and Policy* 43, no. 1 (2021): 458–64; Gabrielle Martins Van Jaarsveld, "The Effects of COVID-19 Among the Elderly Population: A Case for Closing the Digital Divide," *Frontiers in Psychiatry* 11 (2020): 1211.

Chapter Six: A Pivotal Moment

1 Katie Thomas, David Gelles, and Carl Zimmer, "Pfizer's Early Data Shows Vaccine is More Than 90 percent Effective," *New York Times*, November 9, 2020, https://www.nytimes.com/2020/11/09/health/covid-vaccine-pfizer.html?smid=tw-share.

2 Thomas, Gelles, and Zimmer, "Pfizer's Early Data Shows Vaccine is More Than 90 percent Effective."

3 "Moderna's COVID-19 Vaccine Candidate Meets Its Primary Efficacy Endpoint in the First Interim Analysis of the Phase 3 COVE Study," Press Release, November 16, 2020.

4 "FDA Takes Key Action," *FDA News Release*; "Moderna Announces FDA Authorization," *Moderna Press Release*.

5 Feuer, Will. U.S. Administers First Shots of Pfizer's Covid Vaccine, Launching a Historic Rollout." *CNBC*. December 14, 2020, https://www.cnbc.com/2020/12/14/us-administers-first-shots-of-pfizers-covid-vaccine-launching-a-historic-rollout.html.

6 Jennifer Kates, Jennifer Tolbert, and Josh Michaud, "The COVID-19 "Vaccination Line": An Update on State Prioritization Plans," Kaiser Family Foundation, January 11 (2021): 2021, https://www.kff.org/coronavirus-covid-19/issue-brief/the-covid-19-vaccination-line-an-update-on-state-prioritization-plans/.

7 "Johnson & Johnson COVID-19 Vaccine Authorized by U.S. FDA For Emergency Use—First Single-Shot Vaccine in Fight Against Global Pandemic," *Our Company*, Press Release, Johnson & Johnson, February 27, 2021, https://www.jnj

.com/johnson-johnson-covid-19-vaccine-authorized-by-u-s-fda-for-emergency-usefirst-single-shot-vaccine-in-fight-against-global-pandemic.

8 Jack Healy, "'It's Like Buying Bruce Springsteen Tickets': The Hunt to Find a Vaccine Shot," *New York Times*, March 4, 2021, https://www.nytimes.com/2021/03/03/us/covid-vaccine-appointment.html.

9 The Associated Press, "Want a Shot Quicker? Volunteer to Work at Vaccine Sites," *Nextstar Media Wire*, March 9, 2021, https://www.myarklamiss.com/news/national-news/want-the-covid-shot-quicker-volunteer-to-work-at-vaccine-sites/.

10 Amelia G. Johson, Lauren Linde, Akilah R. Ali, Allison DeSantis, Minchan Shi, Carolyn Adam, Brandy Armstrong et al., "COVID-19 Incidence and Mortality Among Unvaccinated and Vaccinated Persons Aged≥ 12 Years by Receipt of Bivalent Booster Doses and Time Since Vaccination—24 US Jurisdictions, October 3, 2021–December 24, 2022," *Morbidity and Mortality Weekly Report* 72, no. 6 (2023): 145, https://www.cdc.gov/mmwr/volumes/72/wr/mm7206a3.htm#F1_down.

11 "What's the nation's progress on vaccinations?" *USA Facts*, May 3, 2023, https://usafacts.org/visualizations/covid-vaccine-tracker-states.

12 "COVID-19 Vaccinations in the United States," *COVID Data Tracker*, CDC, May 9, 2023, https://covid.cdc.gov/covid-data-tracker/#vaccinations_vacc-total-admin-rate-total.

13 "COVID-19 Vaccinations in the United States," *COVID Data Tracker*,

14 Andrea Hsu, "Thousands of Workers Were Fired Over Vaccine Mandates. For Some, the Fight Goes On," *NPR*, December 27, 2022, https://www.npr.org/2022/12/27/1144323505/vaccine-mandates-lifted-sanitation-new-york-city-workers.

15 Sihong Zhao, Simeng Hu, Xiaoyu Zhou, Suhang Song, Qian Wang, Hongqiu Zheng, Ying Zhang, and Zhiyuan Hou, "The Prevalence, Features, Influencing Factors, and Solutions for COVID-19 Vaccine Misinformation: Systematic Review," *JMIR Public Health and Surveillance* 9, no. 1 (2023): e40201.

16 David Heath, *The Inside Story of the Race for a COVID-19 Vaccine*, 2022, Center Street.

17 Cary P. Gross and Kent A. Sepkowitz, "The Myth of the Medical Breakthrough: Smallpox, Vaccination, and Jenner Reconsidered," *International Journal of Infectious Diseases* 3, no. 1 (1998): 54–60.

18 Edward Jenner, An Inquiry into the Causes and Effects of the Variole Vaccine, A Disease Discovered in Some of the Western Counties of England, Particularly Gloucestershire, and Known by the name of the Cow Pox. London: Sampson Low, 1798; Jenner, Edward. Instructions for Vaccine Inoculation, Commonly Called Vaccination. 1807. Philadelphia.

19 Martin Kaufman, "The American Anti-Vaccinationists and their Arguments," *Bulletin of the History of Medicine* 41, no. 5 (1967): 463–78.

20 Alexandra J. Stewart and Phillip M. Devlin, "The History of the Smallpox Vaccine," *Journal of Infection* 52, no. 5 (2006): 329–34.

21 John Illo, "Pasteur and Rabies: an Interview of 1882," *Medical History*. 40, no. 3 (1996): 373–77.

22 "Vaccine Timeline: Before Jenner and After COVID-19," *History of Vaccines*, https://historyofvaccines.org/history/vaccine-timeline/timeline; Barbara J. Hawgood, "Waldemar Mordecai Haffkine, CIE (1860–1930): prophylactic vaccination against cholera and bubonic plague in British India." Journal of Medical Biography 15, no. 1 (2007): 9–19; Ernest Kuchar, M. Karlikowska-Skwarnik, S. Han, and A. Nitsch-Osuch, "Pertussis: History of the Disease and Current Prevention Failure," *Pulmonary Dysfunction and Disease* (2016): 77–82.

23 Marcia Meldrum, "'A Calculated Risk': The Salk Polio Vaccine Field Trials of 1954," *BMJ* 317, no. 7167 (1998): 1233–236.

24 Jane S. Smith, *Patenting the Sun: Polio and the Salk Vaccine* (New York: William Morrow and Company, 1990).

25 "Vaccine Timeline: Before Jenner and After COVID-19," *History of Vaccines*, https://historyofvaccines.org/history/vaccine-timeline/timeline.

26 "Smallpox Eradication Programme—SEP (1966–1980)," *Feature stories/Detail/*, WHO, May 1, 2010, https://www.who.int/news-room/feature-stories/detail/the-smallpox-eradication-programme---sep-(1966-1980).

27 Kaufman, "The American Anti-vaccinationists and Their Arguments."

28 Kaufman, "The American Anti-vaccinationists and Their Arguments."

29 Kim Tolley, "School Vaccination Wars: The Rise of Anti-Science in the American Anti-Vaccination Societies, 1879–1929," History of Education Quarterly 59, no. 2 (2019): 161–94.

30 Foss, *Constructing the Outbreak*.

31 "Measles, Mumps, and Rubella Vaccines," *Smithsonian*, https://www.si.edu/spotlight/antibody-initiative/mmr; "Vaccine Timeline: Before Jenner and After COVID-19," *History of Vaccines*, https://historyofvaccines.org/history/vaccine-timeline/timeline.

32 "Immunization Prevents Death Worldwide," *Data and Statistics*, CDC, April 20, 2023, https://www.cdc.gov/globalhealth/immunization/data/fast-facts.html#:~:text=Immunization percent20Prevents percent20Death percent20Worldwide,save percent20nearly percent2019 percent20million percent20lives.

33 A. J. Wakefield, "MMR Vaccination and Autism," *The Lancet*, *354*, no. 9182 (1999): 949–50.

34 Robert M. Wolfe, Lisa K. Sharp, and Martin S. Lipsky, "Content and Design Attributes of Antivaccination Web Sites," *JAMA* 287, no. 24 (2002): 3245–248.

35 Paul Davies, Simon Chapman, and Julie Leask, "Antivaccination Activists on the World Wide Web," *Archives of Disease in Childhood* 87, no. 1 (2002): 22–25.

36 Xiaoyi Yuan, Ross J. Schuchard, and Andrew T. Crooks, "Examining Emergent Communities and Social Bots Within the Polarized Online Vaccination Debate in Twitter," *Social Media & Society* 5, no. 3 (2019): 2056305119865465.

37 Schuchard Yuan and Crooks, "Examining Emergent Communities."

38 Savannah Santos, "Fighting the Rise of the Anti-Vaccination Movement," ESSAI 17, no. 1 (2019): 36.

39 Joshua M. Sharfstein, "Vaccines and the Trump Administration," *JAMA*, April 4, 2017, https://jamanetwork.com/journals/jama/fullarticle/2614172.

40 Johanna Goldfarb, "Measles: A Dangerous Vaccine-Preventable Disease Returns," *Cleveland Clinic Journal of Medicine* 86, no. 6 (2019): 393.

41 "Vaccination Coverage for Selected Diseases Among Adolescents Aged 13–17 Years, by Selected Characteristics: United States, selected years 2008–2019," *Health, United States, 2020–2021*. CDC. 2020–2021, https://www.cdc.gov/nchs/data/hus/2020-2021/VaxTn.pdf.

42 Heath, *The Inside Story of the Race for a COVID-19 Vaccine*.

43 Donald G. McNeil Jr., "New Tools to Hunt New Viruses," *New York Times*, May 28, 2013, https://www.nytimes.com/2013/05/28/health/new-tools-to-hunt-new-viruses.html?searchResultPosition=1.

44 McNeil Jr., "New Tools to Hunt New Viruses."

45 "3 to 4 Years Needed to Develop Vaccine for Wuhan Pneumonia Strain," *Channel News Asia*, January 5, 2020, https://www.channelnewsasia.com/news/singapore/3-to-4-years-needed-to-develop-vaccine-for-wuhan-pneumonia-12235570.

46 Gerry Shih and Lena H. Sun, "China Identifies New Strain of Coronavirus as Source of Pneumonia Outbreak," *Washington Post*, January 9, 2020.

47 Jonathan Lambert, "What We Know—And Don't Know—About a New Virus Causing Pneumonia in China," *ScienceNews*, January, 10, 2020, https://www.sciencenews.org/article/what-we-know-about-new-virus-causing-pneumonia-outbreak-china.

48 Lindy Washburn, "JFK to Check Those Arriving from Chinese City For Virus." *Daily Record*. January 18, 2020; Ross Lydall, "Passengers on China Flights Checked for Deadly Virus," *Evening Standard*, January 22, 2020; Associated Press, "Concern Spreads About Coronavirus," *Democrat and Chronicle*, January 23, 2020.

49 Jesper Pallesen, Nianshuang Wang, Kizzmekia S. Corbett, Daniel Wrapp, Robert N. Kirchdoerfer, Hannah L. Turner, Christopher A. Cottrell et al., "Immunogenicity And Structures of a Rationally Designed Prefusion MERS-Cov Spike Antigen," *Proceedings of the National Academy of Sciences* 114, no. 35 (2017): E7348-E7357; Heath, *The Inside Story of the Race for a COVID-19 Vaccine*.

50 John Bacon and Grace Hauck, "1st Case of Coronavirus Reported in US," *The Naples Daily News*, January 22, 2020.

51 "Moderna Announces Funding Award from CEPI to Accelerate Development of Messenger RNA (MRNA) Vaccine Against Novel Coronavirus," Press Release, Moderna, January 23, 2020, https://investors.modernatx.com/news/news-details/2020/Moderna-Announces-Funding-Award-from-CEPI-to-Accelerate-Development-of-Messenger-RNA-mRNA-Vaccine-Against-Novel-Coronavirus/default.aspx.

52 Bloomberg, "Virus Vaccine Plans Boost Drugmakers, But Time is Short," *Atlanta Constitution*, January 24, 2020; Zak Vescera, "U of S Scientists Working on Vaccine

for Coronavirus," *The Leader-Post*, January 24, 2020; Stacey Burling, "$9M Grant to Develop Coronavirus Vaccine," *Philadelphia Inquirer*. January 24, 2020.

53 George Roberts, "Coronavirus Vaccine Research to Include Team from Queensland," *ABC News*, Australia, January 23, 2020, https://www.abc.net.au/news/2020-01-24/coronavirus-vaccine-work-starts-with-queensland-researchers/11896346.

54 Hannah Devlin, "Lessons From Sars Outbreak Help in Race for Coronavirus Vaccine," *The Guardian*. January 24, 2020, https://www.theguardian.com/science/2020/jan/24/lessons-from-sars-outbreak-help-in-race-for-coronavirus-vaccine.

55 "Cambridge's Moderna Therapeutics Ramps Up Search for Coronavirus Vaccine," *CBS News Boston*, January 24, 2020, https://www.cbsnews.com/boston/news/coronavirus-vaccine-moderna-therapeutics-cambridge-norwood-massachusetts-cbs-news/; Sara Gilgore, "Different Outbreak, Same Strategy: Inside Novavax's Plans for a Coronavirus Vaccine," *Washington Business Journal*, January 24, 2020.

56 "Safety Trial for Coronavirus Vaccine May Happen Within Three Months," *CNBC*, shared on *YouTube!*. January 24, 2020, https://www.youtube.com/watch?v=vcTJd8WU488&t=238s.

57 "Coronavirus: Death Toll Climbs, and So Does the Number of Infections," *New York Times*, January 28, 2020 (Updated March 9, 2020) https://www.nytimes.com/2020/01/28/world/asia/china-coronavirus.html?searchResultPosition=2.

58 Sophie Scott, Penny Timms, and Loretta Florance, "Australian Lab First Outside of China to Copy Coronavirus, Helping Vaccine Push," *ABC News* Australia, Updated January 31, 2020, https://www.abc.net.au/news/2020-01-29/wuhan-coronavirus-created-in-australian-lab-outside-of-china/11906390?pfmredir=sm&sf229100222=1.

59 Jocelyn Garcia, "'We Thought We Had Three Years': UQ Team To Fast-Track Coronavirus Vaccine," *Brisbane Times*, January 24, 2020, https://www.brisbanetimes.com.au/national/queensland/we-thought-we-had-three-years-uq-team-to-fast-track-coronavirus-vaccine-20200124-p53udl.html.

60 Meghan Fitzgerald, "Novavax Exec: Making a Coronavirus Vaccine Could Take a Long Time," *Yahoo!Finance*. January 24, 2020, https://finance.yahoo.com/news/timeline-for-a-coronavirus-vaccine-could-be-extensive-says-novavax-president-of-rd-210355032.html.

61 "Wuhan Coronavirus Vaccine Could Take Years," January 24, 2020, https://www.onenewspage.com/video/20200125/12661009/Wuhan-Coronavirus-Vaccine-Could-Take-Years.htm.

62 Ken Alltucker, "Drugmakers are Rushing to Create and Test a Coronavirus Vaccine. Here's How They're Doing It," *USA Today*, January 24, 2020, https://www.usatoday.com/story/news/health/2020/01/24/national-institutes-health-has-partnered-boston-area-company-moderna-vaccine-targeting-novel-coronav/4568266002/.

63 Xinhua News Agency, "Coronavirus Vaccine May Be Ready in Months," *Financial Express*, January 24, 2020, https://thefinancialexpress.com.bd/health/coronavirus-vaccine-may-be-ready-in-months-scientists-1579863809.

64 https://twitter.com/ScienceAlert/status/1220888383150592002.
65 Jessica Bursztynsky, "J&J Scientific Officer 'Pretty Confident' They Can Create Coronavirus Vaccine as Outbreak Widens," *CNBC*, January 27, 2020, https://www.cnbc.com/2020/01/27/jj-pretty-confident-it-can-create-china-coronavirus-vaccine.html?__source=sharebar percent7Ctwitter&par=sharebar.
66 Carolyn Y. Johnson, "Coronavirus Vaccine Research is Moving at Record Speed," *Washington Post*, January 30, 2020.
67 Aubree Gordon and Florian Krammer, "When Will There be a Coronavirus Vaccine? Five Questions Answered," *The Conversation*, January 28, 2020, https://theconversation.com/when-will-there-be-a-coronavirus-vaccine-5-questions-answered-130590.
68 Bloomberg, "Virus Vaccine Plans Boost Drugmakers, But Time is Short."
69 https://twitter.com/Bagsy/status/1221128147120410625.
70 https://twitter.com/Forbes/status/1225090459929841665.
71 Lim Ruey Yan, "Jackie Chan offers reward of $197,000 for Antidote to Coronavirus," *The Straits Times*, February 5, 2020, https://www.straitstimes.com/lifestyle/entertainment/jackie-chan-offers-reward-of-197000-for-antidote-to-coronavirus.
72 https://twitter.com/DocMom_TX/status/1220892556730535941.
73 https://twitter.com/agirlcalledlina/status/1220877317486104576.
74 https://twitter.com/dendrades/status/1220984652975919104.
75 https://twitter.com/ThaSouth/status/1221273139826634752.
76 Ashish Joshi, "Coronavirus: 'Significant Breakthrough' in Race for Vaccine Made by UK Scientists," *Sky News*, February 5, 2020, https://news.sky.com/story/coronavirus-significant-breakthrough-in-race-for-vaccine-made-by-uk-scientists-11926469?dcmp=snt-sf-twitter.
77 https://twitter.com/htTweets/status/1225687416091992065.
78 Neda Iranpour, "San Diego Lab Discovers Coronavirus Vaccine in 3 Hours," *KVUE*, February 14, 2020, https://www.kvue.com/article/news/health/coronavirus/coronavirus-vaccine-san-diego/509-e18e37f6-347c-4b08-ad33-910968abb04f.
79 "Moderna Ships MRNA Vaccine Against Novel Coronavirus (MRNA-1273) for Phase 1 Study," Press Release, Moderna, February 24, 2020, https://investors.modernatx.com/news/news-details/2020/Moderna-Ships-mRNA-Vaccine-Against-Novel-Coronavirus-mRNA-1273-for-Phase-1-Study/default.aspx.
80 Paige Winfield Cunningham, and Paulina Firozi, "The Health 202: Drugmakers are Developing a Coronavirus Vaccine. That's a Sign the Disease will be Around a Long Time," *Washington Post*, February 19, 2020, https://www.washingtonpost.com/news/powerpost/paloma/the-health-202/2020/02/19/the-health-202-drugmakers-are-developing-a-coronavirus-vaccine-that-s-a-sign-the-disease-will-be-around-a-long-time/5e4c5169602ff16b163b1a2b/.
81 Amanda Terkel, "Trump Said Coronavirus Would 'Miraculously' Be Gone by April. Well, It's April," *HuffPost*, April 2, 2020, https://www.huffpost.com/entry/trump-coronavirus-gone-april_n_5e7b6886c5b6b7d8095959c2.
82 https://twitter.com/eugenegu/status/1232059599567540224.

83 https://twitter.com/eugenegu/status/1232059599567540224.

84 "Remarks by President Trump, Vice President Pence, and Members of the Coronavirus Task Force in Press Conference," Press Briefings, February 27, 2020, https://trump whitehouse.archives.gov/briefings-statements/remarks-president-trump-vice-president-pence-members-coronavirus-task-force-press-conference/.

85 https://twitter.com/QTRResearch/status/1232280425416056832.

86 "Remarks by President Trump, Vice President Pence, and Members of the Coronavirus Task Force in Press Conference." Press Briefings.

87 https://twitter.com/SenSchumer/status/1232819154866069504.

88 https://twitter.com/janschakowsky/status/1230537703701336064.

89 Lisa Du, "70 Coronavirus Vaccines Are Under Development, with 3 in Human Trials, WHO Says," *Time*, April 13, 2020, https://time.com/5819887/coronavirus-vaccines-development-who/.

90 Knuvl Sheikh and Katie Thomas, "Researchers are Racing to Make a Coronavirus Vaccine. Will It Help?" *New York Times*, January 28, 2020, Updated June 10, 2020, https://www.nytimes.com/2020/01/28/health/coronavirus-vaccine.html.

91 "BioNTech and Pfizer Announce Completion of Dosing for First Cohort of Phase 1/2 Trial of COVID-19 Vaccine Candidates in Germany." *Newsroom.* Pfizer Press Release. April 29, 2020, https://www.pfizer.com/news/press-release/press-release-detail/biontech-and-pfizer-announce-completion-dosing-first-cohort; "Pfizer and BioNTech Dose First Participants in the U.S. as Part of Global COVID-19 mRNA Vaccine Development Program." *Newsroom.* Press Release. May 5, 2020, https://www.pfizer.com/news/press-release/press-release-detail/pfizer_and_biontech_dose_first_participants_in_the_u_s_as_part_of_global_covid_19_mrna_vaccine_development_program.

92 Lisa Du, "70 Coronavirus Vaccines are Under Development, with 3 in Human Trials, WHO Says," *Time*, April 13, 2020, https://time.com/5819887/coronavirus-vaccines-development-who/.

93 "Oxford COVID-19 Vaccine Begins Human Trial Stage." *News & Events.* University of Oxford. April 23, 2020, https://www.ox.ac.uk/news/2020-04-23-oxford-covid-19-vaccine-begins-human-trial-stage.

94 Li Crystal Jiang, Tsz Hang Chu, and Mengru Sun, "Characterization of Vaccine Tweets During the Early Stage of the COVID-19 Outbreak in the United States: Topic Modeling Analysis," *JMIR Infodemiology* 1, no. 1 (2021): e25636.

95 Jiang, Chu, and Sun. "Characterization of Vaccine Tweets."

96 See *Trump Twitter Archive*, https://www.thetrumparchive.com/?searchbox=percent22vaccine percent22&dates= percent5B percent222020-01-05 percent22 percent2C percent222021-12-31 percent22 percent5D&results=1.

97 Philippe Gautret, Jean-Christophe Lagier, Philippe Parola, Line Meddeb, Morgane Mailhe, Barbara Doudier, Johan Courjon et al., "Hydroxychloroquine and Azithromycin as a Treatment of COVID-19: Results of an Open-Label Non-Randomized Clinical Trial," *International Journal of Antimicrobial Agents* 56, no. 1 (2020): 105949; Joffrey Fuhrer and Florian Cova, "'Quick and dirty': Intuitive

Cognitive Style Predicts Trust in Didier Raoult and His Hydroxychloroquine-Based Treatment Against COVID-19," *Judgment and Decision Making* 15, no. 6 (2020): 889–908.

98 "Remarks by President Trump, Vice President Pence, and Members of the Coronavirus Task Force in Press Briefing." *Remarks*, Press Briefing, March 19, 2020, https://trumpwhitehouse.archives.gov/briefings-statements/remarks-president-trump-vice-president-pence-members-coronavirus-task-force-press-briefing-6/.

99 *Google Trends*, Retrieved May 18, 2023, https://trends.google.com/trends/explore?date=2020-03-01 percent202020-08-01&q=hydroxychloroquine; Tessa R. Englund, Alan C. Kinlaw, and Saira Z. Sheikh, "Rise and Fall: Hydroxychloroquine and COVID-19 Global Trends: Interest, Political Influence, and Potential Implications," ACR open rheumatology 2, no. 12 (2020): 760–66.

100 Berkeley Lovelace Jr. and Kevin Breuninger, "Trump Says He Takes Hydroxychloroquine to Prevent Coronavirus Infection Even Though It's an Unproven treatment," *CNBC*, May 18, 2020, https://www.cnbc.com/2020/05/18/trump-says-he-takes-hydroxychloroquine-to-prevent-coronavirus-infection.html.

101 Kacper Niburski and Oskar Niburski, "Impact of Trump's Promotion of Unproven COVID-19 Treatments and Subsequent Internet Trends: Observational Study." *Journal of Medical Internet Research* 22, no. 11 (2020): e20044; Madanay, Farrah, Ryan C. McDevitt, and Peter A. Ubel, "Hydroxychloroquine for COVID-19: Variation in Regional Political Preferences Predicted New Prescriptions after President Trump's Endorsement," *Journal of Health Politics, Policy and Law* 47, no. 4 (2022): 429–51.

102 Madanay, McDevitt, and Ubel, "Impact of Trump's Promotion of Unproven COVID-19 Treatments."

103 "Remarks by President Trump, Vice President Pence, and Members of the Coronavirus Task Force in Press Briefing." *Remarks*. Press Briefing. April 23, 2020, https://trumpwhitehouse.archives.gov/briefings-statements/remarks-president-trump-vice-president-pence-members-coronavirus-task-force-press-briefing-31/.

104 Briana M. Trifiro, Chris Wells, and Alex Rochefort. "The Disinfectant Diversion: The Use of Narratives in Partisan News Media." *Mass Communication and Society* 25, no. 6 (2022): 764–85.

105 EJ Dickson, "What Would Actually Happen to Your Body If You Actually Injected Bleach?" *Rolling Stone*, April 24, 2020, https://www.rollingstone.com/culture/culture-news/trump-coronavirus-injecting-bleach-uv-light-covid-19-989605/.

106 Robert Glatter, "Calls To Poison Centers Spike After The President's Comments About Using Disinfectants To Treat Coronavirus," *Forbes*, April 25, 2020, https://www.forbes.com/sites/robertglatter/2020/04/25/calls-to-poison-centers-spike--after-the-presidents-comments-about-using-disinfectants-to-treat-coronavirus/?sh=562b5d4d1157.

107 Trifiro, Wells, and Rochefort, "The Disinfectant Diversion."

108 Trifiro, Wells, and Rochefort, "The Disinfectant Diversion."

109 Jennifer Jacobs and Drew Armstrong, "Trump's 'Operation Warp Speed' Aims to Rush Coronavirus Vaccine," *Bloomberg News*, April 29, 2020.

110 Jacobs and Armstrong, "Trump's 'Operation Warp Speed' Aims to Rush Coronavirus Vaccine."

111 Brett Samuels, "Trump administration launches 'Operation Warp Speed' to Accelerate Vaccine Development," *The Hill*, April 29, 2020, https://thehill.com/policy/healthcare/495315-trump-administration-pushing-for-accelerated-vaccine-development/.

112 David E. Sanger, "Trump Seeks Push to Speed Vaccine, Despite Safety Concerns," *New York Times*, April 29, 2020.

113 Sanger, "Trump Seeks Push to Speed Vaccine, Despite Safety Concerns."

114 Eden Engel-Rebitzer, Daniel C. Stokes, Zachary F. Meisel, Jonathan Purtle, Rebecca Doyle, and Alison M. Buttenheim, "Partisan Differences in Legislators' Discussion of Vaccination on Twitter During the COVID-19 Era: Natural Language Processing Analysis," *JMIR Infodemiology* 2, no. 1 (2022): e32372.

115 Engel-Rebitzer, Stokes, Meisel, Purtle, Doyle, and Buttenheim, "Partisan Differences in Legislators' Discussion of Vaccination."

116 Jon Cohen, "Unveiling 'Warp Speed,' the White House's America-first Push for a Coronavirus Vaccine," *Science*, May 12, 2020, https://www.sciencemag.org/news/2020/05/unveiling-warp-speed-white-house-s-america-first-push-coronavirus-vaccine; Alec Tyson, Courtney Johnson, and Cary Funk, " U.S. Public Now Divided Over Whether to Get COVID-19 Vaccine," *Science & Society*, Pew Research Center, September 17, 2020, https://www.pewresearch.org/science/2020/09/17/u-s-public-now-divided-over-whether-to-get-covid-19-vaccine/.

117 "Recommendation Regarding the Use of Cloth Face Coverings, Especially in Areas of Significant Community-Based Transmission." *Coronavirus Disease 2019 (COVID-19)*. CDC. April 3, 2020. Accessed through *Wayback Machine*, https://web.archive.org/web/20200404022600/https://www.cdc.gov/coronavirus/2019-ncov/prevent-getting-sick/cloth-face-cover.html.

118 "CDC calls on Americans to wear masks to prevent COVID-19 spread." CDC. July 14, 2020, https://www.cdc.gov/media/releases/2020/p0714-americans-to-wear-masks.html.

119 Jacobs, Philip, and Arvi P. Ohinmaa. "The Enforcement of Statewide Mask Wearing Mandates to Prevent COVID-19 in the US: An Overview." *F1000Research* 9 (2020).

120 Jacobs and Arvi, "The Enforcement of Statewide Mask Wearing Mandates."

121 Kevin Brueninger, "Trump Says Face Masks Are 'Patriotic' After Months of Largely Resisting Wearing One," *CNBC News*, July 20, 2020, https://www.cnbc.com/2020/07/20/trump-says-coronavirus-masks-are-patriotic-after-months-of-largely-resisting-wearing-one.html; Libby Cathey, "Trump, Downplaying Virus, Has Mocked Wearing Masks for Months," *ABC News*, October 2, 2020, https://abcnews.go.com/Politics/trump-downplaying-virus-mocked-wearing-masks

-months/story?id=73392694; Daniel Victor, Lew Serviss, and Azi Paybarah, "In His Own Words, Trump on the Coronavirus and Masks," *New York Times*, October 2, 2020, https://www.nytimes.com/2020/10/02/us/politics/donald-trump-masks.html.

122 Libby Cathey, "Trump, Downplaying Virus, Has Mocked Wearing Masks for Months," *ABC News*, October 2, 2020, https://abcnews.go.com/Politics/trump-downplaying-virus-mocked-wearing-masks-months/story?id=73392694; Daniel Victor, Lew Serviss, and Azi Paybarah, "In His Own Words, Trump on the Coronavirus and Masks," *New York Times*, October 2, 2020,

123 Dannagal G. Young, Huma Rasheed, Amy Bleakley, and Jessica B. Langbaum, "The Politics of Mask-Wearing: Political Preferences, Reactance, and Conflict Aversion During COVID," *Social Science & Medicine* 298 (2022): 114836.

124 Lauren Camera, "GOP Governors Double Down on Orders Barring Mask Man dates in Schools," *U.S. News and World Report*, August 10, 2021, https://www.usnews.com/news/education-news/articles/2021-08-10/gop-governors-double-down-on-orders-barring-mask-mandates-in-schools.

125 Aaron Blake, "Timeline: Trump's Pressure Campaign to Overturn the 2020 Election," *Washington Post*, October 7, 2021, https://www.washingtonpost.com/politics/2021/08/06/trumps-brazen-attempt-overturn-2020-election-timeline/.

126 Aaron Blake, "Timeline: Trump's Pressure Campaign to Overturn the 2020 Election," *Washington Post*. October 7, 2021, https://www.washingtonpost.com/politics/2021/08/06/trumps-brazen-attempt-overturn-2020-election-timeline/.

127 Elizabeth Dwoskin and Rachel Lerman, "'Stop The Steal' Supporters, Restrained by Facebook, Turn to Parler to Peddle False Election Claims," *Washington Post*, November 13, 2020, https://www.washingtonpost.com/technology/2020/11/10/facebook-parler-election-claims/.

128 Katie Thomas, "New Pfizer Results: Coronavirus Vaccine is Safe and 95 percent Effective," *New York Times*, November 14, 2020, https://www.nytimes.com/2020/11/18/health/pfizer-covid-vaccine.html.

129 Fernando P. Polack, Stephen J. Thomas, Nicholas Kitchin, Judith Absalon, Alejandra Gurtman, Stephen Lockhart, John L. Perez et al., "Safety and efficacy of the BNT162b2 mRNA COVID-19 Vaccine," New England Journal of Medicine 383, no. 27 (2020): 2603–615.

130 Associated Press, "Pfizer Says COVID-19 Vaccine is Looking 90 percent Effective," *Black Hills Pioneer* and other newspapers, November 9, 2020; "Get Hawaii Ready for the Vaccine," *Our View. Honolulu Star-Advertiser*. November 9, 2020, A10; Carolyn Y. Johnson, "Trial Vaccine Shows 90 Percent Effectiveness," *Washington Post* and other newspapers, November 10, 2020; Katie Thomas and David Gelles, "Vaccine Shows Promise in Trial: Pfizer's Early Data Reveal 90 Percent Efficacy, But Details Sparse and Questions Abound on Long-term Safety, Protection," *New York Times* (and *Boston Globe*), November 10, 2020; Liz Goodwin, "Vaccine Shows Promise in Trial: As Transition Delay Ensues, Virus Worsens," *Boston Globe*, November 10, 2020; Kay Lazar, "Experts Sound a Note Of Caution: Masks,

Distancing May Be Needed Well Into 2021, Some Say," *Boston Globe*, November 10, 2020, A1; Lauren Neergaard, "What's ahead for COVID-19 Vaccines?" Associated Press, November 10, 2020. A7; Karen Weintraub, "Pfizer's Candidate for Vaccine Raises Hopes," *USA Today* (appearing in The Tennessean and other outlets), November 10, 2020. A1.

131 Joe Murphy, "Vaccine Joy: 'Great Day for Humanity," *Evening Standard*, November 9, 2020. A1; "Pfizer Denies Trump Admin Credit for the Vaccine," *Newsmax*, November 10, 2020; "Harris, Cuomo have balked at COVID vaccine under Trump. What about now?" *Fox News*, November, 10, 2020. "Trump, Biden celebrate Pfizer revealing coronavirus vaccine progress," *Fox News*, November 10, 2020, https://web.archive.org/web/20201110004317/https://www.foxnews.com/.

132 Lindsey R. Baden, Hana M. El Sahly, Brandon Essink, Karen Kotloff, Sharon Frey, Rick Novak, David Diemert et al., "Efficacy and Safety of The Mrna-1273 SARS-CoV-2 Vaccine," *New England Journal of Medicine* 384, no. 5 (2021): 403–16.; Denise Grady, "Moderna Applies for Emergency F.D.A. Approval for Its Coronavirus Vaccine," *New York Times*, November 30, 2020, https://www.nytimes.com/2020/11/30/health/covid-vaccine-moderna.html?searchResultPosition=1; "FDA Takes Additional Action in Fight Against COVID-19 By Issuing Emergency Use Authorization for Second COVID-19 Vaccine," FDA News Release, December 18, 2020, https://www.fda.gov/news-events/press-announcements/fda-takes-additional-action-fight-against-covid-19-issuing-emergency-use-authorization-second-covid.

133 Benjamin Mueller, "Why the U.K. Approved a Coronavirus Vaccine First," *New York Times*, December 2, 2020, https://www.nytimes.com/2020/12/02/world/europe/uk-covid-vaccine-pfizer.html; Michelle Roberts, "COVID-19: Pfizer/BioNTech Vaccine Judged Safe for Use in UK," *BBC News*, December 2, 2020, https://www.bbc.com/news/health-55145696.

134 "FDA Takes Key Action in Fight Against COVID-19 By Issuing Emergency Use Authorization for First COVID-19 Vaccine," *FDA News Release*, U.S. Food & Drug Administration, December 11, 2020, https://www.fda.gov/news-events/press-announcements/fda-takes-key-action-fight-against-covid-19-issuing-emergency-use-authorization-first-covid-19; "FDA Takes Additional Action in Fight Against COVID-19 By Issuing Emergency Use Authorization for Second COVID-19 Vaccine," *FDA News Release*, December 18, 2020, https://www.fda.gov/news-events/press-announcements/fda-takes-additional-action-fight-against-covid-19-issuing-emergency-use-authorization-second-covid.

135 "Johnson & Johnson COVID-19 Vaccine Authorized by U.S. FDA For Emergency Use—First Single-Shot Vaccine in Fight Against Global Pandemic," Press Release, Johnson & Johnson, February 27, 2021, https://www.jnj.com/johnson-johnson-covid-19-vaccine-authorized-by-u-s-fda-for-emergency-usefirst-single-shot-vaccine-in-fight-against-global-pandemic.

136 Sara Berg, "What Doctors Wish Patients Knew About the Johnson & Johnson

Vaccine," *Public Health*, American Medical Association, November 4, 2021, https://www.ama-assn.org/delivering-care/public-health/what-doctors-wish-patients-knew-about-johnson-johnson-vaccine.

137 Alexander Tin, "Omicron Deaths of Johnson & Johnson Recipients Were Double the Rate of Other Vaccinated Americans, New Data Show," *CBS News*, March 25, 2022, https://www.cbsnews.com/news/covid-omicron-johnson-johnson-vaccine/; Deidre McPhillips, "J&J COVID-19 Vaccine No Longer Available in The US," *CNN Health*, May 15, 2023, https://www.cnn.com/2023/05/15/health/johnson-johnson-covid-vaccine-end/index.html.

138 Ben Guarino, Ariana Eunjung Cha, Josh Wood, and Griff Witte, "'The Weapon That Will End the War': First Coronavirus Vaccine Shots Given Outside Trials In U.S.," *Washington Post*, December 14, 2020, https://www.washingtonpost.com/nation/2020/12/14/first-covid-vaccines-new-york/.

139 Alic Park, Jamie Ducharme, and W.J. Hennigan, "How the First COVID-19 Vaccinations Rolled Out at Hospitals Across the U.S," *Time*, December 14, 2020, https://time.com/5921608/covid-19-vaccine-rollout-hospitals/.

140 Liz Hamel, Ashley Kirzinger, Cailey Muñana, and Mollyann Brodie, "KFF COVID-19 Vaccine Monitor: December 2020," *Coronavirus (COVID-19)*, Kaiser Family Foundation, December 15, 2020, https://www.kff.org/coronavirus-covid-19/report/kff-covid-19-vaccine-monitor-december-2020/.

141 Netana H. Markovitz, Arianna L. Strome, and Payal K. Patel, "Commentary: "The Vaccine Selfie" and Its Influence on COVID-19 Vaccine Acceptance," *Vaccine* 40, no. 23 (2022): 3085.

142 Markovitz, Strome, and Payal, "Commentary: "The Vaccine Selfie.""

143 Jennifer Kates, Josh Michaud, and Jennifer Tolbert, "How are States Prioritizing Who Will Get the COVID-19 Vaccine First?" *Policy Watch*, Kaiser Family Foundation, December 14, 2020, https://www.kff.org/policy-watch/how-are-states-prioritizing-who-will-get-the-covid-19-vaccine-first/.

144 Emily Anthes, Madeleine Ngo, and Eileen Sullivan, "Adults in all U.S. states are now eligible for vaccination, hitting Biden's target. Half have had at least one dose." *New York Times*. April 19, 2021, https://www.nytimes.com/2021/04/19/world/adults-eligible-covid-vaccine.html.

145 Anthes, Ngo, and Sullivan. ""Adults in all U.S. states are now eligible for vaccination."

146 Zee Krstic, "35 Vaccine Selfie Captions That People Are Using to Share Their News," *Good Housekeeping*, May 19, 2021, https://www.goodhousekeeping.com/life/a36357526/vaccine-instagram-caption-ideas-social-media/; Rachel Chapman, "Your Vaccine Selfie Deserves A Clever Caption, So Here's Your Shot," *Elite Daily*, April 12, 2021, https://www.elitedaily.com/p/these-40-clever-vaccine-selfie-instagram-captions-deserve-a-shot-on-your-feed-72323124; Raleigh McCool, "How to Find the Caption for Your COVID Vaccine Selfie," *Medium*, April 5, 2021, https://raleighmccool.medium.com/how-to-find-the-caption-for-your-covid-vaccine-selfie-7ee755ef5262.

147 Jessica Guynn, "How to Add 'I Got My COVID Vaccine' Frame to Your

Facebook Profile," *USA Today*, April 1, 2021, https://www.usatoday.com/story/tech/2021/04/01/facebook-covid-vaccine-profile-frames/4829274001/.

148 Andrew Hutchinson, "Facebook Launches New Stickers to Encourage COVID-19 Vaccination on Instagram, Facebook and WhatsApp," *Social Media Today*, April 7, 2021, https://www.socialmediatoday.com/news/facebook-launches-new-stickers-to-encourage-covid-19-vaccination-on-instagr/598015/.

149 "CDC Director Statement on Pfizer's Use of COVID-19 Vaccine in Adolescents Age 12 and Older," May 12, 2021, https://www.cdc.gov/media/releases/2021/s0512-advisory-committee-signing.html.

150 "Student Vaccine Ambassador," Dallas County Health Department, https://communityed.waukeeschools.org/volunteer/student-vaccine-ambassador/; "Vaccine Ambassadors Help Facilitate COVID-19 Vaccination among Three Disproportionately Affected Populations," *Health Equity in Action Projects*, CDC, January 16, 2023, https://www.cdc.gov/healthequity/whatis/healthequityinaction/topics/vaccine-ambassadors.html.

151 "Featured Topics & Resources," *COVID-19 Public Education Campaign*, U.S. Department of Health and Human Services, June 5, 2023, https://wecandothis.hhs.gov/featured-topics-and-resources.

152 #CAMBRIACRUSHESCOVID, "In This Together," https://inthistogethercambria.com/stories/cambriacrushescovid/.

153 "Vaccinate Alabama TikTok Contest," *COVID-19 Vaccine*, Alabama Public Health, March 14, 2023, https://web.archive.org/web/20230326213340/https://www.alabamapublichealth.gov/covid19vaccine/tiktok.html.

154 "TikTok Stars Address Vaccine Hesitancy, Misinformation," *ABC News*, August 24, 2021, https://www.youtube.com/watch?v=Bz4XIaoLuno.

155 Tyler Perry, "COVID-19 and the Black Community: A Tyler Perry Special," TylerPerryStudios, January 28, 2021, https://www.youtube.com/watch?v=M56q6TIJ890; Buckley, Cara. "Tyler Perry Gets COVID-19 Vaccine on TV to Reassure Black Skeptics." *New York Times*. January 30, 2021, https://www.nytimes.com/2021/01/28/arts/tyler-perry-covid-vaccine-skeptics.html.

156 Elizabeth Weise and Aleszu Bajak, "People Hospitalized With COVID-19 Now Have One Overwhelming Thing In Common. They're Not Vaccinated," *USA Today*, June 16, 2021, https://www.usatoday.com/story/news/health/2021/06/16/majority-covid-19-hospital-patients-us-now-unvaccinated-younger/7684857002/?gnt-cfr=1.

157 "FDA Approves First COVID-19 Vaccine." *FDA News Release*. August 23, 2021, https://www.fda.gov/news-events/press-announcements/fda-approves-first-covid-19-vaccine.

158 Wilson Wong, "N.Y.C. Becomes First Major U.S. City to Mandate Vaccination Proof for Indoor Dining, Gyms," *NBC News*, August 3, 2021, https://www.nbcnews.com/news/us-news/nyc-becomes-first-major-u-s-city-mandate-vaccination-proof-n1275807.

159 Evan Castillo, "What Colleges Require the COVID-19 Vaccine?" *Best Colleges*,

Updated June 1, 2023, https://www.bestcolleges.com/news/2021/10/11/list-of-colleges-that-require-covid-19-vaccine/.

160 Haley Messenger, "From Mcdonald's To Goldman Sachs, Here Are The Companies Mandating Vaccines for All or Some Employees," *NBC News*, August 3, 2021, https://www.nbcnews.com/business/business-news/here-are-companies-mandating-vaccines-all-or-some-employees-n1275808.

161 Haley Messenger, "From Mcdonald's to Goldman Sachs, Here Are the Companies Mandating Vaccines for All or Some Employees," *NBC News*, August 3, 2021, https://www.nbcnews.com/business/business-news/here-are-companies-mandating-vaccines-all-or-some-employees-n1275808; Alexis Benveniste, "List of Companies Requiring Vaccinations Is Growing, from Google to Twitter." *WRAL TechWire*. July 29, 2021, https://wraltechwire.com/2021/07/29/list-of-companies-requiring-vaccinations-is-growing-from-google-to-twitter/.

162 David Bauder, "Fox's Vaccine Criticism Focuses Attention on its Own Policy," *Associated Press*, September 16, 2021, Fox's vaccine criticism focuses attention on its own policy | AP News.

163 Grace Sparks, Lunna Lopes, Alex Montero, Liz Hamel, and Mollyann Brodie, "KFF COVID-19 Vaccine Monitor: April 2022," *Polling*, Kaiser Family Foundation, April 2022, https://www.kff.org/coronavirus-covid-19/poll-finding/kff-covid-19-vaccine-monitor-april-2022/.

164 "Summary of data publicly reported by the CDC. Date: 5/3/23," *Children and COVID-19 Vaccination Trends*, American Academy of Pediatrics, Last updated May 3, 2023, https://www.aap.org/en/pages/2019-novel-coronavirus-covid-19-infections/children-and-covid-19-vaccination-trends/.

165 "Summary of data publicly reported by the CDC. Date: 5/3/23." *Children and COVID-19 Vaccination Trends*. American Academy of Pediatrics. Last updated May 3, 2023, https://www.aap.org/en/pages/2019-novel-coronavirus-covid-19-infections/children-and-covid-19-vaccination-trends/.

166 Liz Hamel, Lunna Lopes, Grace Sparks, Ashley Kirzinger, Audrey Kearney, Mellisha Stokes, and Mollyann Brodie, "KFF COVID-19 Vaccine Monitor: October 2021," *Polling*, Kaiser Family Foundation, October 28, 2021, https://www.kff.org/coronavirus-covid-19/poll-finding/kff-covid-19-vaccine-monitor-october-2021/; Mildred F. Perreault and Katherine Foss, "Parents' News Consumption and COVID Sources in Their Decisions to Vaccinate," *Journal of Applied Research on Children: Informing Policy for Children at Risk* 13, no. 2 (2022): 3, https://digitalcommons.library.tmc.edu/cgi/viewcontent.cgi?article=1520&context=childrenatrisk.

167 Cynthia Cox, Krutika Amin, Jennifer Kates, and Josh Michaud, "Why Do Vaccinated People Represent Most COVID-19 Deaths Right Now?" *Policy Watch*, Kaiser Family Foundation, November 30, 2022, https://www.kff.org/policy-watch/why-do-vaccinated-people-represent-most-covid-19-deaths-right-now/; "Rates of COVID-19 Cases and Deaths by Vaccination Status," *COVID Data Tracker*, Last updated May 2023, https://covid.cdc.gov/covid-data-tracker/#rates-by-vaccine-status.

168 "Daily Updates of Totals by Week and State." *COVID-19 Death Data and Resources*.

CDC. May 23, 2023, https://www.cdc.gov/nchs/nvss/vsrr/COVID19/index.htm.

169 Arriel Benis, Abraham Seidmann, and Shai Ashkenazi, "Reasons for Taking the COVID-19 Vaccine by US Social Media Users," Vaccines 9, no. 4 (2021): 315.

170 Ashley Kirzinger, Grace Sparks, and Mollyann Brodie, "KFF COVID-19 Vaccine Monitor: In Their Own Words, Six Months Later," *Polling*, Kaiser Family Foundation, July 13, 2021, https://www.kff.org/coronavirus-covid-19/poll-finding/kff-covid-19-vaccine-monitor-in-their-own-words-six-months-later/.

171 "Older Adults, Democrats, College Graduates, and Those with Higher Incomes Remain Most Likely To Be Vaccinated and Have Received Their COVID-19 Booster Dose," *KFF COVID-19 Vaccine Monitor*, April 13–26, 2022, https://www.kff.org/coronavirus-covid-19/dashboard/kff-covid-19-vaccine-monitor-dashboard/.

172 Kaylin Dodson, Jacquelyn Mason, and R. Smith, "COVID-19 Vaccine Misinformation and Narratives Surrounding Black Communities on Social Media," *First Draft* (2021).

173 Ashley Kirzinger, Marley Presiado, Isabelle Valdes, Liz Hamel, and Mollyann Brodie, "Three Years of KFF Polling," May 7, 2023, The COVID-19 Pandemic: Insights from Three Years of KFF Polling | KFF; Kaylin Dodson, Jacquelyn Mason, and R. Smith, "COVID-19 Vaccine Misinformation and Narratives Surrounding Black Communities on Social Media," *First Draft* (2021). Tyler Perry, "COVID-19 and the Black Community: A Tyler Perry Special," TylerPerryStudios, January 28, 2021, https://www.youtube.com/watch?v=M56q6TIJ890.

174 Ashley Kirzinger, Marley Presiado, Isabelle Valdes, Liz Hamel, and Mollyann Brodie, "Three Years of KFF Polling," May 7, 2023, The COVID-19 Pandemic: Insights from Three Years of KFF Polling | KFF.

175 Julie A. VanDusky-Allen, Stephen M. Utych, and Michael Catalano, "Partisanship, Policy, And Americans' Evaluations Of State-Level COVID-19 Policies Prior To The 2020 Election," *Political Research Quarterly* 75, no. 2 (2022): 479–96.

176 John Carey, Brendan Nyhan, Joseph B. Phillips, and Jason Reifler. "Partisanship Unmasked? The Role of Politics and Social Norms in COVID-19 Mask-Wearing Behavior," *Journal of Experimental Political Science* (2022): 1–14; Joshua Clinton, Jon Cohen, John Lapinski, and Marc Trussler, "Partisan Pandemic: How Partisanship and Public Health Concerns Affect Individuals' Social Mobility During COVID-19," *Science Advances* 7, no. 2 (2021): eabd7204.

177 Michael L. Barnett, Marema Gaye, Anupam B. Jena, and Ateev Mehrotra, "Association of County-level Prescriptions for Hydroxychloroquine and Ivermectin with County-Level Political Voting Patterns in the 2020 US Presidential Election," *JAMA Internal Medicine* 182, no. 4 (2022): 452–54.

178 Heath, *The Inside Story of the Race for a COVID-19 Vaccine.*

179 "U.S. Public Now Divided Over Whether to Get COVID-19 Vaccine," *Coronavirus Disease (COVID-19)*, Pew Research Center, September 17, 2020, https://www.pewresearch.org/science/2020/09/17/u-s-public-now-divided-over-whether-to-get-covid-19-vaccine/.

180 Matt Motta and Dominik Stecula, "The Effects of Partisan Media in the Face of Global Pandemic: How News Shaped COVID-19 Vaccine Hesitancy," *Political Communication* (2023): 1–22.

181 Michael K. Hauer, Alexander Jenkins, Janna MacPherson, Qingyue Sun, and Marianne Swain, "Tweeting About the COVID-19 Vaccine: A Content Analysis," *Atlantic Journal of Communication* (2023): 1–13.

182 Motta, and Stecula, "The Effects of Partisan Media in the Face of Global Pandemic"; Axel Bruns, Stephen Harrington, and Edward Hurcombe, "Coronavirus Conspiracy Theories: Tracing Misinformation Trajectories from the Fringes to the Mainstream," *Communicating COVID-19: Interdisciplinary Perspectives* (2021): 229–49; Sarah Evanega, Mark Lynas, Jordan Adams, Karinne Smolenyak, and Cision Global Insights, "Coronavirus Misinformation: Quantifying Sources and Themes in the COVID-19 'Infodemic'," *JMIR Preprints* 19, no. 10 (2020).

183 Tyler Monroe and Rob Savillo, "Fox has Undermined Vaccines Nearly Every Day in the Last Six Months." *Report*, Media Matters for America, October 15, 2021, https://www.mediamatters.org/coronavirus-covid-19/fox-has-undermined-vaccines-nearly-every-day-last-six-months.

184 Harrison Ray, "Tucker Carlson's Fox News Show Undermined Vaccines 99 Percent of the Days It Covered Them Since Biden Became President," *Report*, Media Matters for America, December 29, 2021, https://www.mediamatters.org/tucker-carlson/tucker-carlsons-fox-news-show-undermined-vaccines-99-days-it-covered-them-biden.

185 Annalise Baines, Muhammad Ittefaq, and Mauryne Abwao. "# Scamdemic,# Plandemic, or# Scaredemic: what Parler Social Media Platform Tells Us About COVID-19 Vaccine." *Vaccines* 9, no. 5 (2021): 421; Carrie Blazina, and Galen Stocking, "Key Facts About Parler," *Social Media*, Pew Research Center, October 20, 2022, https://www.pewresearch.org/short-reads/2022/10/20/fast-facts-about-parler-as-kanye-west-reportedly-plans-acquisition-of-site/.

186 Jasmin Choi, Sarah A. Lieff, Gabriella Y. Meltzer, Margaux M. Grivel, Virginia W. Chang, Lawrence H. Yang, and Don C. Des Jarlais. "Anti-Vaccine Attitudes Among Adults in the US During the COVID-19 Pandemic After Vaccine Rollout," *Vaccines* 10, no. 6 (2022): 933.

187 David Lazer, Jon Green, Katherine Ognyanova, Matthew Baum, Jennifer Lin, James Druckman, Roy Perlis, Mauricio Santillana, and Ata Uslu, "The COVID States Project #57: Social Media News Consumption and COVID-19 Vaccination Rates." (2021).

188 Lazer, Ognyanova, Baum, Lin, Druckman, Perlis, Santillana, and Uslu, "The COVID States Project #57."

189 Stephen R. Neely, Christina Eldredge, Robin Ersing, and Christa Remington. "Vaccine hesitancy and exposure to misinformation: a survey analysis." *Journal of General Internal Medicine* (2022): 1–9.

190 Lazer, Ognyanova, Baum, Lin, Druckman, Perlis, Santillana, and Uslu, "The COVID States Project #57."

191 Lazer, Ognyanova, Baum, Lin, Druckman, Perlis, Santillana, and Uslu, "The COVID States Project #57."

192 Matteo Pinna, Léo Picard, and Christoph Goessmann, "Cable News and COVID-19 Vaccine Uptake," *Scientific Reports* 12, no. 1 (2022): 16804; Jeanette B. Ruiz and Robert A. Bell, "Predictors of Intention to Vaccinate Against COVID-19: Results of a Nationwide Survey," *Vaccine* 39, no. 7 (2021): 1080–86; Motta and Stecula, "The Effects of Partisan Media in the Face of Global Pandemic"; Choi, Lieff, Meltzer, Grivel, Chang, Yang, and Des Jarlais, "Anti-vaccine Attitudes Among Adults."

193 Motta and Stecula, "The Effects of Partisan Media in the Face of Global Pandemic."

194 Mark Jurkowitz and Amy Mitchell, "Americans Who Relied Most on Trump for COVID-19 News Among Least Likely to be Vaccinated," *Coronavirus (COVID-19)*, Pew Research Center, September 23, 2021, https://www.pewresearch.org/short-reads/2021/09/23/americans-who-relied-most-on-trump-for-covid-19-news-among-least-likely-to-be-vaccinated/.

195 Lynas Evanega, Adams Smolenyak, and Cision Global Insights, "Coronavirus Misinformation: Quantifying Sources and Themes in the COVID-19 'Infodemic;'" Sheryl Gay Stolberg and Noah Weiland, "Study Finds 'Single Largest Driver' of Coronavirus Misinformation: Trump," *New York Times*, Updated October 6, 2021, https://www.nytimes.com/2020/09/30/us/politics/trump-coronavirus-misinformation.html.

196 "Vaccinated Adults Highly Confident in COVID-19 Vaccine R&D Process," *Research Topics*, Pew Research Center, September 17, 2021, https://www.pewresearch.org/ps_2021-09-15_covid19-restrictions_00-024/.

197 Nicholas Francis Havey, "Partisan Public Health: How Does Political Ideology Influence Support for COVID-19 Related Misinformation?." *Journal of Computational Social Science* 3, no. 2 (2020): 319–42.

198 Janessa Griffith, Husayn Marani, and Helen Monkman, "COVID-19 Vaccine Hesitancy in Canada: Content Analysis of Tweets Using the Theoretical Domains Framework," *Journal of Medical Internet Research* 23, no. 4 (2021): e26874.; Daniel Joseph E. Berdida, Franchesca Mae C. Franco, Xyllyne Allyah G. Santos, Camille B. Dacol, Michaela Dimaano, Erika S. Del Rosario, and Charlotte Christianne Lantin, "Filipinos' COVID-19 Vaccine Hesitancy Comments in Tiktok Videos: A Manifest Content Analysis," *Public Health Nursing* 40, no. 1 (2023): 135–43.

199 Josh Holder, "Tracking Coronavirus Vaccinations Around the World."

200 Josh Holder, "Tracking Coronavirus Vaccinations Around the World."

201 Josh Holder, "Tracking Coronavirus Vaccinations Around the World."

202 Josh Holder, "Tracking Coronavirus Vaccinations Around the World."

203 "COVID-19 Vaccinations in the United States," *COVID Data Tracker*. CDC. May 9, 2023, https://covid.cdc.gov/covid-data-tracker/#vaccinations_vacc-total-admin-rate-total; Hsu, "Thousands of Workers were Fired Over Vaccine Mandates."

204 Jeffrey V. Lazarus, Katarzyna Wyka, Trenton M. White, Camila A. Picchio, Lawrence O. Gostin, Heidi J. Larson, Kenneth Rabin, Scott C. Ratzan, Adeeba

Kamarulzaman, and Ayman El-Mohandes, "A Survey of COVID-19 Vaccine Acceptance Across 23 Countries in 2022," *Nature Medicine* (2023): 1–10.

205 Yam B. Limbu and Bruce A. Huhmann, "Why Some People Are Hesitant to Receive COVID-19 Boosters: A Systematic Review," *Tropical Medicine and Infectious Disease* 8, no. 3 (2023): 159.

206 Ashley Kirzinger, Grace Sparks, and Mollyann Brodie, "KFF COVID-19 Vaccine Monitor: In Their Own Words, Six Months Later," *Polling*, Kaiser Family Foundation, July 13, 2021, https://www.kff.org/coronavirus-covid-19/poll-finding/kff-covid-19-vaccine-monitor-in-their-own-words-six-months-later/.

207 Oliver J. Watson, Gregory Barnsley, Jaspreet Toor, Alexandra B. Hogan, Peter Winskill, and Azra C. Ghani, "Global Impact of the First Year of COVID-19 Vaccination: A Mathematical Modelling Study," *The Lancet Infectious Diseases* 22, no. 9 (2022): 1293–302; Megan C. Fitzpatrick, S. M. Moghadas, A. Pandey, and A. P. Galvani, "Two Years of US COVID-19 Vaccines Have Prevented Millions of Hospitalizations and Deaths," To the Point (blog), Commonwealth Fund, December 13 (2022).

Chapter Seven: Depicting the "New Normal"

1 Liz Shackleton, "Lights, Camera, Inaction: Hong Kong and China Film Industry in Lockdown," *HKDC Research*, May 20, 2020, https://research.hktdc.com/en/article/NDI5NjcxNjA5.

2 Mohammed Hamza, "COVID-19's Impact on Europe's TV Networks and Production Landscape," *S & P Global Market Intelligence*, April 8, 2020, https://www.spglobal.com/marketintelligence/en/news-insights/research/covid-19s-impact-on-europes-tv-networks-and-production-landscape.

3 Mohammed Hamza, "COVID-19's Impact on Europe's TV Networks and Production Landscape," *S & P Global Market Intelligence*, April 8, 2020, https://www.spglobal.com/marketintelligence/en/news-insights/research/covid-19s-impact-on-europes-tv-networks-and-production-landscape ; Naman Ramachandran, "India Suspends Film and TV Production Amid Coronavirus Fears," *Variety*, March 16, 2020, https://variety.com/2020/film/news/coronavirus-india-halt-film-tv-production-1203535244/.

4 Richard Procter, "Remember When? Timeline Marks Key Events in California's Year-long Pandemic Grind," *Cal Matters*, March 4, 2021, https://calmatters.org/health/coronavirus/2021/03/timeline-california-pandemic-year-key-points/.

5 History.com Editors. Broadway goes dark due to COVID-19 pandemic. *History.com*, February 23, 2021, https://www.history.com/this-day-in-history/broadway-goes-dark-covid19-pandemic.

6 Office of Governor Gavin Newsom, Governor Gavin Newsom Issues Stay at Home Order, Executive Order N-33–20, https://www.gov.ca.gov/wp-content/uploads/2020/03/EO-N-33-20-COVID-19-HEALTH-ORDER-03.19.2020-002.pdf;

Judy Lin, "Gov. Gavin Newsom Orders All of California to Shelter in Place," *Cal Matters*. March 20, 2020, https://calmatters.org/health/coronavirus/2020/03/california-coronavirus-half-of-californians-gavin-newsom-donald-trump/.

7 Jiachuan Wu, Savannah Smith, Mansee Khurana, Corky Siemaszko, and Brianna DeJesus-Banos, "Stay-at-Home Orders Across the Country," *NBC News*, April 29, 2020, https://www.nbcnews.com/health/health-news/here-are-stay-home-orders-across-country-n1168736.

8 Krystie Lee Yandoli, "How the Coronavirus is Changing Television Production," *BuzzFeed News*, April 25, 2020, https://www.buzzfeednews.com/article/krystiey-andoli/coronavirus-kardashians-walking-dead-virtual-production; Mary Honkus, "Food Network Is Airing 5 New Episodes of *The Pioneer Woman* Shot by Ree Drummond's Daughters," *People*, April 8, 2020, https://people.com/food/the-food-network-airing-special-pioneer-woman-staying-home-episodes-shot-by-family/.

9 LaToya Ferguson, "'Saturday Night Live' Review: SNL at Home' Says Goodbye for the Season," *IndieWire*, https://www.indiewire.com/2020/05/snl-review-at-home-kristen-wiig-1202230374/.

10 Krystie Lee Yandoli, "How the Coronavirus is Changing Television Production," *BuzzFeed News*, April 25, 2020, https://www.buzzfeednews.com/article/krystiey andoli/coronavirus-kardashians-walking-dead-virtual-production.

11 Scott Roxborough, As Europe Begins to Reopen for Film and TV Shoots, Safety Requirements Vary. *The Hollywood Reporter*. May 15, 2020, https://www.hollywoodreporter.com/news/general-news/starting-production-europe-coronavirus-guide-by-country-1294732/.

12 *The Safe Way Forward: A Joint Report of the DGA, SAG-AFTRA, IATSE and Teamsters' Committees for COVID-19 Safety Guidelines*, June 2020, https://www.sagaftra.org/files/sa_documents/ProductionSafetyGuidelines_June2020EditedP.pdf.

13 Matt Stevens, "TV Production Adapted to Weather the Pandemic. Now What?" *New York Times*, April 28, 2021, https://www.nytimes.com/2021/04/28/arts/television/tv-production-coronavirus.html.

14 Faith Karimi, "Some TV Shows Are Telling Stories About The Pandemic. Some Viewers Wish They Wouldn't," *CNN*, February 23, 2021, https://www.cnn.com/2021/02/23/media/television-shows-coronavirus-trnd/index.html.

15 Dennis Bingham, *Whose lives are they anyway?*, Rutgers University Press, 2010.

16 Dennis Bingham, *Whose lives are they anyway?*, Rutgers University Press, 2010; Custen, George Frederick, and George Custen. *Bio/pics: How Hollywood constructed public history*. Rutgers University Press, 1992.

17 Lee Margulies, "Episode to Air March 9 : 'Punky' Deals with Shuttle Tragedy," *Los Angeles Times*, February 19, 1986, https://www.latimes.com/archives/la-xpm-1986-02-19-ca-9722-story.html.

18 Lynn Spigel, "Entertainment Wars: Television Culture After 9/11," In *The Selling of 9/11*, 119–54. Palgrave Macmillan, New York, 2005.

19 Spigel, "Entertainment Wars: Television Culture After 9/11."

20 Rachel Dean-Ruzicka, "Vengeance, Healing and Justice: Post 9/11 Culture Through the Lens of *CSI*," *Quarterly Review of Film and Video* 26, no. 2 (2009): 118–30.

21 Adam Bryant, "*CSI: NY* 9/11 Tribute Episode Shows a New Side of Mac," *TV Guide*, September 23, 2011, https://www.tvguide.com/news/csi-ny-premiere-1038029/.

22 Christoph Classen and Kirsten Wächter, "Balanced Truth: Steven Spielberg's *Schindler's List* Among History, Memory, and Popular Culture," *History and Theory* 48, no. 2 (2009): 77–102.

23 Solange Davin, "Healthy Viewing: The Reception of Medical Narratives," *Sociology of Health & Illness* 25, no. 6 (2003): 662–79; Candace Cummins Gauthier, "Television Drama and Popular Film As Medical Narrative," *The Journal of American Culture* 22, no. 3 (1999): 23–25; Beth L. Hoffman, Robert Hoffman, Charles B. Wessel, Ariel Shensa, Michelle S. Woods, and Brian A. Primack, "Use of Fictional Medical Television in Health Sciences Education: A Systematic Review," *Advances in Health Sciences Education* 23, no. 1 (2018): 201–16; Truls Østbye, Bill Miller, and Heather Keller, "Throw That Epidemiologist Out of the Emergency Room! Using the Television Series ER as a Vehicle for Teaching Methodologists About Medical Issues," *Journal of Clinical Epidemiology* 50, no. 10 (1997): 1183–186.

24 Rebecca L. Collins, Marc N. Elliott, Sandra H. Berry, David E. Kanouse, and Sarah B. Hunter, "Entertainment Television as a Healthy Sex Educator: The Impact of Condom-Efficacy Information in an Episode of Friends," *Pediatrics* 112, no. 5 (2003): 1115–121.

25 Donald Horton and R. Richard Wohl, "Mass Communication and Para-Social Interaction: Observations on Intimacy at a Distance," *Psychiatry* 19, no. 3 (1956): 215.

26 Holger Schramm and Werner Wirth, "Testing A Universal Tool for Measuring Parasocial Interactions Across Different Situations and Media," *Journal of Media Psychology* (2010), 27.

27 Richard Dyer, 1999, "Entertainment and Utopia," In *The Cultural Studies Reader*, Edited by: During, Simon. 373. London and New York: Routledge.

28 Stuart Hall, "Encoding, Decoding," In *The Cultural Studies Reader*, Edited by: During, Simon. 509. London and New York: Routledge.

29 Irene Cambra-Badii, Elena Guardiola, and Josep-E. Baños, "The COVID-19 Pandemic in Serial Medical Dramas," *JAMA* 327, no. 1 (2022): 20–22.

30 Marc Shapiro, "One Year Later: Are Front-line Workers Still 'Heroes?'" *Johns Hopkins Medicine News & Publications*, May 25, 2021, https://www.hopkinsmedicine.org/news/articles/one-year-later-are-front-line-workers-still-heroes.

31 "3607 US Healthcare Worker Deaths," *Lost on the Frontline*, a partnership between *The Guardian* and *Kaiser Health News*, April 2021, https://www.theguardian.com/us-news/ng-interactive/2020/aug/11/lost-on-the-frontline-covid-19-coronavirus-us-healthcare-workers-deaths-database.

32 "3607 US Healthcare Worker Deaths," *Lost on the Frontline*.

33 "3607 US Healthcare Worker Deaths," *Lost on the Frontline*.

34 John Eligon, Audra D. S. Burch, Dionne Searcey, and Richard A. Oppel Jr., "Black Americans Face Alarming Rates of Coronavirus Infection in Some States," *Washington Post*, April 7, 2020, https://www.nytimes.com/2020/04/07/us/coronavirus-race.html.

35 Latoya Hill and Samantha Artiga, COVID-19 Cases and Deaths by Race/Ethnicity: Current Data and Changes Over Time, *Kaiser Family Foundation*, February 22, 2022, https://www.kff.org/coronavirus-covid-19/issue-brief/covid-19-cases-and-deaths-by-race-ethnicity-current-data-and-changes-over-time/#:~:text=These percent20age percent2Dstandardized percent20data percent20show,19 percent20infection percent20than percent20White percent20people.

36 Katherine A. Foss, *Television and Health Responsibility in an Age of Individualism* (New York: Lexington Books, 2014).

37 Mohammed, Ibrahim, Areej Nauman, Pradipta Paul, Sanjith Ganesan, Kuan-Han Chen, Syed Muhammad Saad Jalil, Shahd H. Jaouni et al., "The Efficacy And Effectiveness of The COVID-19 Vaccines in Reducing Infection, Severity, Hospitalization, and Mortality: A Systematic Review," *Human Vaccines & Immunotherapeutics* (2022): 1–20.

38 Falk, Gene, Romero, Paul D., Nicchitta, Isaac A., and Nyhof, Emma C. Unemployment Rates During the COVID-19 Pandemic. *Congressional Research Service*. August, 20, 2021, https://sgp.fas.org/crs/misc/R46554.pdf.

39 Tracking the COVID-19 Economy's Effects on Food, Housing, and Employment Hardships. *COVID Hardship Watch*. Center on Budget and Policy Priorities. September 23, 2021, https://www.cbpp.org/research/poverty-and-inequality/tracking-the-covid-19-economys-effects-on-food-housing-and#:~:text=The percent20unemployment percent20rate percent20jumped percent20in,2021 percent20than percent20in percent20February percent202020.

40 Spigel, "Entertainment Wars: Television Culture After 9/11."

41 Wu, Smith, Khurana, Siemaszko, and DeJesus-Banos, "Stay-at-Home Orders Across the Country."

42 Jane Tyska, Photos: San Diego Protest Against Coronavirus Shelter-in-Place Restrictions, *The Mercury News*, April 27, 2020, https://www.mercurynews.com/2020/04/26/photos-san-diego-protest-against-coronavirus-shelter-in-place-restrictions/.

43 Camila Saggioro de Figueiredo, Poliana Capucho Sandre, Liana Catarina Lima Portugal, Thalita Mázala-de-Oliveira, Luana da Silva Chagas, Ícaro Raony, Elenn Soares Ferreira, Elizabeth Giestal-de-Araujo, Aline Araujo Dos Santos, and Priscilla Oliveira-Silva Bomfim, "COVID-19 Pandemic Impact on Children and Adolescents' Mental Health: Biological, Environmental, and Social Factors," *Progress in Neuro-Psychopharmacology and Biological Psychiatry* 106 (2021): 110171.

44 Anousha Sakoui, "New Back-to-Work Deal Requires Boosters for Vaccinated Film Crews," *Los Angeles Times*, February 16, 2022, https://www.latimes.com

/entertainment-arts/business/story/2022-02-16/vaccinated-workers-hollywood-boosters-covid-crews-back-to-work.

45 David Bauder, Fox's Vaccine Criticism Focuses Attention on its Own Policy, *ABCNews*, September 16, 2021, https://abcnews.go.com/Entertainment/wireStory/foxs-vaccine-criticism-focuses-attention-policy-80067696.

46 Mike Ives, "Two Actors Leave the Soap Opera 'General Hospital' Over Its Vaccine Mandate," *New York Times*, November 24, 2021; Nellie Andreeva, "Rockmond Dunbar Exists '9-1-1' Over Covid Vaccine Mandate After Pursuing Medical & Religious Exemptions," *Deadline*. November 16, 2021, https://deadline.com/2021/11/rockmond-dunbar-exits-911-covid-vaccine-mandate-medical-religious-exemptions-1234874927/; Jones, Marcus. *Run the World* star Andrea Bordeaux Exits Series Over Vaccine Mandate. *Entertainment Weekly*. February 4, 2022, https://ew.com/tv/andrea-bordeaux-exits-run-the-world-vaccine-mandate/.

47 Andrea Wurzburger, "Celebrities We Lost to COVID-19," *People*, January 4, 2022, https://people.com/health/celebrity-coronavirus-deaths/.

48 Liz Shackleton, "Lights, Camera, Inaction: Hong Kong and China Film Industry in Lockdown," *HKDC Research*, May 20, 2020, https://research.hktdc.com/en/article/NDI5NjcxNjA5; Hamza, Mohammed. COVID-19's Impact on Europe's TV Networks and Production Landscape. *S & P Global Market Intelligence*. April 8, 2020, https://www.spglobal.com/marketintelligence/en/news-insights/research/covid-19s-impact-on-europes-tv-networks-and-production-landscape.

49 "Forever Changed: COVID-19's Lasting Impact on the Entertainment Industry," Consumer Study, United Talent Agency, June 2021, https://unitedtalent.app.box.com/s/j4ijgxd8169jpgkxji8eqxnyqc7lszy2.

50 "Forever Changed: COVID-19's Lasting Impact on the Entertainment Industry," United Talent Agency.

Chapter Eight: Life After Crisis

1 Joseph R. Biden, "A Proclamation on Remembering the 1,000,000 Americans Lost to COVID-19," *Statements and Releases*, The White House, May 12, 2022, https://www.whitehouse.gov/briefing-room/statements-releases/2022/05/12/statement-from-president-joe-biden-marking-one-million-american-lives-lost-to-covid-19/.

2 "WHO Coronavirus (COVID-19) Dashboard." WHO.

3 "U.S. and World Population Clock." United States Census. July 2, 2023. Population Clock (census.gov) "WHO Coronavirus (COVID-19) Dashboard." WHO; https://covid19.who.int/.

4 "Track COVID-19 in the U.S.," *New York Times*, July 1, 2023, https://www.nytimes.com/interactive/2023/us/covid-cases.html.

5 "Track COVID-19 in the U.S.," *New York Times*.

6 "Track COVID-19 in the U.S," *New York Times*, July 1, 2023, https://www.nytimes.com/interactive/2023/us/covid-cases.html.

7 "WHO Coronavirus (COVID-19) Dashboard." WHO; "2022 Nationwide

COVID-19 Infection- and Vaccination-Induced Antibody Seroprevalence (Blood donations)," *COVID Data Tracker*, CDC, July 2023, https://covid.cdc.gov/covid-data-tracker/#nationwide-blood-donor-seroprevalence-2022?ftag=YHF4eb9d17; Alexander Tin, " How Many Americans Still Haven't Caught COVID-19? CDC Publishes Final 2022 Estimates," *CBS News*, July 3, 2023, https://www.cbsnews.com/news/how-many-americans-havent-caught-covid-cdc-estimates/.

8 "Children and COVID-19: State-Level Data Report," *Critical Updates on COVID-19*, American Academy of Pediatrics, May 16, 2023, https://www.aap.org/en/pages/2019-novel-coronavirus-covid-19-infections/children-and-covid-19-state-level-data-report/.

9 Alice Burns, "Long COVID: What do the Latest Data Show?" *Policy Watch*, Kaiser Family Foundation, January 26, 2023, https://www.kff.org/policy-watch/long-covid-what-do-latest-data-show/.

10 Foss, *Constructing the Outbreak.*

11 Joshua Zeitz, "Rampant Lies, Fake Cures and Not Enough Beds: What the Spanish Flu Debacle Can Teach Us About Coronavirus." *Politico.* March 17, 2020, https://www.politico.com/news/magazine/2020/03/17/spanish-flu-lessons-coronavirus-133888; Hannah Hagemann, "The 1918 Flu Pandemic Was Brutal, Killing More Than 50 Million People Worldwide," *NPR*, April 2, 2020, https://www.npr.org/2020/04/02/826358104/the-1918-flu-pandemic-was-brutal-killing-as-many-as-100-million-people-worldwide; Becky Little, " How the Flu Pandemic Changed Halloween in 1918," *History.com*, October 19, 2020, https://www.history.com/news/halloween-1918-flu-pandemic; Christine Hauser, "The Mask Slackers of 1918," *New York Times*, December 10, 2020, https://www.nytimes.com/2020/08/03/us/mask-protests-1918.html.

12 "COVID-19: Tracking the Impact," Nielsen.

13 Foss, *Constructing the Outbreak.*

14 Liaquat Hossain, D. Kam, F. Kong, R. T. Wigand, and Terence Bossomaier, "Social Media in Ebola Outbreak," *Epidemiology & Infection* 144, no. 10 (2016): 2136–143; Jeanine PD Guidry, Yan Jin, Caroline A. Orr, Marcus Messner, and Shana Meganck, "Ebola on Instagram and Twitter: How Health Organizations Address the Health Crisis in their Social Media Engagement," *Public relations review* 43, no. 3 (2017): 477–86.

15 Kim Yi Dionne and Fulya Felicity Turkmen, "The Politics of Pandemic Othering: Putting COVID-19 in Global and Historical Context," *International Organization* 74, no. S1 (2020): E213-E230.

16 Niall PAS Johnson and Juergen Mueller, "Updating the Accounts: Global Mortality of the 1918–1920" Spanish" influenza pandemic." *Bulletin of the History of Medicine* (2002): 105–15; Owen Dyer, "COVID-19: Study Claims Real Global Deaths Are Twice Official Figures," *BMJ: British Medical Journal (Online)* 373 (2021).

17 Foss, *Constructing the Outbreak.*

18 "WHO Coronavirus (COVID-19) Dashboard." WHO.

19 Singh, McNab, Olson, Bristol, Nolan, Bergstrøm, Bartos et al., "How An Outbreak Became a Pandemic."

20 Singh, McNab, Olson, Bristol, Nolan, Bergstrøm, Bartos et al., "How An Outbreak Became a Pandemic."

21 From February 2020 on, international dashboards kept count. The Johns Hopkins University "COVID-19 Dashboard" was one of the earliest. CDC and WHO had dashboards. *New York Times*, *Washington Post*, and other media outlets also offered dashboards for cases, deaths, and later, vaccinations.

22 "WHO Coronavirus (COVID-19) Dashboard," WHO; Watson, Barnsley, Toor, Hogan, Winskill, and Ghani, "Global Impact of the First Year of COVID-19 Vaccination: A Mathematical Modelling Study"; C. Meagan Fitzpatrick, S. M. Moghadas, A. Pandey, and A. P. Galvani, "Two Years of US COVID-19 Vaccines Have Prevented Millions of Hospitalizations and Deaths," To the Point (blog), Commonwealth Fund. December 13 (2022).

23 Tanya Lewis, "How the U.S. Pandemic Response Went Wrong—and What Went Right—during a Year of COVID," *Scientific American*, March 11, 2021, https://www.scientificamerican.com/article/how-the-u-s-pandemic-response-went-wrong-and-what-went-right-during-a-year-of-covid/; Lawrence O. Gostin, "The Coronavirus Pandemic 1 Year on—What Went Wrong?" *JAMA* 325, no. 12 (2021): 1132–133; Stolberg and Weiland, "Experts See Lessons for Next Pandemic as Covid Emergency Comes to an End," *New York Times*, May 11, 2023, https://www.nytimes.com/2023/05/11/us/politics/covid-response-lessons.html.

24 Bo Bian, Jingjing Li, Ting Xu, and Natasha Z. Foutz, "Individualism During Crises," *Review of Economics and Statistics* 104, no. 2 (2022): 368–85; Samuel Bazzi, Martin Fiszbein, and Mesay Gebresilasse, "'Rugged Individualism' and Collective (In)action During the COVID-19 Pandemic," *Journal of Public Economics* 195 (2021): 104357.

25 Rebekah H. Nagler, Rachel I. Vogel, Sarah E. Gollust, Alexander J. Rothman, Erika Franklin Fowler, and Marco C. Yzer, "Public Perceptions of Conflicting Information Surrounding COVID-19: Results from a Nationally Representative Survey of US Adults," *Plos One* 15, no. 10 (2020): e0240776.

26 K. David Patterson and Gerald F. Pyle, "The Geography and Mortality of the 1918 Influenza Pandemic," *Bulletin of the History of Medicine* 65, no. 1 (1991): 4–21.

27 Foss, *Constructing the Outbreak.*

28 Hannah R. Stevens, Yoo Jung Oh, and Laramie D. Taylor, "Desensitization to Fear-Inducing COVID-19 Health News on Twitter: Observational Study," *JMIR Infodemiology* 1, no. 1 (2021): e26876; Steven Taylor, Geoffrey S. Rachor, and Gordon JG Asmundson, "Who Develops Pandemic Fatigue? Insights from Latent Class Analysis," *PLoS One* 17, no. 11 (2022): e0276791.

29 "Coronavirus Pandemic," Gallup Poll. 2022, https://news.gallup.com/poll/308222/coronavirus-pandemic.aspx.

30 Daniel Burke, "Coronavirus Preys on What Terrifies Us: Dying Alone," *CNN*, March 29, 2020, https://www.cnn.com/2020/03/29/world/funerals-dying-alone-coronavirus/index.html.

31 Huibertha B. Mitima-Verloop, Trudy Mooren, Maria E. Kritikou, and Paul A. Boelen, "Restricted Mourning: Impact of the COVID-19 Pandemic on Funeral Services, Grief Rituals, and Prolonged Grief Symptoms," *Frontiers in psychiatry* 13 (2022): 878818.

32 Elisa Shearer and Emily Tomasik, "After Increasing in 2020, Layoffs at Large U.S. Newspapers and Digital News Sites Declined in 2021," *Media Layoffs & Employment*, Pew Research Center, October 13, 2022, Layoffs at large newspapers and digital news sites fell considerably in 2021 | Pew Research Center; Abernathy, *The Expanding News Desert*.

33 "The Nielsen Total Audience Report: April 2020," *Insights*, Nielsen, April 2020, https://www.nielsen.com/insights/2020/the-nielsen-total-audience-report-april-2020/; Koeze and Popper, "The Virus Changed the Way We Internet"; Isabel Cabrera, "World Reading Habits in 2020," *Global English Editing*, November 6, 2020, https://geediting.com/world-reading-habits-2020/.

34 Katerina Eva Matsa and Kirsten Worden, "Local Newspapers Fact Sheet," *State of the News Media (Project)*, Pew Research Center, May 26, 2022, Local Newspapers Fact Sheet | Pew Research Center; News organizations drop paywall for coronavirus information, *Associated Press*, March 19, 2020, News organizations drop paywall for coronavirus information | AP News.

35 Michael Barthel, "6 key takeaways about the state of the news media in 2020," *State of the News Media (Project)*, Pew Research Center, July 27, 2021, The state of the news media industry in 2020: 6 key takeaways | Pew Research Center.

36 Elisa Shearer, Jacob Liedke, Katerina Eva Matsa, Michael Lipka, and Mark Jurkowitz, "Podcasts as a Source of News and Information," *Audio, Radio & Podcasts*, Pew Research Center, April 18, 2023, How Americans Use Podcasts To Get News and Information | Pew Research Center.

37 Mason Walker and Katerina Eva Matsa, "News Consumption Across Social Media in 2021," *Social Media & the News*, Pew Research Center, September 30, 2021, News Consumption Across Social Media in 2021 | Pew Research Center; Katerina Eva Matsa, "More Americans are getting news on TikTok, bucking the trend on other social media sites," *TikTok*, Pew Research Center, October 21, 2022, More Americans are getting news on TikTok, bucking social media trend | Pew Research Center.

38 Emily Saks and Alec Tyson, "Americans Report More Engagement with Science News Than in 2017, *Science News & Information*, Pew Research Center, November 10, 2022, Americans are more engaged with science news than in 2017 | Pew Research Center.

39 Katerina Eva Matsa, "More Americans are Getting News on TikTok, Bucking the Trend on Other Social Media Sites," *TikTok*, Pew Research Center, October 21, 2022, More Americans are getting news on TikTok, bucking social media trend | Pew Research Center; Mason Walker and Katerina Eva Matsa, "News Consumption Across Social Media in 2021," *Social Media & the News*, Pew Research Center, September 30, 2021, News Consumption Across Social Media in 2021 | Pew

Research Center; Naomi Forman-Katz and Katerina Eva Matsa, "News Platform Fact Sheet," *News Platforms & Sources*, Pew Research Center, September 20, 2022, https://www.pewresearch.org/journalism/fact-sheet/news-platform-fact-sheet/.

40 "How Americans Navigated the News in 2020: A Tumultuous Year in Review." *Politics in Media*. February 22, 2021, https://www.pewresearch.org/journalism/2021/02/22/about-a-quarter-of-republicans-democrats-consistently-turned-only-to-news-outlets-whose-audiences-aligned-with-them-politically-in-2020/.

41 "How Americans Navigated the News in 2020," *Politics in Media*.

42 "How Americans Navigated the News in 2020," *Politics in Media*.

43 "How Americans Navigated the News in 2020," *Politics in Media*.

44 Yunjuan See Luo and Yang Cheng, "The Presumed Influence of COVID-19 Misinformation on Social Media: Survey Research from Two Countries in the Global Health Crisis," *International Journal of Environmental Research and Public Health* 18.11 (2021): 5505; Levi Uchechukwu Osuagwu, "COVID-19: A Global Challenge–Misinformation, Misconceptions and Myths," *Journal of the Nigerian Optometric Association* 23, no. 1 (2021): 2–3; Bruns, Harrington, and Hurcombe, "Coronavirus Conspiracy Theories: Tracing Misinformation Trajectories from the Fringes to the Mainstream"; Alfonso J. Rodriguez-Morales and Oscar H. Franco, "Public Trust, Misinformation and COVID-19 Vaccination Willingness in Latin America and the Caribbean: Today's Key Challenges," *The Lancet Regional Health–Americas* 3 (2021); Meeyoung Cha, Chiyoung Cha, Karandeep Singh, Gabriel Lima, Yong-Yeol Ahn, Juhi Kulshrestha, and Onur Varol. "Prevalence of Misinformation and Factchecks on the COVID-19 Pandemic in 35 Countries: Observational Infodemiology Study." *JMIR human factors* 8, no. 1 (2021): e23279.

45 Aimei Yang, Jieun Shin, Alvin Zhou, Ke M. Huang-Isherwood, Eugene Lee, Chuqing Dong, Hye Min Kim et al., "The Battleground of COVID-19 Vaccine Misinformation on Facebook: Fact Checkers Vs. Misinformation Spreaders," *Harvard Kennedy School Misinformation Review* (2021).

46 Ramez Kouzy, Joseph Abi Jaoude, Afif Kraitem, Molly B. El Alam, Basil Karam, Elio Adib, Jabra Zarka, Cindy Traboulsi, Elie W. Akl, and Khalil Baddour, "Coronavirus Goes Viral: Quantifying the COVID-19 Misinformation Epidemic on Twitter," *Cureus* 12, no. 3 (2020); Tony Room, "Facebook, Google and Twitter Scramble to Stop Misinformation about Coronavirus," *Washington Post*, January 27, 2020, https://www.washingtonpost.com/technology/2020/01/27/facebook-google-twitter-scramble-stop-misinformation-about-coronavirus/.

47 Rachel Lerman, "Facebook Says It Has Taken Down 7 Million Posts for Spreading Coronavirus Misinformation," *Washington Post*, August 11, 2020, Facebook and Instagram removed 7 million posts for coronavirus misinformation—The Washington Post (archive.org).

48 Kouzy, Jaoude, Kraitem, El Alam, Karam, Adib, Zarka, Traboulsi. Akl, and Baddour. "Coronavirus Goes Viral"; Tony Room, "Facebook, Google and Twitter Scramble to Stop Misinformation About Coronavirus."

49 J. Scott Brennen, Felix M. Simon, Philip N. Howard, and Rasmus Kleis Nielsen, "Types, Sources, and Claims of COVID-19 Misinformation," PhD diss., University of Oxford, 2020; Vosoughi, Soroush, Deb Roy, and Sinan Aral. "The Spread of True and False News Online," *Science* 359, no. 6380 (2018): 1146–151.

50 "The Disinformation Dozen: Why Platforms Must Act on Twelve Leading Online Anti-Vaxxers," Center for Countering Digital Hate (2021, March 24), https://252f2edd-1c8b-49f5-9bb2-cb57bb47e4ba.filesusr.com/ugd/f4d9b9_b7cedc0553604720b7137f8663366ee5.pdf; Yang, Shin, Zhou, Huang-Isherwood, Lee, Dong, Kim et al. "The Battleground of COVID-19 Vaccine Misinformation on Facebook."

51 Mark Jurkowitz and Amy Mitchell, "Cable TV and COVID-19: How Americans Perceive the Outbreak and View Media Coverage Differ by Main News Source," *Pew Research Center* (2020); P. Sol Hart, Sedona Chinn, and Stuart Soroka. (2020). Politicization and Polarization in COVID-19 News Coverage. *Science Communication*, 1075547020950735.

52 Stolberg and Weiland, "Study Finds 'Single Largest Driver' of Coronavirus Misinformation: Trump."

53 Sheera Frenkel and Davey Alba, "Trump's Disinfectant Talk Trips Up Sites' Vows Against Misinformation," *New York Times*, April 30, 2020, https://www.nytimes.com/2020/04/30/technology/trump-coronavirus-social-media.html.

54 Search of "Donald J. Trump" and "Fake News," *The American Presidency Project*, https://www.presidency.ucsb.edu/advanced-search?field-keywords= percent22fake+news percent22&field-keywords2=&field-keywords3=&from percent5B date percent5D=01-01-2020&to percent5Bdate percent5D=12-31-2020&person2=200301&items_per_page=100.

55 Motta, Matt, Dominik Stecula, and Christina Farhart, "How Right-Leaning Media Coverage of COVID-19 Facilitated the Spread of Misinformation in the Early Stages of the Pandemic in the US," *Canadian Journal Of Political Science/ Revue Canadienne De Science Politique* 53, no. 2 (2020): 335–42.

56 Owen, Laura Hazard. "Older People and Republicans are Most Likely to Share COVID-19 Stories from Fake News Sites on Twitter." *Audience and Social.* Nieman Lab. October 26, 2020. Older people and Republicans are most likely to share Covid-19 stories from fake news sites on Twitter | Nieman Journalism Lab (niemanlab.org).

57 Havey, "Partisan Public Health: How Does Political Ideology Influence Support for COVID-19 Related Misinformation?"; Kakkar, Hemant and Asher Lawson. "We Found the One Group of Americans Who Are Most Likely to Spread Fake News." *Politico.* January 14, 2022, https://www.politico.com/news/magazine/2022/01/14/we-found-the-one-group-of-americans-who-are-most-likely-to-spread-fake-news-526973; Lawson, M. Asher, and Hemant Kakkar. "Of Pandemics, Politics, and Personality: The Role of Conscientiousness and Political Ideology in the Sharing of Fake News." *Journal of Experimental Psychology: General* 151, no. 5 (2022): 1154.

58 Sahil Loomba, Alexandre de Figueiredo, Simon J. Piatek, Kristen de Graaf, and

Heidi J. Larson, "Measuring the Impact of COVID-19 Vaccine Misinformation on Vaccination Intent in the UK and USA," *Nature Human Behaviour* 5, no. 3 (2021): 337–48; Ciara Greene and Gillian Murphy, "Can Fake News Really Change Behaviour? Evidence From a Study of COVID-19 Misinformation." (2020).

59 Jurkowitz and Mitchell, "Cable TV and COVID-19: How Americans Perceive the Outbreak"; Hart, Chinn, and Soroka, "Politicization and Polarization in COVID-19 News Coverage."

60 Vanessa Romo, "Poison Control Centers are Fielding a Surge of Ivermectin Overdose Calls," *NPR* (2021, September 4), https://www.npr.org/sections/coronavirus-live-updates/2021/09/04/1034217306/ivermectin-overdose-exposure-cases-poison-control-centers; Ben Collins, "Covid Vaccine Hold Outs are Caving to Mandates—Then Scrambling to 'Undo' Their Shots," *NBC News*, (2021, November 12), https://www.nbcnews.com/tech/tech-news/covid-vaccine-mandates-push-holdouts-get-shot-detox-rcna4859.

61 Jay Amol Bapaye and Harsh Amol Bapaye, "Demographic Factors Influencing the Impact of Coronavirus-Related Misinformation on WhatsApp: Cross-sectional Questionnaire Study," *JMIR Public Health and Surveillance* 7, no. 1 (2021): e19858; Jon Roozenbeek, Claudia R. Schneider, Sarah Dryhurst, John Kerr, Alexandra LJ Freeman, Gabriel Recchia, Anne Marthe Van Der Bles, and Sander Van Der Linden, "Susceptibility to Misinformation About COVID-19 Around the World," *Royal Society Open Science* 7, no. 10 (2020): 201199; Shuhei Nomura, Akifumi Eguchi, Daisuke Yoneoka, Takayuki Kawashima, Yuta Tanoue, Michio Murakami, Haruka Sakamoto et al., "Reasons for Being Unsure or Unwilling Regarding Intention to Take COVID-19 Vaccine Among Japanese People: A Large Cross-Sectional National Survey," *The Lancet Regional Health–Western Pacific* 14 (2021): 100223.

62 Dustin P. Calvillo, Bryan J. Ross, Ryan J.B. Garcia, Thomas J. Smelter, and Abraham M. Rutchick, "Political Ideology Predicts Perceptions of the Threat of COVID-19 (and Susceptibility to Fake News About It)," *Social Psychological and Personality Science* 11, no. 8 (2020): 1119–128.

63 Calvillo, Ross, Garcia, Smelter, and Rutchick, "Political Ideology Predicts Perceptions of the Threat of COVID-19."

64 "How Americans Navigated the News in 2020," *Politics in Media.*

65 "How Americans Navigated the News in 2020," *Politics in Media.*

66 Brian Kennedy, Alec Tyson, and Cary Funk, "Americans Value U.S. Role as Scientific Leader, But 38 percent Say Country Is Losing Ground Globally," *Trust in Science*, Pew Research Center, October 25, 2022, Americans Value U.S. as Scientific Leader, but 38 percent Say Country Is Losing Ground Globally | Pew Research Center; Michelle Faverio, "Majority of U.S. Twitter Users Say They've Taken a Break from the Platform in the Past Year," *Twitter*, Pew Research Center, May 17, 2023, https://www.pewresearch.org/short-reads/2023/05/17/majority-of-us-twitter-users-say-theyve-taken-a-break-from-the-platform-in-the-past-year/.

67 Gottfried, Jeffrey, Amy Mitchell, Mark Jurkowitz, and Jacob Liedke, "Journalists and the Public Differ on How Journalists Are Doing, How Connected They Are,"

Media Industry, Pew Research Center, June 14, 2022, https://www.pewresearch.org/journalism/2022/06/14/journalists-and-the-public-differ-on-how-journalists-are-doing-how-connected-they-are/.

68 Gottfried, Mitchell, Jurkowitz, and Liedke. "Journalists and the Public Differ on How Journalists are Doing."

69 For example, see "YouGov Survey: 2023 U.S. Trust in Media Poll." 2023, https://docs.cdn.yougov.com/91fpeaaosh/2023 percent20U.S. percent20Trust percent20in percent20Media percent20Poll_poll_results.pdf.

70 Sapna Maheshwari and Amanda Holpuch, "Why Countries Are Trying to Ban TikTok," *New York Times*, May 23, 2023, https://www.nytimes.com/article/tiktok-ban.html; Kate Conger and Lauren Hirsch, "Elon Musk Completes $44 Billion Deal to Own Twitter," *New York Times*, October 27, 2022, https://www.nytimes.com/2022/10/27/technology/elon-musk-twitter-deal-complete.html; Belle Wong, "Top Social Media Statistics and Trends Of 2023," *Forbes*, May 18, 2023, https://www.forbes.com/advisor/business/social-media-statistics/.

71 Jessica Gall Myrick, Robin L. Nabi, and Nicholas J. Eng, "Consuming Memes During the COVID Pandemic: Effects of Memes and Meme Type on COVID-Related Stress and Coping Efficacy," *Psychology of Popular Media* 11, no. 3 (2022): 316.

72 Saad, Lydia. "At Year Three, Americans Split on Whether Pandemic Is Over." *Politics*. Gallup. March 9, 2023, https://news.gallup.com/poll/471734/year-three-americans-split-whether-pandemic.aspx.

73 Saad, "At Year Three, Americans Split on Whether Pandemic Is Over."

74 Saad, "At Year Three, Americans Split on Whether Pandemic Is Over."

75 Saad, "Americans' COVID-19 Concerns Rise, but Still Restrained." *Wellbeing*. Gallup. September 21, 2023, Americans' COVID-19 Concerns Rise, but Still Restrained (gallup.com).

76 Saad, "Americans' COVID-19 Concerns Rise, but Still Restrained."

77 Jeffery Ho, Sabir Hussain, and Olivier Sparagano, "Did the COVID-19 Pandemic Spark a Public Interest in Pet Adoption?" *Frontiers in Veterinary Science* 8 (2021): 647308; New ASPCA Survey Shows Overwhelming Majority of Dogs and Cats Acquired During the Pandemic are Still in Their Homes," *Press Releases*, ASPCA. May 26, 2021, https://www.aspca.org/about-us/press-releases/new-aspca-survey-shows-overwhelming-majority-dogs-and-cats-acquired-during.

78 Kim Parker, "About a Third of U.S. Workers Who Can Work from Home Now Do So All the Time," *Coronavirus (COVID-19)*, Pew Research Center, March 30, 2023, https://www.pewresearch.org/short-reads/2023/03/30/about-a-third-of-us-workers-who-can-work-from-home-do-so-all-the-time/.

79 Daniel Furtner, Salil Prakash Shinde, Manmohan Singh, Chew Hooi Wong, and Sajita Setia, "Digital Transformation in Medical Affairs Sparked by the Pandemic: Insights and Learnings From COVID-19 Era and Beyond." *Pharmaceutical Medicine* 36, no. 1 (2022): 1–10; Jitendra Singh, Keely Steele, and Lovely Singh, "Combining the Best of Online and Face-To-Face Learning: Hybrid and

Blended Learning Approach for COVID-19, Post Vaccine, & Post-Pandemic World," *Journal of Educational Technology Systems* 50, no. 2 (2021): 140–71; Madeline Fitzgerald, "How Online Learning Is Reshaping Higher Education," *U.S. News & World Report*, February 15, 2022, https://www.usnews.com/news/education-news/articles/2022-02-15/how-online-learning-is-reshaping-higher-education.

80 Ben Casselman, "Start-Up Boom in the Pandemic is Growing Stronger," *New York Times*, April 19, 2021, https://www.nytimes.com/2021/08/19/business/startup-business-creation-pandemic.html.

81 "Seasonally Adjusted Business Applications." *Business and Industry*. The United States Census Bureau. July 5, 2023, https://www.census.gov/econ/currentdata/?programCode=BFS&startYear=2004&endYear=2023&categories[]=TOTAL&dataType=BA_BA&geoLevel=US&adjusted=1&notAdjusted=1&errorData=0#line024.

82 Jillian Kramer, "How COVID-19 Vaccines May Lead to New Shots for Other Deadly Viruses," *National Geographic*, January 29, 2021, https://www.nationalgeographic.com/science/article/how-covid-vaccines-may-lead-to-new-shots-for-other-deadly-viruses; Thomas Calder, Tina Tong, Dale J. Hu, Jerome H. Kim, Karen L. Kotloff, Richard A. Koup, Mary A. Marovich et al., "Leveraging Lessons Learned from the COVID-19 Pandemic for HIV," *Communications Medicine* 2, no. 1 (2022): 110.

83 Sinéad Harmey and Gemma Moss, "Learning Disruption or Learning Loss: Using Evidence from Unplanned Closures to Inform Returning to School After COVID-19," *Educational Review* 75, no. 4 (2023): 637–56; Bastian A. Betthäuser, Anders M. Bach-Mortensen, and Per Engzell, "A Systematic Review and Meta-Analysis of the Evidence on Learning During the COVID-19 Pandemic," *Nature Human Behaviour* 7, no. 3 (2023): 375–85.

84 Claudia Andrade, Martie Gillen, José Alberto Molina, and Melissa J. Wilmarth, "The Social and Economic Impact of COVID-19 on Family Functioning and Well-Being: Where Do We Go from Here?" *Journal of Family and Economic Issues* 43, no. 2 (2022): 205–12; Rakesh Kochhar and Stella Sechopoulos, "COVID-19 Pandemic Pinches Finances of America's Lower- and Middle-Income Families," *COVID-19 & the Economy*, Pew Research Center, April 20, 2022, https://www.pewresearch.org/social-trends/2022/04/20/covid-19-pandemic-pinches-finances-of-americas-lower-and-middle-income-families/.

85 John Gramlich, "Mental Health and the Pandemic: What U.S. Surveys Have Found." *Coronavirus (COVID-19)*. Pew Research Center, March 2, 2023, https://www.pewresearch.org/short-reads/2023/03/02/mental-health-and-the-pandemic-what-u-s-surveys-have-found/.

86 Zelalem Mengesha, Esther Alloun, Danielle Weber, Mitchell Smith, and Patrick Harris. "'Lived the Pandemic Twice': A Scoping Review of the Unequal Impact of the COVID-19 Pandemic on Asylum Seekers and Undocumented Migrants." *International Journal of Environmental Research and Public Health* 19, no. 11 (2022): 6624; Tumaini R. Coker, Tina L. Cheng, and Marci Ybarra, "Addressing the Long-term Effects of the COVID-19 Pandemic on Children and Families: A

Report from the National Academies of Sciences, Engineering, and Medicine," *JAMA* 329, no. 13 (2023): 1055–56.

87 Hill, Ndugga, and Artiga, "Key Data on Health and Health Care by Race and Ethnicity."

88 Hill, Ndugga, and Artiga, "Key Data on Health and Health Care by Race and Ethnicity."

89 Kiana Cox and Khadijah Edwards, "Black Americans Have a Clear Vision for Reducing Racism but Little Hope It Will Happen," *Black Americans*, Pew Research Center, August 30, 2022, https://www.pewresearch.org/race-ethnicity/2022/08/30/black-americans-have-a-clear-vision-for-reducing-racism-but-little-hope-it-will-happen/; Andrew Daniller, " Majorities of Americans See at Least Some Discrimination Against Black, Hispanic And Asian people in the U.S.," *Racial Bias & Discrimination*, Pew Research Center, March 18, 2021, https://www.pewresearch.org/short-reads/2021/03/18/majorities-of-americans-see-at-least-some-discrimination-against-black-hispanic-and-asian-people-in-the-u-s/; Nina Totenberg and Sarah McCammon, "Supreme Court Overturns Roe V. Wade, Ending Right to Abortion Upheld for Decades," *NPR*, June 24, 2022, https://www.npr.org/2022/06/24/1102305878/supreme-court-abortion-roe-v-wade-decision-overturn; "What anti-trans bills passed in 2023?" *Trans Legislation Tracker*, Accessed July 5, 2023, https://translegislation.com/bills/2023/passed; "ACLU Comment on Supreme Court's Ruling Against Harvard and UNC's Affirmative Action Policies." *Press Release*. American Civil Liberties Union. June 29, 2023, https://www.aclu.org/press-releases/aclu-comment-on-supreme-courts-ruling-against-harvard-and-uncs-affirmative-action-policies; Negro, Giacomo, Williams, Melissa J., Lopiano, Gabrielle, Petion, Ashlei R., and Roemerman, Ryan M. "LGBTQ Institute Southern Survey: A Snapshot on the Conditions and Life Experiences of LGBTQ Southerners." LGBTQ Institute. April 2023, https://www.lgbtqsouthernsurvey.org/; Martell, Michael E., and Leanne Roncolato. "Economic Vulnerability of Sexual Minorities: Evidence from the US Household Pulse Survey." *Population Research and Policy Review* 42, no. 2 (2023): 28.

90 David A. Weaver, "The Mortality Experience of Disabled Persons in the United States During The COVID-19 Pandemic," *Health Affairs Scholar* (2023); Divya Goyal, Xanthe Hunt, Hannah Kuper, Tom Shakespeare, and Lena Morgon Banks, "Impact of the COVID-19 Pandemic on People with Disabilities and Implications for Health Services Research," *Journal of Health Services Research &* Policy 28, no. 2 (2023): 77–79; WHO, Global Report on Health Equity for Persons with Disabilities, WHO, 2022.

91 Lee, Kett, Mohammed, Frogner, and Sabin," "Inequitable Care Delivery."

92 Jonathan Franklin, "More Than 600,000 White Flags on the National Mall Honor Lives Lost To COVID," *NPR*, September 17, 2021, https://www.npr.org/sections/coronavirus-live-updates/2021/09/17/1037011493/covid-national-mall-white-flags-art-exhibit-memorial-pandemic-dead.

93 "COVID Memorial Quilt: Honoring Those Lost to COVID-19." 2023, https://

covidquilt2020.com/; "COVID-19 Memorial Mural." City of Knoxville, https://www.knoxvilletn.gov/government/mayors_office/c_o_v_i_d-19___coronavirus_/c_o_v_i_d-19_memorial_mural; "COVID-19 Memorial Public Art Project." *Commission on Arts and Sciences*. Baltimore County Government. 2023, https://www.baltimorecountymd.gov/departments/arts-sciences/covid19-memorial-project; Bruce Shriner, "Kentucky dedicates memorial to honor those lost to COVID-19"; Associated Press, May 24, 2023, https://apnews.com/article/covid-pandemic-memorial-kentucky-7f9286569a55cbdf10c44a40b0fa03da.

94 Foss, *Constructing the Outbreak*.

95 Mario Coccia, "Sources, Diffusion and Prediction in COVID-19 Pandemic: Lessons Learned To Face Next Health Emergency," *AIMS Public Health* 10, no. 1 (2023): 145; Lewis, "How the U.S. Pandemic Response Went Wrong—and What Went Right"; Gostin, "The Coronavirus Pandemic 1 Year On—What Went Wrong?"; Sheryl Gay Stolberg and Noah Weiland, "Experts See Lessons for Next Pandemic as Covid Emergency Comes to an End," *New York Times*, May 11, 2023, https://www.nytimes.com/2023/05/11/us/politics/covid-response-lessons.html.

96 Melissa Tully, Adam Maksl, Seth Ashley, Emily K. Vraga, and Stephanie Craft, "Defining and conceptualizing news literacy," *Journalism* (2021): 14648849211005888; Emily K. Vraga, Melissa Tully, and Leticia Bode, "Empowering Users to Respond to Misinformation about COVID-19," *Media and Communication* 8, no. 2 (2020): 475–79.

Index

FSC
www.fsc.org
MIX
Papier | Fördert
gute Waldnutzung
FSC® C083411

Kolibri 360 GmbH
Ferdinand-Jühlke-Straße 7
99095 Erfurt, Deutschland
produktsicherheit@kolibri360.de